AAV-9366
VC - Lib Stud

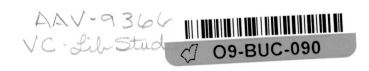
O9-BUC-090

Please remember that this is a library book,
and that it belongs only temporarily to each
person who uses it. Be considerate. Do
not write in this, or any, library book.

WITHDRAWN

CHILDREN IN FAMILIES AT RISK

WITHDRAWN

CHILDREN IN FAMILIES AT RISK
Maintaining the Connections

Edited by

Lee Combrinck-Graham, MD

Foreword by Theodora Ooms

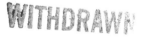

THE GUILFORD PRESS
New York   London

©1995 The Guilford Press
A Division of Guilford Publications, Inc.
72 Spring Street, New York, NY 10012

All rights reserved

No part of this book may be reproduced, stored in a retrieval
system, or transmitted, in any form or by any means, electronic,
mechanical, photocopying, microfilming, recording, or otherwise,
without written permission from the Publisher.

Printed in the United States of America

This book is printed on acid-free paper.

Last digit is print number: 9 8 7 6 5 4 3 2 1

Library of Congress Cataloging-in-Publication Data

Children in families at risk : maintaining the connections / edited
by Lee Combrinck-Graham.
        p.   cm.
    Includes bibliographical references and index.
    ISBN 0-89862-852-0
    1. Child mental health.   2. Family—Mental health.
I. Combrinck-Graham, Lee.
RJ499.C4893   1995
362.7′686—dc20   95-8793
                                                                         CIP

Contributors

Cynthia Archacki-Stone, MS, Family Builders Program, Meadville Medical Center, Meadville, PA

Markus Bartell, MEd, Graber Elementary School, Hutchinson, KS

Gerald Bereika, PhD, Mentor Clinical Care, Boston, MA

Lindsay Bicknell-Hentges, PhD, Department of Psychology, Chicago State University, Chicago, IL

Stephen Christian-Michaels, LCSW, MA, Mental Health Division, DuPage County Health Department, Wheaton, IL

Rocco A. Cimmarusti, MSW, Life Concerns, Skokie, IL

Lee Combrinck-Graham, MD, Mental Health Systems Consultant, Stamford, CT

Raymond X. De Maio, EdD, New Jersey Center of Family Therapy, Springfield, NJ

Marcia A. Eckstein, BA, Continuum Foster Care Program, New Life Services, Inc., Cincinnati, OH

Judith A. Falk, MSW, Sisters of St. Francis, Syracuse, NY

Francine Feinberg, ACSW, PsyD, Meta House Program, Our Home Foundation, Inc., Milwaukee, WI

Michael R. Fox, MD, Private Practice, Baltimore, MD

Laura H. Fraser, LCSW, MSW, Eastfield Ming Quong, Campbell, CA

Barbara King, MEd, Graber Elementary School, Hutchinson, Kansas

Faye A. Koop, MS, Marriage and Family Therapy Program, Kansas State University, Manhattan, KS

Karen Gail Lewis, ACSW, PhD, Private Practice, Washington, DC

Daniel R. Lord, PhD, Department of Marriage and Family Therapy, Friends University, Wichita, KS

Vickie Burgess McArthur, MS, Home-Based Services, Friends University, Wichita, KS

William A. McKay, MSW, Graber Elementary School, Hutchinson, KS

Julie McKenzie, MEd, McKenzie and Associates, Boston, MA

Edwin J. Mikkelsen, MD, Mentor Clinical Care, Boston, MA

Patricia Minuchin, PhD, Family Studies, Inc., New York, NY

Donald Monack, MSW, MBA, Mentor Clinical Care, Boston, MA

James Nelson, PhD, Change, Inc., Minneapolis, MN

Lora Randolph, MEd, Graber Elementary School, Hutchinson, KS

Steven W. Rathbun, PhD, Department of Marriage and Family Therapy, Friends University, Wichita, KS

John Sargent, MD, Philadelphia Child Guidance Center, Philadelphia, PA

Wayne Stelk, PhD, Mentor Clinical Care, Boston, MA

Foreword

As a former therapist, I found many of the theoretical ideas in these chapters thought provoking, and the clinical stories fascinating and inspiring. But I believe the significance of the book lies in the broader policy context. It offers us both hope and challenge during a time of deepening distrust in government programs.

The public is seriously disturbed by the escalating symptoms of family and community disintegration and by the failure of decades of government spending to solve them. Daily reports in the media of increases in youth violence, child and spousal abuse, substance abuse, foster care and residential placement, and so on serve to fuel public distrust of and frustration with, the government. Powerful political voices argue that the solution is to spend less on federal programs and to transfer responsibility for dealing with these problems to the states and communities.

No one disagrees that the present categorical, fragmented, and rule-bound system of health and social services is ineffective, wasteful, and does not respond to the needs and problems of today's families. But the answer lies not in mindless cutbacks but in making major changes in the way we deliver services.

For several decades dedicated public officials have been working with program administrators, front line human service professionals, and sometimes families themselves, to design and implement major changes in financing, organization, and the delivery of services in order to improve outcomes for poor children and families. At the same time clinicians have been crafting new approaches to treatment that build on family systems and ecological theory. Community based family support programs, home-based programs, and family scholars have identified new concepts of family strengths and family empowerment.

It has been fascinating to watch the new services paradigm emerging at the confluence of these rivers of reforms. The new paradigm cuts across many program areas. There is a quite astonishing consensus on its guiding principles, repeated so often they constitute a "mantra." Child and family services must be "comprehensive, flexible, individually tailored, family-centered, community based, culturally competent and outcome-oriented." These principles are embedded in several landmark pieces of legislation—for example the Part H IDEA early intervention services for infants and toddlers, the Child and Adolescent Service System Program (CASSP) in the mental health sector, and, most recently, the Family Preservation and Support Services Program in child welfare.

Many sceptics acknowledge the promise of this new rhetoric but doubt that the bold new vision will ever become reality. To me, the excitement and importance of this book is that it disproves the sceptics and confounds the critics. The seventeen examples that Lee Combrinck-Graham has masterfully assembled here are convincing evidence that the new paradigm's principles are being applied in real situations, and, therefore, that public monies can be used effectively and humanely.

The book's challenge to all of us arises from its refusal to promise a quick fix to these complicated family and community problems. Successful approaches require complicated, multi-level interventions, low caseloads, time, and an infrastructure of sustained training, supervision, and administrative support. In the short run these approaches are clearly not cheap, but there is some tantalizing evidence given—though we need much more—that in the long run they are cost effective. Documentation and evaluation are important because as many of the authors make clear, if the programs are to survive and flourish they need the understanding and support of a wide range of stakeholders—public and private funders, collaborating agencies, managed care providers, and ultimately the public—the tax payers. This, ultimately, is our challenge.

THEODORA OOMS

Preface

This volume started as a collection of pieces on family preservation, probably the single most significant movement in the evolution of services for all aspects of child welfare (safety, mental health, education, and civics) in the last 2 decades. But by including programs that work with children in family settings other than their own, we have also considered a broader implication of keeping children connected with families.

Many of the discussions presented in this book explicitly acknowledge the mother–child "bond" as a force and resource. For example, using mothers' attachments and commitments to making their children's lives different has a significant role in the treatment of addicted mothers, and in motivating the rehabilitation of incarcerated mothers. The reciprocal, child–mother "bond" also draws attention, as we see children constantly opting for less than optimal situations in order to defend, protect, or simply stay connected to the mother.

But this dyadic thinking about family connectedness does not begin to do justice to the larger sense of a magnetic force that families exert on their members—a force that can lead families to destruction and devastation, but also the force that sustains families through humiliation, poverty, crises, and degradation. As we see in the instances where parents may have disappeared, siblings' relationships to each other can sustain this healing force, and the sibling subsystem can accomplish a great deal to move the family back together.

What we have learned, and these chapters reinforce this knowledge, is that family connectedness often sustains families, in spite of the "helpers" who think that helping is best done by removing family members, whether by taking dysfunctional adults away from their children or taking children away to presumably better situations in the hope that they will become part of more functional child–adult relationships. It does not happen that way, and such actions inevitably step up the family members' desperate attempts to make meaning out of their connections. Of course, there are situations when families cannot live safely together. We have several examples of parents and children living apart—mothers in prison, children in hospitals or foster care. The vital effort here, even so, is to keep the children connected with their families; the outcomes are astonishing.

The programs described here are still exceptional, though there is now legislation in many states mandating family preservation services. They are exceptional because the balance of opinion about the possibility of families being able to handle their children versus children being better cared for by experts is still weighted in favor of experts. Child professionals' confidence in families is complicated by the rise in awareness of child exploitation and neglect within families that seems to contradict the assertions of those who maintain that families are their children's best hope. Well, perhaps some families, the professionals aver, but not *these* families—not these families that have chosen drugs over relationships or who have exploited their children for sex, money, or a sense of personal power and control; not these mothers who subject their children to abuse in order to maintain a relationship with a man; not these families who clearly cannot manage their children's aggressive, suicidal, or other destructive impulses. Yet it is just these families about whom we have written in these chapters.

When a closer, sympathetic look at a family that appears to have neglected and injured their child reveals that the child was accidentally injured in a fight between the father and mother, readers may conclude that that is a different situation from the exploiters and abusers. I submit that it is not. It is the kind of thing that one finds in such families when one approaches the inquiry with the assumption that the families, too, are concerned about how their lives are unfolding and would be willing to change the course, if they could.

To believe in these possibilities is a professional step that must be taken. A chapter on training child welfare workers is included in order to illustrate some of the processes and difficulties encountered when trying to change professionals' minds. In addition, in each chapter the authors raise the question, how do we get stakeholders to buy into this approach? Even after professionals have taken this step, however, there is a massive challenge in persuading families that this opportunity is for real. Most of the chapters address this process. This fact, that we have to convince professionals and families that these approaches are not "business as usual" is the saddest commentary on the extraordinary social welfare developments of our century. We still have a few years to make this adjustment. It is beginning.

To begin this display of extraordinary programs based on a sense of family connectedness is an unusual program that takes the concept of family from the households we usually imagine when thinking of "family" to tribes reminiscent of the families in communities and clans that were commonplace only two generations ago. These tribal families are still most evident among Native Americans, but James Nelson, who ran The City, Inc., in Minneapolis for 15 years, allows the idea of connection to inform the sense of responsibility for community that can emerge in youth in the inner city. In doing so, he framed and tracked the relationships between youths, including their families, so that, being perceived as viable and valuable components of a community, they began to assume these responsibilities. The goal is keeping children and families connected to each other and to their communities.

For some years I have been promoting the idea that four "giant steps"—conceptual leaps for mental health professionals—must be taken in order to have a positive impact on children's mental health. The first step is to recognize that meanings are constructed in interpersonal contexts (in "conversation"). In this book, one often finds a clash between agency meaning and family meaning, with the helping professionals dancing on a bridge that links them. Nelson, for example, contrasts the type of organizational and outcome information required by the United Way (an important source of financial support) with the meaningful chaos of conversations from the many voices in his community. Cimmarusti describes how difficult it is for child welfare workers to work on a positive family image when the agency administrators are more comfortable with a "save the child" approach.

The second conceptual giant step is that events occur in a patterned relationship to one another that is not simple cause and effect. This step challenges the professional to ask, "What patterns are these? How am I participating in perpetuating old, destructive patterns? How am I contributing to the development of new, constructive patterns?" Minuchin's approach addresses head-on the age-old suspicion and antagonism between foster and natural parents by having the "professional" step aside in order to let these parties, both concerned about caring for children, work together. Fraser's work constantly reflects on how the workers may become a part of the patterned problem.

The third giant step is the recognition that all systems, no matter how dysfunctional, exploitative, neglectful, or, whatever, have competence. Every chapter in this book begins with this premise. For families who are threatened with separation of children and parents, this competence may be utilized to accomplish the often heroic tasks of changing in order for parents to keep their children with them, or to get their children back; alternatively, it may be used to recognize that their children may be better off in another's care. With this approach, rarely is it necessary for an outside agent to make a unilateral decision about someone else's children.

The fourth giant step is a definition of mental health, something we often fail to reflect on our day-to-day thinking. But if we don't think about what mental health is, how can we be sure that we are mental health professionals who are contributing to positive outcomes in mental health? Mental health can be found in systems that are organized for the mutual benefit of their parts. The system in which a mother maintains her attachment to a man at the expense of her children is not healthy. But neither is the system where the welfare worker is constantly under criticism by the press and so-called public advocates. In the first instance, the mother may allow her children to be abused or neglected in order to sustain the relationship. In the second instance, the welfare worker may violate the family by arbitrarily removing children in order to prevent the punishing reaction of the press should a child come to harm or injury.

Many of the authors explicitly consider the question of safety—how do we insure safety while still advocating for families?

The authors of this book are working people. Each one is actively engaged in the work described in these chapters, and it has been our aim to tell the stories of these programs and some of the people served in them, so that others may get ideas and confidence from the experiences set down here.

Many of the authors employ family systems thinking in conceptualizing their programs, but some do not. The crucial element of family systems thinking that works in these approaches is the sense that families have competence and capacity for being a family and caring for one another. All of these approaches are contextual, looking for resourceful contexts. All of these approaches are realistic, not forcing families and children together beyond their abilities to manage each other. Mothers do not stay out of jail just because they have children; children are not brought home from placement just because the family is willing; mothers do not give up drug habits just because they have children; the police do not trust inner-city gang youth just because they have been defined as a tribe; school personnel do not ignore children's adaptation to peers and learning just because their families are involved in working on difficulties; children are not left at home just because there is a family preservation program, and so on.

It is pretty clear to me after looking at programs that emphasize keeping children in their families or returning them to their natural families that this approach can be as dangerous as removing them in the belief that some other environment can effectively replace the family. Both are sometimes important policies; neither is always appropriate. There is no replacing the family—even for a child adopted at birth there is the fantasy of the "real" family. It may be possible, however, to provide a safer, more consistent, and more hopeful environment than the family could have provided, and then the challenge becomes how does this setting supplement the fundamental relationships and support connectedness.

This book is about connection between children and families and the strength that these connections lend to the development of the children and the effectiveness of their parents.

The assembly of this book is also about connection. Though I have corresponded with all of the authors and spoken with most on the telephone, there are some authors I have never met. How did I get to know them? Riding on an airplane, chatting with a colleague about the idea of the book; knowing I wanted a chapter on a certain topic, and asking around; hearing someone present and wanting him or her to do a chapter; telling an audience at a workshop about the book, and having someone say to me, "Don't you need a chapter on x?" I think the book grew in the way these movements grow, by chance, by casual acquaintance, by keeping one's eyes open, by being open to possibilities, and by being committed to families as children's most significant resources.

Contents

I

CHANGING THE WAYS
WE THINK
ABOUT ENGAGING
FAMILIES

The chapters in the first part of this volume aim to change how we think about families and how we work with them, especially when they are families under siege. Most mental health and child care professionals, themselves besieged by a stream of difficult children and seemingly inaccessible families, probably need to step back and think about how these experiences make them feel about this population, and to further reflect on how their expectations may elicit family behavior that may confirm the professionals' attitudes. This circular process perpetuates discouragement of both professionals and families. Fundamental to the chapters in this part, and, indeed, in the whole volume, is the belief that families love their children and do the best they can, most of the time. When problems arise, professionals need to identify resources, strengthen families' areas of competence, and work collaboratively with families to achieve goals within the scope of the families' social, cultural, and economic circumstances.

Jim Nelson's chapter is about finding or defining the families of youth gangs in the customs of the many Native American youth who are a part of gang life in Minneapolis. Defining these gangs–tribes–families is but one example of changes in thinking required to provide a trustworthy and effective resource to these youth.

Steve Rathbun and colleagues have developed an approach to court-ordered assessments that involves the family in reviewing the data and participating in the resulting disposition. Their assessment has a mixture of scientific instruments and clinical feel: The former lends an air of science to the evaluation that may impress those who make decisions, the latter is used to persuade the family to assist in the process. The outcome of family involvement, however, is the remarkable participation of the family in the recommended plan — because they have been part of the process of forming it!

Stephen Christian-Michaels describes a system of care that works. This system has been evolving since the late 1980s and, as Christian-Michaels demonstrates, has had a remarkable impact on reducing the numbers of children placed out of their homes while increasing the the effectiveness of the family and community supports for seriously disturbed children.

Remembering that there are other supportive relationship systems than nuclear families, remembering to involve the family in assessing and planning, especially if it involves the future of a child member of that family, and being able to serve a child and family with a range of services available in a rich system of care all make it possible to engage people in a positive way.

1

Working with Inner-City Tribes: Collaborating with the Enemy or Finding Opportunities for Building Community?

James Nelson

The purpose of this chapter is to share some of the experiences of an inner-city agency that grew, in part, from the assumptions and values of family and community life in inner-city Minneapolis. As a family therapist, I have been impressed by the applicability of systems theory and related thinking to the experiences of this organization. It should be noted that the discussion and framework(s) offered for consideration are informed by my perspective/role, since 1974, as a family practitioner and chief executive officer of The City, Inc. (hereafter referred to as The City), and, therefore, this account suffers from all the pitfalls of a biased informant.

In Europe, Asia, Africa, Latin America, and the inner-city United States, one hears that the "traditional" infrastructures are under siege, as societies splinter along the lines of race, ethnicity, language, socioeconomic status, and other differences. In the midst of this battle, there is a lot of fear about regressing to tribalism, because tribalism is primitive and primitive is bad, or so the argument goes. Proponents of this view are adamant about protecting or restoring the cultural values and institutions being challenged. When a society and its institutions begin to break down, it seems to me that one response is to become desperately sure about what should be done; those who have the most to lose seem to be the most emphatic, as their sense of security and predictability begins to diminish. Curiosity about what other communities of people have to offer is one of the first casualties, and certainty about one's own solutions carries the day in an uneasy atmosphere of continuous and growing failures arising from the status quo.

In our society, consider the institution of the family, with record out-of-home placements of children, teen suicide, drug abuse, and growing, debilitating poverty — crumbling families, crumbling communities, and a crumbling nation. Lynn Hoffman (1990) noted that "the individual must fit within the family, the family must fit within the community, and all must fit within the larger ecology" (p. 6). In reflecting on this statement, Hoffman later commented that she sounded like an "ecological fascist" (p. 6). I think she backed off too quickly from what people's intuition tells them about the interacting ecologies of life: Healthy individuals do seem to live in healthy, family-like organizations, and healthy, family-like organizations do seem to thrive in healthy communities. If we focus on the "healthy" in this vision, we have the challenge of operationalizing its definition, searching for health within the "crumbling" structures of society. Where are there visions of health? To whom can we go for help? The answer, from the experiences of this author and The City, is into communities and their cultures. The intent of this chapter is to offer up experiences of working within communities that may at first appear foreign, but upon closer scrutiny may be seen to hold an ancient and time-honored set of experiences and competencies that resonate with our collective "common sense." The experiences of these communities may even provide some traditional reminders about how to keep children and families together in the larger society.

Adopting or accepting alternative perspectives of healthy functioning on a societal level is different in a cultural context dominated by a "them" versus "us" mentality, as mainstream and inner-city communities become pitted against each other as they lose contact with each other. University of Chicago sociologist William Julius Wilson (1987) characterizes inner-city "underclass" communities as socially isolated from mainstream America. From a traditional research standpoint (Taylor, Chatters, Tucker, & Lewis, 1990), we know next to nothing about the involvement of African American men in family life, yet the popular media and politicians seldom lack opinions about what to do for these communities. When the powerful media and its many relatives, representing a dominant culture and class perspective, rely on second- and third-hand information about the inner city, powerful stereotypes can go unchallenged. For example, cultural commentator Robert Bly (1990) demonstrates his lack of knowledge about gangs when he declares that they are young men without fathers. Bly's knowledge of gangs more accurately reflects his social class and its biases. The membership of the national associations called gangs, with which I am familiar, includes ages representing the entire life cycle: sons, daughters, mothers, and fathers. Bly's curiosity was satisfied simply by using a police chief as sole source of information. Historically, the results of uninformed opinions held by those in power have been, for example, vigorous and vengeful pursuits to destroy the tribal life of American Indians (only recently were American Indians legally allowed to practice their religious rites) and the promotion of stereotypical fear at the mere mention of African American gangs in our inner cities. Our stereotyping of people into enemies to be feared or strangers to be misunderstood obscures an appreciation of the simple act of one person caring for another or whole communities caring for each other. I have found that most people, regardless of their background, can speak of experiences in their lives in which they were cared for by another person even though those experiences may seem foreign or unlikely and therefore threatening to the "sensibilities" of others.

An approach based on curiosity rather than on isolation, ignorance, and fear would be more productive. For example, what if urban tribal life and the so-called "gang phenomenon" represent a group of associations socially adapted to provide the basic building blocks of community, relationships, and culture? What if these phenomena represent a cost-effective place to begin a transformation of the quality of life in our inner cities? An analogous situation exists in the scientific realm when mainstream science neglects ancient folk wisdom. Ethnobiologist Wade Davis (1988) implores us to not be so quick to jeopardize the centuries of herbal knowledge, and those tribal communities that hold that knowledge, by further destruction of our rain forests. In a similar vein, Eugene Linden wrote in *Time* magazine, that "when native cultures disappear, so does a trove of scientific and medical wisdom," adding that the "prevailing attitude has been that Western science, with its powerful analytical tools, has little to learn from tribal knowledge" (p. 48). This has been equally true in the cultural sphere. Yet how can we afford to turn our modern backs to tribal networks and structures without first knowing what potential contributions we may be ignoring? This chapter is an attempt to explore some of the contributions that American Indian tribal life and African American gang affiliation may make to community building.

While there have been some exceptions (Attneave, 1982; Aponte, 1986; Minuchin, Montalvo, Guerney, Rosman, & Schmer, 1967), the field of family therapy, based on an awareness and appropriation of the mutual and defining influences between people and their significant relationships, has had surprisingly little use for the substantive influences of the community. Perhaps it is because of the field's focus on the interiority of the family coupled with definitional debates about what is and is not community. In any case, there are an abundance of resources available through relationships and associations that surround inner-city families in their neighborhoods and communities. I am aware of this because part of my job has been to find what is necessary to do the job of caring, and I have found that what is necessary has been there all along. John McKnight (1989a) indicates that an overwhelming reliance on professionals and "deficit-oriented" services, particularly within inner-city communities, blocks an appreciation and appropriation of what is possible with community resources in addressing the "emptiness" that many feel in their inner-city neighborhoods. He suggests that communities hold the opportunity for members, "to express and share their gifts, skills, capacities, and abilities with friends, neighbors, and fellow citizens. As deficiency-oriented service systems obscure this fact, they inevitably harm their client *and* the community by preempting the relationship between them" (p. 7).

If one takes the time to look up close, one will discover within inner-city communities the presence of those functional skills and talents that create and sustain relational networks. These strengths have been overlooked by those politicians and social scientists who would dismiss "the problem with inner-city communities" with correct but simplistic emphases on values of self-discipline and responsibility taking. Rather than assuming an absence of values, we might want to start by joining in building up the already present capacity of these communities, but that assumes some kind of conversation, relationship, and invitation.

The City has had such opportunities and has experienced the positive contributions of community networks of urban American Indians as well as gangs in African American communities. There may well be some parallels between American Indian tribal life in inner cities and national African American associations — or gangs — but the loss, through slavery, of a land base, language, and tribal culture have posed a challenge to African American communities that contrasts with the battle of American Indians to hold on to their lands, languages, and cultures. Differences notwithstanding, both of these groups are, in their understanding of themselves, carriers of culture. What is this culture? What are the collective visions and wish dreams of these social networks? Is help needed for these groups to be more effective in their efforts? These questions might be appropriate to ask before outside groups assume what program efforts would be helpful to whom.

PHILOSOPHY

I am providing two descriptions of the philosophy and theoretical frame-works that underlie the approach of The City to augment the context of some of the issues and experiences I will describe. The first set I call "personal" because it consists of some ruminations as a therapist (Gurnoe & Nelson, 1989; Nelson, 1994; Nelson & Shelledy, 1980, 1982). The second set is the product of the collective efforts of our management team and organizational leadership. We use some of this statement in proposals.

Personal Assumptions

In the spirit of social construction (Berger & Luckman, 1967), ecosystemic theory (Keeney, 1983), and cultural anthropology (Marcus & Fischer, 1986), I consciously offer this presentation as a contextual confession, a "passing theory" (Rorty, 1989) informed by the dialogical, emergent emphasis of anthropologists like Stephen Tyler (1987), who notes that "discourse" is privileged over "text," that the ethnographer benefits from the "cooperative and collaborative," and that the "mutual dialogical production of a discourse" replaces the "observer-observed" ideology. As a result, "the form itself should emerge out of the joint work of the ethnographer and his native partner . . . that provides a negotiated text for the reader to interpret" (pp. 126–127).

This background has led me to several points that are crucial to my cross-cultural work in the programs and procedures of The City:

1. Relationships are key.
2. Reality is a complex process of social construction.
3. Generally, flexibility and diversity denote health.
4. A stance of "functional paranoia" is pragmatic for the change agent.

Relationships Are Key

People change within the context of a relationship with an "other." Being curious (Cecchin, 1987) seems to promote interactions or conversations between people, and these interactions, in turn, promote sharing of self (selves) or, more generically, confession. As a change agent generalist, I have found utility in the skill and value of enactment (Minuchin, 1974), that is, getting people to talk with each other. Curiosity, conversation and confessions, over time, will also produce conflict—a critical but too often avoided dimension in "real" relationships—and they may also lead to a personal experience of the culture of orientation of the other. In fact, cur-

iosity, conversation, confession, conflict, and culture are crucial to relationship and community building.

Reality Is a Complex Process of Social Construction

The phrase "objective reality" really means that a group of people has
agreed on what is real. Cultures, societies, groups, families, and individuals
use these definitions of reality to manage their own sense of well-being
and to persuade or coerce others to behave in accordance with these notions of reality. Those in control of a particular society get edgy when
their views about what is real are threatened by other, emerging and competing, realities. From my point of view, what has been defined as "objective reality" is emergent from the complexities of relationships between
people. At the individual level, reality emerges from these relationships
based on perceptions and distinctions that stand out, distinguishing themselves in the mind's eye from other possible perceptions and distinctions.
In its simplest form, change in reality potentially begins with some kind
of contrast. Technically, the processes of framing and reframing experiences (Bateson, 1972; Goffman, 1974) have been helpful to introduce
change in perceived reality.

Generally, Flexibility and Diversity Denote Health

Systems that have developed rigidly repeated responses, rituals, or reactions to the exclusion of other options are at greatest risk for developing
"pathologies," as defined by a particular group. This notion is similar to
the biological concept of "climax system" (Keeney, 1983; Krebs, 1972;
Smith, 1966), wherein the system that "tolerates" diversity of species appears to be the most resilient to disease. This assumption is also in the
spirit of cybernetician W. Ross Ashby's (1956) "law of requisite variety,"
focusing on capacity of "regulation and control" (more realistically, influence) as being tied to one's "capacity as a channel of communication"
(p. 211).

A Stance of "Functional Paranoia" Is Pragmatic for the Change Agent

In response, being careful about one's own conclusions about perceptions
seems appropriate given the complexity of life. Drawing on the relational
emphasis of curiosity, that reality in the world is socially defined, and the
notion that rigidity of response or pattern may reflect pathology suggests
that an agent of change should continuously question what he or she per-
ceives or believes about the world.

One's curiosity provides the foundation for maintaining a stance of functional paranoia. In answering the question "What encourages the development of multiple perspectives and voices?" Cecchin (1987) notes: "We again return to the idea that curiosity facilitates the development of multiplicity and polyphony" (p. 407). Clinically, the questioning of certainty, realizing that other perspectives and voices are possible, depends on one's curiosity.

Program Philosophy

In operationalizing our mission, The City has developed a series of "strategies" to indicate our evolving program philosophy. While the operating philosophy of The City can be as important as the specific programs, this philosophy is to be understood as "what we're currently working on" rather than as a recipe.

Building on The City's historical emphasis on relationships and community since 1967, the organization continues to wrestle with moving beyond managing problems through service provision to solving problems through community building. Our current strategies in building community are developing (1) a sense of history and place; (2) relationships and making relatives; (3) the utility of culture; (4) comprehensive, community solutions; (5) advocacy and institutional opposition; and (6) a commitment to reflection: experimentation and research.

A Sense of History and Place

The City remembers its history—an emphasis on inner-city Minneapolis, young people and their families, the criminal justice system, culture, and pluralism—in stories both written and oral, and passes on these stories to new generations of staff and board. This remembering keeps us centered on our mission as well as on a sense of how we got here. Over time values emerge, "mistakes" can be corrected, and a sense of connection takes place from this retelling, this reminding. Our collective sense is that without a sense of history and place, a community is virtually nonexistent.

Relationships and Making Relatives

The importance of and ability to make and keep friendships drives all that The City does. Trusting relationships require mutuality—"we will have an effect on each other." To promote relationship making and keeping, all of The City's activities are intended to reduce social isolation, promoting social interaction with young people and families; therefore, The City attempts to hire staff with relational values and skills. If an individual student or family member can be brought to trust in a single relationship, that person can begin to take advantage of and contribute to the greater family network of The City and its many relatives. These relatives are not narrowly understood as biological, but rather, broadly as those with whom there are relations and interactions. A community's ability to care for itself and its members is predicated, in part, on its collective ability to make and keep relatives.

The Utility of Culture

We have embraced the notion, along with Charles Waldegrave (1990), that "culture is probably the most influential determinant of meaning in people's lives" (p. 15). As a result of a history of experiencing the profound healing influences of culture, The City has developed an organizational competence that is reflected in the development of culturally specific approaches to our activities. This competence is predicated on the ability to appropriate culture through relationships with those that "hold and" carry the culture, that is, tribes, churches, traditional teachers, and healers. As a result, The City advocates the legitimation of alternative certifications in both educational and therapeutic endeavors, hires staff from within its community and has developed strong preferences for cultural and communal solutions rather than institutional solutions to problems and issues.

McKnight's (1987, 1989a, 1989b) notion that inner-city communities have been marked by an overreliance on consumption, particularly of educational and social services, has underscored our advocacy. The City attempts to reverse this trend of creating "client communities" by focusing on opportunities for production of educational and therapeutic services through the identification and hiring of community teachers and healers.

Comprehensive Community Solutions

While acknowledging that individuals face substantial challenges, from being labeled by some as members of "dysfunctional families" to having repeated personal "failures," The City also examines the contributions of structural—economic, social, spiritual, and political—dynamics. To focus on individual and family explanations while excluding broader social structures and contexts is not only incomplete but distorted and insensitive.

The City's response to these issues not only emphasizes the importance of context and perspective but utilizes the strengths inherent within the community we serve. A 25-year organizational preference and success in hiring staff from the community has underscored the fact of these strengths. The implications are then not only in addressing the "whole person" but in appropriating the "whole life cycle" in that effort.

The City's commitment to community-based programming stems from an experientially based belief that keeping people in their community of support and with family members has independent positive and therapeutic benefits. There are positive and healing social forces in these communities that remain untapped by most conventional approaches — the power of friends and neighbors, the value of churches, the healing influences of extended families or relational communities, and cultural traditions, all the elements of the social control that are provided by the informal network. These many positive resources remain unknown without relationship.

Advocacy and Institutional Opposition

Dominant-culture institutions controlled by mainstream and corporate interests tend to create solutions dictated by the interests and values of the dominant culture — solutions that often do not work well for affected families and neighborhoods. Families and young people who are involved with The City know, through the experience of relationships, that staff will fight for them and stick up for them.

All of our staff persons have strong track records in advocating for young people and families in the judicial system and other systems. Increasingly, the community that we serve comes to know us by our advocacy on their behalf, both in practical matters and around important issues. The City realizes there is a strong need for articulation of alternative or oppositional perspectives as part of public policy debates and intends to play a forceful role in those presentations.

Somebody, it is felt, needs to advocate from the perspectives of local neighborhoods, the nondominant culture, kids outside the economic mainstream, and families alienated from educational and social service organizations.

A Commitment to Reflection: Experimentation and Research

The City has a long history of experimentally developing new approaches to chronic problems, beginning with its school program in the 1960s, the family therapy program in the '70s, street outreach initiatives with youth gangs in the '80s and ideally, small but successful economic development efforts in the '90s.

The City believes that reflection and feedback are critical to the health of a community, family, individual, and organization. In response, The

City continues to be a "reflective practitioner" (Schon, 1983), participating in formal and informal program and performance evaluations, creating various opportunities to "re-search" our efforts, and conducting a strategic thinking process annually.

THE MODEL

"Model building" is a dangerous but necessary enterprise. Recipes for models run the risk of making us less curious, overdependent on formulas, and blind to important differences. Perhaps, this is no more profoundly evident then when considering cultural and class issues in educational and social model building. All models are cultural artifacts, products of the interacting symbols, meaning systems, and values of the builders. From a culturally sensitive viewpoint, an important part of this process might well include an attempt by the builder to confess the cultural and class values embodied in the system.

Given the issues facing inner-city communities, it seems prudent to converse about working models of hope and how they are imagined to work. This tension, between the need to know effective models and the danger of formulas, necessitates attending to the constructivists (Atkinson & Heath, 1987) who emphasize "giving it up," confessing limitations, the intended and unintended, and convening a dialogue that places the assumptions of a particular model in conversation with others, again à la Tyler (1987): "the mutual dialogical production of a discourse, a story of sorts" (p. 126). A part of building and articulating models should include the intentions and limitations of the model builder. These intentions and limitations encourage dialogue about the model and its relationships with other models, resulting in revision of the original design.

The organizational descriptions of The City are, of course, cultural artifacts. I like Karl Weick's (unpublished) "eight punctuations" on organizations and their effectiveness, which suggest that an effective organization is "garrulous, clumsy, haphazard, hypocritical, condones monsters, wandering, grouchy, and octopoidal." Aristophanes suggested that "whirl is King," and I have experienced organizations as importantly conflictual and chaotic, at times defying definition, full of those dynamics Carlos Castaneda (1974) called the *nagual,* the things that can't be named but only experienced. In the midst of this "whirl," conversation and relationships become our organizational linchpins and anchors.

With that in mind, The City emphasizes function over form. Our funders, however, reward organizations for having a "form" that is intelligible to the funders' values, experiences, and perspectives. Since the staff and program participants at The City are primarily comprised of people of color from cultural orientations differing from the dominant society, it is understandable that our organizational preferences and practices would tend to be influenced by those particular cultures rather than just by the culture of our corporate funders.

In the past few years, we have self-reflectively understood our organizational structure as tribal. Consciously borrowing from the Ojibway's (Johnston, 1976) notion of totems—the functional contribution one makes to the community—we speak of five functions in our community organization: leading, healing, teaching, advocating, and sustaining. The City's organizational chart (see Figure 1.1) indicates these functions.

There is an ever-present tension in The City as a community-organization model. When we get caught up in our "organizational aspects," we invariably get pulled up short by the community, and when we get caught up in our "community aspects," organizational requirements intervene. Why is this? The fact that The City receives significant United Way, corporate, and government dollars might more than suggest that The City is an agent of the dominant culture. The fact that The City operates an "organization" and uses organizational language (e.g., personnel policies, budgets, strategic plans) might more than suggest that The City has been infected by the dominant culture of corporate America, the mother ship colonizing the world of the poor. The case could be made

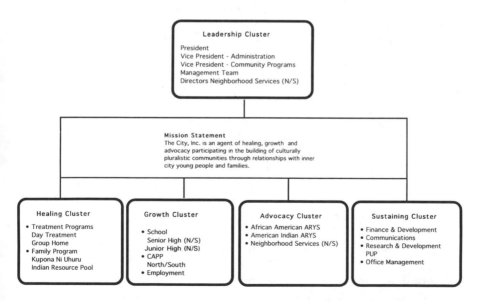

FIGURE 1.1. Organizational chart of The City, Inc.

that this tension is a result of the dominant culture at work, pitting The City as community organization against itself in an ongoing tension that will always represent a functional challenge of organizational self-incapacitation.

Or is this organizational tension simply a challenge to meet the need for both internal coherence and external alliances? This situation may be similar to how the Ojibway describe the functions of the warrior society: protecting the tribe, ever ready for battle, representing an ongoing tension between stability and change within the tribal community. This tension is likely to be ever present, particularly as long as The City has organizational aspects funded by dominant-culture institutions but constituted by inner-city cultures. Again, it is the conversation that centers and keeps the tension—the communal and the organizational. As long as the local community desires resources from the dominant culture, this strategy to create a community organization must contain tension.

Officially, corporate America pays for us to focus on the lives of individuals and families in the inner-city communities of Minneapolis. If one were just to pay attention to that aspect of corporate America's relationship with The City, one would miss the equally important necessities of The City's and corporate America's need for ongoing conversations to create alliances. The energies of an organization which functions, in part, to serve a local community must also capture resources to do the job; this need necessitates attending to the development and empowerment of local community coherence (nurturing and enhancing developing relationships and associations at the community level) and also to the creation of external alliances with those who have the funding.

PERSUADING STAKEHOLDERS

Storytelling is a primary mode by which The City's history and beliefs are communicated. This dynamic is related both to what The City is and who it serves; oral tradition, "the constant exercise of a rich memory" (Lopez, 1978, p. 81), is prized above written tradition within tribal communities. This tradition has given rise to an anecdotal emphasis in The City's process of evaluation. Unfortunately, anecdote does not have a high standing within traditional research.

Just as conversation as a form of communication is emphasized, access to those conversations is valued as equally important. Such access stands the traditional notion of "authority" on its head. Participation and inclusion are important whether in new staff hires, discipline issues, or simple day-to-day matters; families and their children will be a part of the process. Important aspects of these conversations have been getting and giving feedback, reflecting on what has happened, and making adjustments as well as creating and re-creating strategies. Conversations hold a central place throughout the organization, providing an opportunity to persuade as well as be persuaded. In fact, written procedures and structures are strikingly absent from day-to-day activities. These dynamics force new staff as well as members of our board of directors to stick around long enough to "hear" and to interact. But they also cause some *angst* in individuals who expect certain organizational procedures to be readily available in manuals.

Drawing on relationships developed with families and their cultures during the 1970s, The City began to consciously understand the importance of ways of knowing quite different from that of organizational cultures traditional to the United Way system. Having participated in an earlier United Way evaluation project in 1978, The City became concerned about the exclusive emphasis on a management-by-objective form promulgated by the United Way. Weren't there other processes of evaluation that also had credibility? Or, if one uses a different process, is that process less credible?

The need of The City to communicate to two audiences who were from different cultural and class perspectives became apparent. It is important not to overlook the fact that one of these audiences represents the dominant culture and serves as the gatekeeper, who defines what is and is not a "legitimate" inquiry process, to the financial resources of this society. The United Way system looked askance on anecdotal processes as sloppy and too subjective, but the management-by-objective system was given life within the corporate structures across America, not invented by the tribal elders at the Red Lake Reservation or on the streets of inner-city Minneapolis, and therefore did not fit our other audience.

The awareness of cultural and class differences in the determination of what were and were not "legitimate" processes of evaluation (or, minimally, what processes were of equal legitimacy) led The City to emphasize the interaction between belief and persuasion in our healing/counseling processes (Frank, 1961; Lambo, 1978; Lévi-Strauss, 1963; Powers, 1982; Torrey, 1986). Persuasion and belief seem to transcend cultures and classes in the sense that everybody believes some things about their world and utilizes those beliefs to persuade themselves and others about what is and is not real about their world.

Lévi-Strauss (1963, p. 168), in working with South American tribal healers, experienced a relationship between "efficacy of certain magical practices" and the "belief in magic." This relationship requires a combination of the sorcerer's belief in his or her effectiveness and the patient's expectation of the sorcerer's effectiveness, both belief and expectation emerging and held together in the faith of the community. Jerome Frank

(1961) echoes this emphasis on the interplay between patient, healer, and group in *Persuasion and Healing* (p. 53). From whence do these beliefs and expectations necessary to the induction of hope and healing come? Lambo (1978), while indicating that modern techniques fall short, emphasizes the importance of collaborating with native healers to appropriate "the therapeutic practices that already existed in the indigenous culture" (p. 37). For Lambo, "the most important therapeutic factor was the patient's social contacts" (p. 38). The essential connection between community and healing was also noted by the anthropologist Powers (1982) in his work with the Oglala. He observed, "It was neither patient nor the medicine man who really counted in the rhythmic flow of rituals. It was the people—the community, the Oglalas. Everything and everyone else was expendable" (p. 85).

The community holds together and gives definition to this relationship between the healer and healed, teacher and taught, in an ongoing dance of persuasion and belief. It is within this dance that the collective healing needs of the community are shaped, addressed, and evaluated. Accountability exists within the relationship, as the "healer" is dependent on families believing they have been healed and communicating this belief to others within the community. It is the community that sustains these important functions of healing, teaching, advocating, sustaining, and leading.

Persuading stakeholders, funders, and program participants is contingent upon a combination of one's belief in the efficacy of one's own "system and techniques," and one's ability, in consort with the community, to transfer that belief into an expectancy in the mind and heart of the stakeholder, funder, and program participant. In relationship and community, mutuality and reciprocity are a given part of what emerges. Systems of belief and persuasion are key dynamics to what is perceived as reality. These systems emerge from communities.

THE CITY'S EVALUATION PROCESS

In 1980, the United Way of Minneapolis instituted an evaluation system that was designed to provide an opportunity for its member agencies to demonstrate impact and effectiveness in addressing "community problems." While who decides the meaning of "impact" and "effectiveness" is critical, equally important are the questions "impact on what?" and "effectiveness for what?" Because of The City's historical emphasis on relationships and because a large majority of its staff is from the community, the program participants' perspective and meanings about these two questions have been essential. The importance of program participants' definitions is further underscored when considering class and culture issues within the context of racism. Our therapists, our healers, have been able to stay anchored in these discussions by focusing on the question "How do you know, at the end of the day, week, month, or year that you have done a good job?" Critical and implicit to this accountability question is the perspective of the program participant *in community:* As a healer, teacher, or advocate chosen by your community, to what are you paying attention? The assumption is you are paying attention to that which is in the interest of the community that chose and sustains your function. A system that gives frequent feedback to staff members regarding their activity in providing client-community benefit is critical.

Here is where Weick's "messiness" is most evident. We have a lot of staff meetings: Stories are told, numbers shared, criticisms aired, challenges considered, accepted, and rejected. For instance, imagine a large weekly group of family therapists presenting their rationales with video examples as "evidence" of their reality, then having a group deconstruction–reconstruction. The hierarchy created by roles and experience are suspended for the moment as this group becomes the authority. This process is both threatening and affirming. Accountability to community is not easy work.

The staff, board of directors, and as many of our relatives as we can imagine review program participant–community effectiveness on a quarterly and annual basis. In these activities, both anecdotal and quantitative analyses become realistic responses, given The City's challenge to communicate with various cultures and communities. Program participants, staff, board, funder, and wider community are all related in this partnership of reflecting, re-searching, and co-creating strategies for building community in the inner city. In spite of and, yet, because of the corporate value system, The City continues to learn how to communicate more effectively with its funders. Of course, it is important to be vigilant so as to not lose the soul of our work to numbers. Our system of evaluation was created to keep us focused on our mission and niche in order to effectively serve individuals, families, and the inner-city community, as well as to attract those resources necessary to carry out the mission through the process of "the making of relatives." Witness the circle of relationships between healer and healed, teacher and student and their community.

CULTURAL CASE EXAMPLES

The Indian Resource Pool (IRP)

Critical to the understanding of this case study is our experience that relationships opened the door to cultural processes. The history of relationships led to the experience of culture at work in the everyday lives of the young people and families with whom we have been involved. The Indian Resource Pool (IRP) was the first such programmatic venture (Nelson, 1994).

The IRP was formally established in 1980 at the initiation of two American Indian staff in our family counseling program who believed The City had a unique opportunity: American Indian families could have the advantage of receiving services from American Indian staff members. Of course, this required staff members with the vision, access, and competency; leadership was and continues to be one of the most important variables in this endeavor.

The IRP was created for two primary reasons: (1) to provide culturally appropriate "therapy" to American Indian families believing, based on experience, that American Indian traditional therapists and healers can be at least as effective using their methods as their European American counterparts can be using standard counseling techniques, and (2) to establish a training and supervision process directed by American Indians which would attract as well as further enhance the competencies of American Indian therapists and healers.

The IRP provides an effective, working demonstration of the efficacy of cultural healing practices, something American Indians always knew about their cultures. The program also makes economic sense. Consider the dollars a psychiatrist, psychologist, social worker, or family therapist makes, then consider the community where this professional is likely to live and spend those dollars. If it is correct that inner-city communities have been marked as "client communities," with an overwhelming emphasis on consuming rather than producing services, and if the economic concept is correct that the longer a dollar stays in a particular community, the healthier the economics of that community, then it may stand to reason that the dollars a medicine man or woman spends in an inner-city community are economically more contributory to that community than the same dollars given to a psychologist to spend in a suburban community.

Initially, the United Way volunteers who determine what is funded and at what level were concerned about what they called "reverse discrimination." We responded that the importance of culture in healing and community building, coupled with the structural barriers of racism in the field of counseling, outweighed such concerns (actually, we had to bite our tongues). The United Way has supported the IRP from its beginnings. Throughout the negotiations process, the United Way focused on our performance measures and outcomes, without questioning our methodology. This focus is an important, essential consideration in cross-cultural work; if the dominant culture is allowed to dictate both method and outcome, without realization of the its pervasive role in all so-called "professional processes," other cultures do not have a chance.

Currently, The City has medicine people on staff, representing Ojibway, Dakota, and Lakota cultures, whose jobs are to make available their healing gifts and expertise as well as to provide access to the rich range of healing processes of their tribes and cultures. Since the healing accoutrements of these healers do not represent the entire range of healing processes available through their cultures, they also provide referrals. This cultural competency stands alongside of the European and American traditions of social work, family therapy, psychology, and psychiatry.

The IRP's focus is highly correlated with relationships and community. There is a functional community emphasis that centralizes issues of living and quality of life for a urban community bound up in relationships and rituals of the tribe. The tribe—not necessarily its political aspects but its relationship-making aspects—transcends and extends its influence to the inner-city community. It is a source of reconnection to the healing aspects and contributions of the culture. Many who have worked culturally with American Indian communities, when faced with the plight of individuals and families, often inquire when they last had visited their people. Returning for a weekend powwow, sweat, or simply a visit with relatives can be helpful, as such cultural reconnections in and of themselves are healing.

The City, building on these types of experiences, attempts to take advantage of cultural rituals for Indian families who, for whatever reason, find themselves cut off from these connecting opportunities. The springtime ritual of the Sugar Bush, in upper midwestern tribes, is a rigorous but healing opportunity not only to collect maple sugar with extended family and other members of social networks but also to focus on the event of spring, celebrating new life. Annually, The City's staff and students participate in this ceremony as family-in-community therapy.

I have had the honor of participating in both sweat lodge and healing ceremonies. Once, on the Lac Courte Oreilles reservation, I was surprised at the number of recovering alcoholics who had traveled great distances on a weekly basis to participate in this healing ritual; one participant told me that his "life depended on it." These rituals are held by the tribe, the extended relational networks of the community. As Eliade (1964) and Campbell (1988) have written, there is a connection between traditional rituals, the cycles of life, hope, and healing, traditions long forgotten by many European American practitioners.

At-Risk Youth Services (ARYS)

These experiences within the American Indian community opened the door for the development of The City's capacity to access and utilize cultural and community resources. The City found itself in a position to respond to the more recent gang phenomenon in portions of the African American community because it knew organizationally that healing dynamics are embedded within these social networks and can be appropriated and enhanced. Questions arise when one seeks to apply experiences with one community/culture of people to another group. What are the attitudes, predispositions and skills needed to pull off the jobs of accessing and utilizing cultural and community resources? What are the strategies (which encourage coherence) used to identify the relatives internal to that community? What are the strategies (which encourage alliances) used to make relatives external to that community? How are these skills acquired? I think it has something to do with the community dynamic of "generational transmission." It assumes capitalizing on active opportunities to appropriate the human aspects and contributions of the history of a community through the life cycle.

What formal aspects of tribal life are available today for African Americans? Consider the cultural traditions readily practiced and available to the Dakota, Lakota, and Ojibway in the state of Minnesota. There are no parallels, no readily available traditions, for those African Americans of Yoruba, Zulu, or Bushman tribal lineage. In fact, many African Americans have no idea of their tribal heritage nor have the resources to acquire such information. While The City has little idea how many tribes our young people and families represent, we have a healing program, Kipona Ni Uhuru (Swahili for "Healing Is Freedom"), charged with seeking out, developing, and instituting African American healing traditions.

History, however, has numerous examples of functional attempts to preserve cultural knowledge transmitted through adaptive tribal structures. The Maroon and Bizango societies of the Caribbean (Davis, 1988), the history of the African American church (Alexander, 1987), and the so-called gang phenomenon (Dawley, 1992; Vigil, 1988) in inner cities across America are just some of the many examples. When the institutions charged with protecting and serving a particular community are judged by that community, for whatever reasons, as no longer providing those functions, communities have, throughout history, developed their own processes to provide for these needs. Consider Friedman's (1989) comments in *From Beirut to Jerusalem:*

> What all of the associations have in common is the fact that their members are all bound together by a tribe-like spirit of solidarity, a total obligation to one another, and a mutual loyalty that takes precedence over allegiances to the wider community or nation-state. . . . resources were so limited that everyone had to become a wolf and be prepared to survive at the expense of the other tribe. There just weren't enough *resources* to satisfy everyone all the time. . . . These alliances began with the most basic blood association—the family—and then expanded to

the clan, the tribe, and then to other tribes. [Everyone] understood that because of the nature of this world, the bonds of kinship must be honored before all other obligations; anyone who did not behave in this way was totally dishonored. (pp. 87–88)

The dominant culture "accepts" the phenomenon of American Indian tribes but does not understand or accept inner-city gangs. The City has come to understand these social networks as tribes attempting to build community and transmit cultural values in the Beirut-like context of our inner cities.

The City's At-Risk Youth Services (ARYS, pronounced "arise") grew out of the cultural experiences of the IRP and our collective curiosity about tribal communities. Given the media's fascination with so-called "youth gangs," it is instructive to learn that these organizations seldom utilize that moniker to describe themselves, preferring the terms nations, families, people, folks, associations, or sets, and have membership that not only has, in some cases, spanned 40 years but has represented the entire life cycle as well. Upon closer investigation, one discovers that portions of the Vice Lord nation have subscribed to the five principles of Islam and the Disciple family attends to the wisdom found in the Old Testament. The Vice Lords of Chicago have an in-depth history of social and educational action and community development in late 1960s that seldom receives notice (Dawley, 1992).

At-Risk Youth Services (ARYS) was born from the vision of one of our staff persons, a humanitarian with a long term involvement in the civil rights movement in our community. He was very concerned in the early 1980s about an unprecedented rise in gang activity in Minneapolis; the local community did not pay attention. He remarked to me, "If a group of young people was behaving in a certain way, doesn't it make sense that the adult community would go find out what's up?" He further believed that if we were to ever be successful at altering negative gang behavior, we needed to provide opportunities that were every bit as attractive as gang membership. A nagging question was whether or not we, as a society, could afford to continue an enforcement–eradication–suppression–only strategy. The prison population in America has grown 400% since 1970 and is projected to double again by 1994. A single strategy, it seemed to us, would bankrupt this society, particularly with recidivism as high as it is, coupled with the knowledge that prisons do not rehabilitate.

In 1987, The City, through a combination of local foundation support and a federal grant hired gang leadership to work with young people and adults currently involved in this gang activity or at greatest risk for such involvement. In spite of newspaper accounts that said, "The City receives funds to fights gangs," our interest was in working with the young members and their families, which was probable only if we had some kind of relationship with the leadership of these organizations. An essential point was in identifying and hiring leadership chosen by the local community, not by an ideal notion of an homogenized African American community, where the dominant community chooses "leaders" they are comfortable with to represent the entire African American community and its experiences.

Of course, that was no short order. Fortunately, because of our community relationships, we had staff on board who were intimate with the communities where they worked. The relationships developed there would facilitate what we were trying to do organizationally: build communities with others and, in this case, with leaders of organizations called gangs.

From my 20-year perspective of inner-city work, I have serious questions about our national obsession with enforcement strategies, particularly given the exponential growth of our prisons and their substantive lack of effectiveness at much other than warehousing. I have heard it said many times, "Prison's supposed to be a 'carrot-and-stick' issue, but jail time ain't no stick, just three meals a day, a chance to work-out daily, access to sex and drugs and hang out with friends."

Even if one considers these inner-city people an "enemy," one strategy is the engagement of conversation. What one will likely find in these conversations is that the denial of economic opportunity in these inner-city communities is a primary hypothesis that will challenge engagement. Consider this section from *Mpls/St. Paul Magazine:*

> Inadequate family life, poverty, deteriorating neighborhoods, ineffective religion, poor education and lack of recreational facilities. Together they amount to a denial of opportunity so complete it can extinguish hope. And as author James Baldwin once wrote, the most dangerous creature a society can create is one without hope. (Robeson, 1990, p. 68ff.)

Carrying out the strategy becomes a matter of providing that opportunity in hopes that there will be change.

Early on, one of our major funders, out of remarkable curiosity, met with 25 or so gang members from various "sets." The inquiry was simple: "Why do you hang out with each other?" Around the table, stories of support, loyalty, and friendship blotted out any reference to money and drugs and gave way to touching talk of fathers, brothers, and friends — an inner-city answer to extended social and family networks? In the minds of these leaders, their relationships provided real opportunity for friendships, protection, housing, and food.

The City's "covenant" was simple: Leave behind the negative behavior of street crime, get and keep your membership in school, mediate disputes, and promote jobs, and The City will hire you as an outreach worker. *Mpls/St. Paul Magazine,* writing about gangs and our program staff, noted some of the challenge:

> Copeland shares a car, office space and counseling strategies with Farly Cotten, a three-year veteran outreach worker. During the 1980's, Cotten was a guiding force behind the Minneapolis Bloods, a fearsome gang whose stronghold is primarily in south Minneapolis. . . . The relationship between Copeland and Cotten is remarkable because the Disciples and the Vice Lords—the dominant gangs in both Chicago and the Twin Cities—are bitter rivals. The fact that Copeland and Cotten face physical danger for associating with each other lends credence to their claims that they want to move beyond gang violence and become positive role models in the community. (Robeson, 1990, p. 66)

Ranking members of the Bloods, Disciples, Souls, and Vice Lords, hired for their positions as community leaders, kept their positions of persuasion and influence so that their ranks might pause to consider other options to the streets: a chance for a "legitimate" job and a life that might just be a few steps further from death.

The City School was a place for one's "homeys" but also for those who, on the streets, were the enemy. In the first year of the ARYS program, we had a "full bore competition" between the Bloods, Disciples, Souls, and Vice Lords as to what "set" earned more credits or got more of their membership elected to the student board. I am sure it would be hard for people who rely primarily on news accounts for their opinions to imagine two young, street-tough gang members arguing in the hallway of our school over what constituted a sentence—only satisfied when their teacher, as the authority, settled the dispute.

One of our students, a ranking leader in the Disciples as well as president of the student board, took advantage of the opportunity to volunteer in our on-site day care for school credit. He found he had a natural talent in working with infants and toddlers, and upon his graduation, we were in a position to hire him as a child care aide. But "Chill" had to get to school and stay. What kept him at the task of his education? A partnership between teachers and street leadership delicately balanced by their working relationship with each other. The opportunity to learn was supported and made possible through these relationships.

Recently, one of our local newspapers ran an alarming story on the increasingly large numbers of police calls to junior and senior high schools. The City School, with almost 200 students, all with extensive criminal justice system histories, has had no calls for the police in the past 10 years. While knocking on wood, we believe the record is an indication of this relational atmosphere created by the students and staff. Not that conflict is absent, but, rather, it is nestled within relationships that are committed, for this moment, to working things out. Conflict is a given, and negative behavior is best addressed in the day-to-day-relationships where the convenience of "go to the principal's office" is replaced by conversations between two people trying to negotiate a learning environment.

And it is not that guns are not present—they are. It is a safety issue. If young people do not feel safe and you, as an adult, cannot make them feel safe—whether in school, home, or the streets—they are going to carry weapons.[1] Adults need to focus on what they can control, letting go of that which they cannot control. If you focus on gun control, you de-focus education. It is the same with wearing gang colors or hats cocked right or left—it is the wrong thing to focus on and it is based on control: Aren't adolescents suppose to "mess with" control issues as a normal part of development? Historically and by definition, adolescents are quite astute at defying the attempts of the adult community to control their young lives.

Strong words, negative looks, fights, and shootings between two rival groups in the neighborhood threatened the peace and stability of our community and school on the Northside. It took the staff leadership from both groups and, as importantly, the relationship between these leaders, to provide the glue for bringing and keeping the families together for a morning "meeting."

There was a need to fully air the issues, with death as a real option if the need was not addressed. It was important that everyone *felt* heard; this was a part of developing and establishing decency and respect. The words were strong and loud. In the beginning of the meeting, staff often had to forcefully remind everyone of the need for one person speaking at a time. The growing, collective ability to "hang" through the energy and passion without escalation was evidenced throughout the meeting. After the issues were on the table, the staff cautiously had people from the different families talk *with* each other. Sprinkled in between were staff reminders about respect. As time went on, the level of overt conflict and escalating threats began to diminish. The community staff replaced pleas for respect with punctuations of encouragement as conversations began to take on an air of the sacred: "Someone is speaking now."

From my perspective, a new reality was being created through the conversations (enactments) being attempted—new relationships, mirroring the relationships modeled between the staff, who were once enemies, themselves. The possibility occurred to me that the skills of enactment and reframing may be rooted in ancient tribal traditions, as the skills were being naturally and aptly used by the staff with no clinical training: Gang leaders as therapists.

The meeting ended with a concluding homily from the program director, "Is this what this is all about? We're shooting at each other because you didn't like how she looked at you?" A new hope was present only through the success of the conversations over the past 2 hours. Handshakes and slow leave taking until another day—ideally, one with less violence.

A few months later, an angry crowd of 200 or so gang members from two different groups gathered in our parking lot. Shots in the neighborhood at one group by the other had resulted in shooting in our lot. Tempers flared. There was a continued insistence on respect. The inquiry "What did I do to disrespect you? Nothing? Then why you treatin' me this way?" finally got the leaders together to talk out of sight of the crowd. The conversation quickly moved to nobody wanting violence and who was going to do what to guarantee that no violence occurred. One of the most vocal people throughout the incident was a woman we later hired as a "community associate." "Pee Wee" was interested in people respecting each other and "calling out" The City to do more about that by representing all "sets" equally. Clearly, she represented challenging and impassioned leadership, rich with relational skills. These relationships established a beginning context for peace, particularly that night.

The resource of relationship is developed here: this night with gunfire, hostility, groups called gangs, and a community staff. Conversation is about all we had. The opportunity for security from violence—a negotiated community security—is a by-product. This setting is their community and their families' and children's dreams and hopes. These "gang" leaders are their leaders. Finding the incentive to keep communities together is critical. Cops and "others," without community relationships, get nervous about "people and folks"[2] getting together; concluding conspiracy, they invent laws that focus on associations rather than behavior. This is why engagement is important; it can diffuse conspiracy theories and the further objectification of groups of people as problems and threats.

Our road has been rocky and likely will continue to be so. In 1988, three gang members came into our building and shot one of our ARYS staff in the head. In response, a Minneapolis deputy chief of police, who had never been in our building nor met any staff, proclaimed: "I have no time for The City, Inc. I'm not impressed by them. These are some of the people who have done everything they can for 20 years to bilk the community" (Bonner, 1988, p. 1A). In spite of the fact that this was a front page story, the deputy chief's apology was later run on the back page of the paper.

A letter from a person unknown to anyone in Minneapolis but purporting to know our staff received wide circulation in local community newspapers:

These individuals, with dubious pasts, hoodlum mentality, drug users, professional program hustlers, have not made any positive contributions to the Black community. . . . We are particularly concerned about Jim Nelson who has created a hostile and hoodlum atmosphere around the vicinity of The City and is now being used by the white power structure to be the vehicle through which old Black, faded, irresponsible leaders have a chance to regain power. (Boone, 1988, p. 3)

Later, an article appeared in *Mpls/St. Paul Magazine* on gangs:

The At-Risk program attempts to mediate potentially violent gang disputes, truancy and criminality among inner-city youths and counsel those who are considering entering or leaving a gang. It is not without controversy: Both inside and outside various law-enforcement agencies, the outreach aspect of the program is perceived as either one of the few, best hopes for reaching deeply troubled youths or a paid haven and front for some of the most ruthless and influential gang members in the Twin Cities. (Robeson, 1990, p. 65)

Recently, a commentary in the *Minneapolis Star Tribune* took a more positive bent:

When members of a youth gang wanted to dispute the initial police version of Tycel Nelson's death (a 16-year-old African American shot in the back by police) they went to a community agency they trust—for some, perhaps the only one. It's called The City, Inc. . . . The agency hires gang members for its staff; none has been arrested while employed. . . . On issues of troubled youth, The City is truly on society's front line. (Inskip, 1990, p. 23A)

The national philanthropic newspaper *The Chronicle of Philanthropy* ran a special report on nine organizations that were taking risks and had "the best chance of making it through the 1990's":

Employing gang members is part of the organization's effort to build trust with inner-city minority youths and families and to help them build self-sufficient communities. Consistent with that mission, The City has hired people with the same ethnic and racial backgrounds as its clients. While Mr. Nelson is white, 87 per cent of the staff members live in the inner city and are black, Hispanic, or American Indian. The City even hired three medicine men to counsel American Indian families. Seven gang members are on the staff. . . .

But the policy has put the City at odds with the police.

"It's like having the fox guard the chicken coop," says a police officer, . . . a gang-crime specialist with the Minneapolis Police Department. Police officers believe that some gang members hired by The City are still active in illegal activities and that the organization is inadvertently contributing to crime committed by the estimated 3,500 gang members in the Twin Cities. (Hall, 1992, p. 1ff.)

A conference on community and violence sponsored by The City, The Minneapolis Police Department, the Minneapolis Youth Coordinating Board and the U.S. Department of Health and Human Services received play locally as well as nationally (*Chicago Tribune*):

> A ranking Chicago gang member who just served a 10 year murder sentence in Minnesota, began a new career this week as a youth outreach worker. His job: to win over younger gang members to constructive law-abiding lives.
>
> Some police officers wince at the idea. But James Nelson, director of City Inc., the Minneapolis community development agency that hired [staffmember's name] considers him a risk worth taking. . . .
>
> In Minneapolis, City, Inc. focuses on the concept of community building rather than ridding the area of gangs. . . .
>
> But for all their suspicion, several dozen Minneapolis police officers participated in a two-day conference on youth violence with City, Inc. last week. As part of the meeting, the officers were bused to several of Minneapolis' minority ethnic groups. A goal was to get them to feel part of the community, Nelson said.
>
> "Part of the problem," he said " is that the simplicity of what is required gets lost in the shuffle: Caring for each other." (Worthington, 1991, pp. 29, 32)

Over time, ARYS staff, through their relationships, facilitated a gang council:

> A group of self-described gang leaders announced Tuesday that they will join in a group called United for Peace and work to diminish street violence in the Twin Cities.
>
> The announcement appears to commit members of the several gangs that were represented to an unspecified accord that will emphasize "keeping the peace."
>
> Sitting side by side at a news conference at The City Inc., an alternative school and drop-in center for inner-city youth, the five gang leaders told reporters that they plan to meet regularly with the aim of minimizing gang tensions and improving the standing of black youth. (Diaz, 1992, p. 1A)

The *St. Paul Pioneer Press* ran an editorial stating the following:

> The stunning announcement Tuesday by leaders of four rival African-American gangs in Minneapolis that their gangs have joined a new union

United for Peace, is an answer to prayers . . . it is also a tribute to the work of Spike Moss and The City, Inc., a social service agency and alternative school that serves inner-city youth and employs Mr. Moss. The City and Mr. Moss helped build bridges to the gang leaders and encouraged the new direction of non-violence. ("Support Groups' Efforts," 1992, p. 12A)

In the aftermath of the Los Angeles rebellion, Minneapolis had a similar challenge. The ARYS staff were key to restoring order to the community, according to the *Minneapolis Star Tribune*:

Deputy Chief David Dobrotka said about 15 black volunteers, including ministers, gang leaders and staff from The City, Inc., were instrumental in keeping the violence from escalating further.
"If it wasn't for them, I would have had to have 100 cops there," he said. "No doubt in my mind."
On his way to the scene, Dobrotka stopped at The City, Inc.'s northside office and asked for assistance from youth outreach worker Spike Moss and anyone else available. . . . "I give them all the credit in the world," Dobrotka said. "Otherwise we'd have been back to the '60's with all these cops here with helmets and nightsticks and ugly confrontations." ("Teenager's Shooting," 1992, pp. 1A, 12A)

Today, we still employ gang *leaders* who have taken a sabbatical from the negatives of gang behavior to "try on" something else: encouraging their membership to not only get in school but to progress toward graduation as well as find and develop jobs. So far, it is working. The other option is the continued warehousing of groups of people, segregated by race and culture, in programs that have no demonstrated, positive impact yet cost society billions of dollars. Why not invest in building community rather than prisons?

POSTSCRIPT

In early September 1992, we were associated by affiliation with the murder of a police officer. A true tragedy. There was/is a lot of posturing, speculation, and irresponsible talk of guilt by innuendo without due process, something poor communities of color have grown used to. The relationship between the community we serve and the Minneapolis Police Department has been broken. The metaphors of Sisyphus and the roller coaster are apt here. A relational beach head established today erodes tomorrow in this ebb and flow of human successes and failures. The future is wildly fluid and the peacemakers hope for the potential of healing in conversations. . . . all my relatives. . . . Have pity on us. . . .

NOTES

1. If we are aware that a student is "carrying," the weapon is confiscated and turned over to the parent or guardian of the student. The student may be subjected to community consequences, such as a meeting with the student board to discuss the reason for carrying a weapon as well as the threat to the community this action may have posed. Family work is sometimes initiated.

2. This is what two gangs call their groups.

REFERENCES

Alexander, B. (1987). The Black church and community empowerment. In R. Woodson (Ed.), *On the road to economic freedom: An agenda for Black progress* (pp. 45–69). Washington, DC: Regnery Gateway.

Aponte, H. (1986). If I don't get simple, I cry. *Family Process, 25*(4), 531–548.

Ashby, R. (1956). *An introduction to cybernetics.* London: Chapman Hall.

Atkinson, B., & Heath, A. (1987). Beyond objectivism and relativism: Implications for family therapy research. *Journal of Strategic and Systemic Therapies, 6*(1), 8–17.

Attneave, C. (1982). American Indians and Alaska native families: Emigrants in their own homeland. In M. McGoldrick, J. K. Pearce, & J. Giordano (Eds.), *Ethnicity and family therapy* (pp. 55–83). New York: Guilford Press.

Auerswald, E. H. (1968). Interdisciplinary versus ecological approach. *Family Process, 7,* 205–215.

Bateson, G. (1972). *Steps to an ecology of mind: A revolutionary approach to man's understanding of himself.* New York: Ballantine Books.

Berger, L., & Luckmann, T. (1967). *The social construction of reality: A treatise in the sociology of knowledge.* New York: Anchor Books.

Bly, R. (1990). *Iron John, a book about men.* Reading, MA: Addison-Wesley.

Bonner, B. (1988, February 15). Minneapolis shootings revive street gang issue. *St. Paul Pioneer Press,* p. 1A.

Boone, P. (1988, September). They're back. *Northside Residence and Redevelopment Council Review,* p. 3.

Campbell, J. (1988). *Myths to live by.* New York: Bantam Books.

Castaneda, C. (1974). *Tales of power.* New York: Simon & Schuster.

Cecchin, G. (1987). Hypothesizing, circularity, and neutrality revisited: An invitation to curiosity. *Family Process, 26*(4), 405–414.

Davis, W. (1988). *Passage of darkness: The ethnobiology of the Haitian zombie.* Chapel Hill: University of North Carolina Press.

Dawley, D. (1992). *A nation of lords* (2nd ed.). Prospect Heights, IL: Waveland Press.

Diaz, K. (1992, May 6). Five gang leaders unite for peace on area streets. *Minneapolis Star Tribune,* p. 1A.

Eliade, M. (1964). *Shamanism: Archaic techniques of ecstasy.* Princeton, NJ: Princeton University Press.

Frank, J., (1961). *Persuasion and healing: A comparative study of psychotherapy.* Baltimore: Johns Hopkins University Press.

Friedman, T. (1989). *From Beirut to Jerusalem.* New York: Anchor Books.

Goffman, E. (1974). *Frame analysis: An essay on the organization of experience.* New York: Harper Colophon Books.

Gurnoe, S., & Nelson, J. (1989). Two perspectives on working with American Indian families: A constructivist-systemic approach. In E. Gonzales-Santin (Ed.), *Collaboration: The key* (pp. 63–85). Tempe: Arizona State University School of Social Work.

Inskip, L. (1990, December 19). The City Inc.—Building trust on society's front line. *Minneapolis Star Tribune,* p. 23A.

Hoffman, L. (1990). Constructing realities: An art of lenses. *Family Process, 29*(1), 1–12.

Hall, H. (1991, January 15). Taking risks in hard times, The City Inc.: Gang members on staff. *The Chronical of Philanthropy,* pp. 1ff., 6–8.

Johnston, B. (1976). *Ojibway heritage.* Toronto: McClelland & Stewart.

Keeney, B. P. (1983). *Aesthetics of change.* New York: Guilford Press.

Krebs, C. J. (1972). *Ecology: The experimental analysis of distribution and abundance.* New York: Harper & Row.

Lambo, T. A. (1978, March). Psychotherapy in Africa. *Human Nature,* 33–39.

Lévi-Strauss, C. (1963). *Structural anthropology.* New York: Basic Books.

Linden, E. (1991, September 23). Lost tribes, lost knowledge. *Time,* pp. 46–55.

Lopez, B. (1978). *Of wolves and men.* New York: Scribner's.

Marcus, G., & Fischer, M. (1986). *Anthropology as cultural critique: An experimental moment in the human sciences.* Chicago: University of Chicago Press.

McKnight, J. (1987, Winter). Regenerating community. *Social Policy,* 54–58.

McKnight, J. (1989a, Summer). Do no harm: Policy options that meet human needs. *Social Policy,* 5–15.

McKnight, J. (1989b). *The future of low-income neighborhoods and the people who reside there: A capacity-oriented strategy for neighborhood development.* Unpublished manuscript, Center for Urban Affairs and Policy Research, Northwestern University.

Minuchin, S. (1974). *Families and family therapy.* Cambridge, MA: Harvard University Press.

Minuchin, S., Montalvo, B., Guerney, B., Rosman, B., & Schumer, F. (1967). *Families of the slums: An exploration of their structure and treatment.* New York: Basic Books.

Nelson, J. (1994). *Family therapy and the city: An examination of the community's role in healing, 1981–1990.* Unpublished doctoral dissertation, University of Minnesota, Minneapolis. Publication pending in *Dissertation Abstracts International.*

Nelson, J., & Shelledy, J. (1980). The application of structural family therapy with an American Indian family. In Y. Red Horse (Ed.), *Traditional and nontraditional community mental health services with American Indians* (pp. 4–29). Tempe: Arizona State University School of Social Work.

Nelson, J., & Shelledy, J. (1982). Problem-solving for effective parenting: A strategic approach. In J. R. Red Horse (Ed.), *American Indian families: Development strategies and community health* (pp. 1–22). Tempe: Arizona State University.

Powers, W. (1982). *Yuwipi: Vision and experience in Oglala ritual.* Lincoln: University of Nebraska Press.

Robeson, B. (1990, May). Mean streets. *Mpls/St. Paul Magazine,* p. 65ff.

Rorty, R. (1989). *Contingency, irony and solidarity.* Cambridge: Cambridge University Press.

Schon, D. (1983). *The reflective practitioner: How professionals think in action.* New York: Basic Books.

Smith, R. L. (1966). *Ecology and field biology.* New York: Harper & Row.

Support group's efforts to pursue peace. (1992, May 7). *St. Paul Pioneer Press,* p. 12A.

Taylor, R. J., Chatters, L., Tucker, M. B., & Lewis, E. (1990). Developments in research on Black families: A decade review. *Journal of Marriage and the Family, 52*(45), 993–1014.

Teenager's shooting stirs unrest. (1992, May 8). *Minneapolis Star Tribune,* pp. 1A, 12A.

Torrey, E. F. (1986). *Witchdoctors and psychiatrists: The common roots of psychotherapy and its future.* New York: Harper & Row.

Tyler, S. (1987). Post-modern ethnography: From document of the occult to occult document. In J. Clifford & G. Marcus (Eds.), *Writing culture: The poetics and politics of ethnography* (pp. 122–140). Berkeley: University of California Press.

Vigil, J. D. (1988). *Barrio gangs: Street life and identity in Southern California.* Austin: University of Texas Press.

Waldegrave, C. (1990). Just therapy. *Social Justice and Family Therapy: The Dulwich Centre Newsletter,* No. 1, 5–46.

Weick, K. *On pre-punctuating the problem of organization effectiveness.* Unpublished manuscript, Cornell University.

Wilson, W. J. (1980). *The declining significance of race: Blacks and changing American institutions* (2nd ed.). Chicago: University of Chicago Press.

Worthington, R. (1991, December 15). Minneapolis enlists gang members' help. *The Chicago Tribune,* pp. 29, 32.

2

Families in Their Own Evaluations

Steven W. Rathbun
Daniel R. Lord
Faye A. Koop
Vickie Burgess McArthur

The main character in *The Wizard of Oz,* Dorothy, voices a heartfelt sentiment that can be applied to our evaluation efforts. After her journey of high drama and wonder, she concludes her experiences by joyously exclaiming, "There's no place like home!" The Friends University Family Evaluation Project possesses this same conviction that "there's no place like home" to engage and evaluate families. Therefore, we have given up the convenience of our offices in order to meet with families in the place most central to their lives—their homes.

Wanting to produce a different type of evaluation, one that more sufficiently reflected the multidimensional complexities of family life, we ventured into uncharted waters. Although such a headlong plunge has its hazards, the experience nonetheless has been a rewarding one of discovery. Given the present exploratory stage of development, the model is undergoing continuous change and is "emerging" with each new family that we encounter.

Though we did not possess a "standardized model" that clearly mapped the procedures of evaluating families, we did have several guiding objectives that gave direction from the project's inception. First, we were committed to producing a family systems theory-based evaluation project. We believe this paradigm is theoretically robust and clinically rich in its capacity to explain the behavior of individuals and the functioning of their families (Gurman & Kniskern, 1991).

Second, we were committed to working with families and professionals through a collaborative means. Friends University has a strong Quaker heritage that shapes the thinking of this academic community. One of the fundamental ideals of the Society of Friends is an emphasis upon obtaining consensus amongst its members. We believe this is a worthy ideal that makes its own special contribution to the project. Through a collaborative approach we have been able to better secure the confidence of families and professionals alike to our family evaluation project.

Third, we were committed to viewing families' responses to us in the following perspective. Because we are complete strangers to the families, and therefore intruders into their daily routines, their protective responses are viewed as natural and to be respected. Though we receive entrance into their homes, we do not assume this to be an invitation to become deeply involved in their lives. Families often possess the belief in some variant form that they have little to gain and potentially much to lose by participating with yet another "concerned agency." To be accepted as a resource in the family's current crisis requires us to be respectful and patient in the joining process.

THE ORGANIZING FRAMEWORK OF THEORY

Our first step in the evaluation effort was that of clarifying the "family systems" theory that would guide our work. We began by choosing from this expansive field a selection of conceptual models that might offer both breadth and pragmatic use. William Doherty's (Doherty, Colangelo, & Hovander, 1991) Family Fundamental Interpersonal Relational Orientation (FIRO) soon became the primary theory base for our model, supported by specific strengths in the Circumplex (Olson, Russell, & Sprenkle, 1983) and McMaster (Epstein, Bishop, & Baldwin, 1982) models of family functioning.

Doherty's Family FIRO is a revisiting of Schutz's (1958) model of small group behavior developed in the 1950s. Doherty and his colleagues argue quite effectively that this conceptual lens holds promise as an organizing framework for the multitude of factors constituting any ongoing relationship system. As such, it offers several qualities we especially value for our own effort. First, it serves as a bridging language for a variety of systemic models. Second, it offers a needs-based, behavioral description of systemic relational functioning. And third, it serves a pragmatic role in efficient organization of clinical data from family interviews.

Through the Family FIRO, two primary "domains" of interpersonal activity describe the essential relational needs of the human. The first is inclusion. Doherty et al. (1991) describe it as defining "who's in and who's out," thus representing the fundamental matters of "organization and bonding" (p. 229). This domain represents the personal need to accomplish distinctiveness and worth as a member of a valued group. Inclusion is simply and profoundly the need to belong. Three subcategories help to clarify its behavioral expressions: (1) structure, seen through boundaries, roles, hierarchy, rules, and the resulting organizational patterns; (2) connection, observed through the enactment of attachment, nurture, and belonging; and (3) shared meaning, constituting distinctiveness at the group level of family identity through values, beliefs, ritual, and so forth.

The second domain is control. If inclusion is thought of as the accomplishment of interpersonal recognition, control is the activity of interpersonal effectiveness. Here, the Family FIRO recognizes the need of persons to experience a measure of individual influence and power in interaction with significant others. Doherty et al. (1991) describe this domain relative to family conflict, when individuals are most likely to experience their own interests in competition with others. We view it more broadly as the constant activity of negotiating personal authority within the context of significant relational membership (Bray, Williamson, & Malone, 1984). Descriptors such as competence, responsibility, and accountability have important application here. Again, Doherty adds detail by viewing three types of control interactions: (1) dominating, where one person attempts to exert influence over another; (2) reactive, where one person attempts to enact power by countering another's influence; and (3) collaborative, where two persons attempt to enact equal influence in the interaction. The Family FIRO offers a conceptual grid that is extremely useful for organizing the massive relational data rendered by even a single clinical interview (see Table 2.1).

Perhaps the Family FIRO's most clinically relevant features are its two assumptions regarding change. The first is obvious. Change will challenge and disrupt the family's previously existing enactments of inclusion and control processes. This is assumed whether the change be predictable (as in life cycle development), planned (as in accomplishing intentional goals), or unplanned (as in encountering unexpected trauma and distress). Change may alter role allocation and routine (inclusion–structure), the exchange of belonging behaviors (inclusion–connection), and even the family's confidence in the coherence of its group in relation to the world around it (inclusion–shared meaning). A balance of personal agency and family membership once acceptable may no longer be so setting in motion intense conflict (control interaction).

Doherty et al.'s (1991) second assumption demonstrates an epigenetic

TABLE 2.1. Family FIRO Concepts

Categories	Subcategories and descriptive terms		
Inclusion:	*Structure*	*Connectedness*	*Shared meaning*
Interactions	Boundaries	Nurturance	Identity
relating to	Role organization	Involvement	Loyalty
bonding and	Alliance	Commitment	Rituals
organization	Membership	Belonging	Values
	Position	Affiliation	World view
Control:	*Dominating*	*Reactive*	*Collaborative*
Interactions	Confrontation	Resistance	Negotiation
relating to	Coercion	Rebellion	Compromise
influence and	Manipulation	Submission	Balancing
power during	Dictating	Withdrawal	Give and take
conflict	Discipline	Disobedience	Working through
Intimacy:			
Interactions		Mutual sharing of feelings	
relating to		Relating to one another as unique	
open self-		personalities	
disclosure and		Emotionally close sexual interactions	
close personal		Sharing vulnerabilities	
exchanges			

Note. Data from Doherty, Colangelo, and Hovander (1991).

principle within the Family FIRO that is most important in guiding treatment efforts. Doherty is emphatic when he proposes that change is best managed by granting issues of inclusion priority over control process.

This is the core principle for us. Serious conflict following major family change can be viewed as commonly stemming from the family's failure to adapt its role patterns satisfactorily, leaving family members feeling left out or unfairly burdened, from undesired changes in the family's level of connectedness or cohesion, and/or from the family's loss of a sense of coherence about its identity and worldview. Therefore, issues of inclusion have highest priority for successful resolution during family transitions because they are the *sine qua non*s for successful adaptation in the control and intimacy areas.

In our view, this epigenetic principle within the Family FIRO defines the key directive for intervention. The clinician's primary task is to intervene through inclusion behavior rather than control interactions. Once the clinician attempts to force change upon the family, the line is crossed into control interaction and simply one more person is ensnared in the struggle for influence. The clinician's competence must be based in stimulating, engaging, and guiding the family's resources in the domain of inclusion behaviors.

Following this priority upon inclusion, we have drawn two additional family models into our project to add further resources to our own clinical efforts in this domain. Again, we are following Doherty's lead in attempting to enhance the synergistic power of the theory base by bringing relational models of similar concern into conversation through the Family FIRO framework (Doherty & Hovander, 1990).

The strength of the Circumplex model developed by Olson et al. (1983) lies in its cohesion dimension. In this dimension, the model attempts to describe the extent to which a relationship system balances individuality with membership. Where membership demonstrates exaggerated priority, the system is termed *enmeshed*. Where individuality dominates in the extreme, the system is regarded as *disengaged*. The resulting continuum offers a tool for designating a quick reading of a family's general management of this crucial and ever-present relational task. We agree with Doherty and Hovander (1990) that the Circumplex model's cohesion dimension interacts nicely with the Family FIRO's inclusion–connection subdomain. Together, the two concepts allow us to conceptualize both a family's perceived sense of belonging and its characteristic appearance in relational behavior.

The McMaster Model of Family Functioning (MMFF) (Epstein et al., 1982) offers similar enhancement to the Family FIRO. Its three task areas offer a simple grid for organizing stressors confronting the family. The extent to which a family may be encountering difficulty meeting basic life needs while negotiating prominent developmental tasks and being forced to cope with unexpected trauma simultaneously determines the extent of strain upon its inclusion processes. The MMFF's six areas of family functioning then provide useful detail to further describe contextual-based relational behavior. Problem solving and communication assist description of control interactions. Behavior control and role allocation indicate concerns of inclusion–structure. Affective responsiveness and involvement detail useful aspects of inclusion–connection.

Through the power of the Family FIRO to organize relational data, the strengths of both the Circumplex model and the MMFF are aligned for consistent and effective clinical use. This is true for the family therapy theoretical leanings within our evaluation team as well. Our structural family therapy lenses bring the detail of boundary identification across subsystems into the assessment of inclusion–structure. Bowen theory adds perspective to the predictable patterns of emotional reactivity fueling exaggerated control interactions. Our constructivist interests guide us in charting the family's inclusion–shared meaning through dominant narrative, beliefs, and rituals. Data from the vantage points of numerous conceptual systems interact through the common language of the Family FIRO, making our effort both stimulating and efficient.

One last acknowledgment is needed regarding our use of the Family FIRO. The temptation to be overwhelmed with the contextual and behavioral difficulties of the families themselves is constant. When our own sense of adequacy wanes, our presence can easily become coercive, our attitude resentful, and our language either hopeless or blaming. In such moments, the urge is strong to join with the family by blaming the referring agency or support the agency by blaming the family. When our own place and influence is so challenged, it seems almost natural to sacrifice the competence of one group to bolster inclusion in another. To do so, however, simply fuels the fires of control interaction at a larger systemic level, often complicating even more the originally well-intentioned effort to help families in distress.

This recognition has caused us to place priority upon two clinical concerns guiding the overall utilization of our theory base. The first is attention to the self of the therapist throughout our clinical involvement. The theory base just described reminds us to observe first of all our own responses to both the referring agencies and the families with whom we become involved. The Family FIRO helps us to construct and monitor our own roles in the larger, multilayered "therapeutic system." In that process, we have most control over our own behavior and see this as the most important tool of therapeutic change that we have to offer. The Family FIRO serves us well not only in facilitating evaluation of the families we serve but in keeping us accountable for our own thought, emotion, and behavior in relation to our own professional responsibilities.

The second clinical concern is to employ what White and Epston (1990) identify as the text analogy, or narrative, as we seek entry into each subsystem of the larger treatment milieu. We work at simply asking the family to tell us their story regarding both the course of events leading to the current difficulty as well as who they are as persons within their own family world. With the Family FIRO as our conversational guide, we attempt to take a learning position about the family identity and resist the temptation of allowing the referral incident to become the dominant narrative of the therapeutic relationship. If successful, this position and the resulting interaction dampens coercive control processes, promotes inclusion, and equips both the family and the therapeutic system with the potential of constructing a more positive story through the relationships of the treatment system.

While "evaluation" is our primary effort, our conceptual model also defines a specific intervention process. Disruption within a specific family context typically is exaggerated by the attempts of external agencies to assist. The process we attempt to engage is designed to interrupt this all too common expansion of runaway control behaviors. Our efforts to stimulate an inclusion process via the presenting problem holds the potential of creating a collaborative treatment context conducive to second- and third-order change. So far, it has been our observation that such change is promoted not only within the family itself but also within the relational complex of client, social agency, and treatment provider. Ideally, this becomes the larger goal of our work.

INTRODUCTION TO THE FRIENDS UNIVERSITY HOME-BASED FAMILY EVALUATION MODEL

The Friends University Home-Based Family Evaluation Model contains six distinct stages. Each stage is titled by its outcome goal. The description of the stages contains the processes by which we attempt to obtain the objective of each phase. Therefore, this segment of the chapter will focus on the processes engaged in the evaluation procedures rather than specifying the particular steps involved in carrying out the goal.

Stage 1: Establishing a Relationship with the Referring Agency

Establishing a working relationship with the referring agency is an important component of the evaluation project. There are various reasons to adopt this perspective, not the least of which is self-interest in survival. The challenge that is before us is to win the confidence of the various professionals involved with the families we evaluate. This is no small task. The most effective means of securing this relational confidence has been through the invitation to collaborate in a shared initiative to produce an evaluation service more suitable and responsive to the needs of families and agency alike.

Additionally, the collaborative invitation is extended by soliciting the agency's ideas in defining the central purpose of the evaluation being requested. Specifying the purpose is vital, for it gives clarity and direction to the assessment process. To proceed without the benefit of agreed upon objectives is to engage and produce a service potentially off the mark and of little value to the referring agency. Therefore, the time spent facilitating a mutual perspective is an effort well expended. The confidence of both concerned parties is better established, for the one side believes it will obtain a service tailored to its specified needs, while the other accepts the case knowing that it falls within its scope of expertise and practice.

Case Example

The primary referral agency for family services in our community is the Sedgwick County Department of Social Rehabilitation Services (SRS). This unit of government is charged with an impossible range of responsibilities, including child protective services. Stories abound among local clinicians of SRS cases hurried, mishandled, and bungled. At the same time, an emphasis on family preservation and greater cooperation with outside agencies and clinicians was consistently emerging from our county's SRS chief.

After drafting a description of our relational home-based evaluation model, we contacted the SRS chief requesting his agency's feedback to our ideas. In this first contact, we clearly stated our interest in a pilot project that sought to apply the relational expertise of marriage and family therapy to the challenge of determining family services to agency- and/or court-involved family cases. We asked to meet to learn more about the agency's current experience with such families, especially its stated effort to keep families intact, if at all possible, and to receive its critique on our own family evaluation model.

This approach resulted in a series of meetings involving several top SRS administrative and supervisory personnel. Our ideas were discussed, critiqued, and affirmed. We also listened to the agency's leadership critique their own system, voice their frustration with inadequate budgets and overwhelming caseloads, and dream of promoting change in their own ranks. After funding sources were clarified, referral procedures for requesting family evaluation were determined and set in motion. A new relationship system had been defined in which SRS leadership and our Friends University faculty negotiated a purposeful inclusion process.

First contacts with line staff social workers paralleled the relational process experienced with SRS administrators. Although initiated by the social worker, the interaction proceeded by exploring mutual interests, defining concerns, exploring options, and clarifying expectations and roles. The content was now that of a specific family and a specific service rather than an abstract conceptual model. But the interaction clearly demonstrated our attempt to facilitate adequate inclusion processes with the referring social worker.

Referral of the Miller family, described in this chapter, reflected this pattern. The case worker was encouraged by her supervisor to refer the family to our family evaluation pilot project. The social worker was quick to describe the details surrounding Tanya, an 8-year-old African American girl removed from her biological parents and placed with her maternal grandmother. The precipitating incident was the child's report to a teacher of a mark on her chest causing her pain. The girl also had several congenital physical conditions that the teacher felt were not receiving adequate medical attention. When the girl reported that her mother had thrown an object which hit her the night before, causing the mark, SRS was contacted, leading to the out-of-home placement for the child's safety.

During this conversation, details of the case were carefully tended to. However, the primary task for us was defining a relationship with the SRS case worker. Guided by our model, we attempted to craft a relationship built on an offering of respect and collaboration accomplished within the boundary of the treatment system rather than triangled through speculation about the family's incompetence. With this task accomplished, we could agree to proceed with the referral.

Stage 2: Establishing a Relationship with the Family

Historically, individuals have been placed in a rather passive position in the assessment enterprise. They have been asked to meet with an unknown expert, in an unfamiliar location, to take some unknown tests, for unknown purposes, and to conclude the meeting with unknown consequences. Understandably, this approach results in people being situated in personally uncertain positions whereby they feel little control throughout the entirety of the assessment experience. By contrast, our evaluation project intentionally requests people to relate to the assessment domain in a different manner. The way this occurs is through a collaborative effort initiated with the family from the beginning moments of contact. First, the family members are engaged in the familiar surroundings of their home. It has been said that for a family to meet with professionals in their offices requires a relatively high level of relational functioning (L. Combrinck-Graham, personal communication, February, 1993). We agree with this notion, for many of the people we work with have limited personal resources (such as adequate transportation), and it represents a hardship for them to have to access services in an outlying area.

Second, an invitation is extended to the family members to actively participate in the assessment endeavor. This request assures them that their "insider" perspectives are considered to be crucial to a more balanced and fair outcome. We believe this conveys a sense of respect and communicates that their involvement is desired. At times the family's confidence can be promptly accessed. However, we typically find it necessary to be patient in the joining process and allow the family members adequate time to voice any concerns and grievances that they may have. Their agreement must be secured before proceeding to the clinical interview. It has been our experience that when family members sense an authentic invitation to have an active voice in their own evaluation they are less inclined to take protective stances and more willing to involve themselves.

Case Example

This proved to be the case with the Miller family. In the initial phone contacts, both parents were cautious and resistant toward the evaluation team member. Efforts to describe the purpose of the evaluation and our identity separate from SRS were received with suspicion. Attempts to schedule an appointment in their home to begin the evaluation elicited the parents' evasiveness. Our request to include the family's other three children, ages 12, 6, and 4, in the home interview were openly questioned. The parents were skeptical about how a such a meeting, whatever it was called, could be helpful to them.

Our conceptual model provided a useful perspective at this point, interacting with our goal of establishing a collaborative relationship with the family. First, it defined the family's "resistance" as characteristic of control process, simply acknowledging that we had not accomplished a relationship with the parents. Second, it allowed a possibly positive interpretation of the parental behavior as behavior protective of the family's inner sphere. In short, we were strangers. We were "out," not "in." The parents were acting carefully to protect the private realm of their family unit. This perspective helped us to manage our own reactivity in this early stage of contact, allowing us a vital measure of patience in the process.

Several phone conversations were required before terms for an initial meeting in the home were agreed upon. We took the position that proceeding with the evaluation would be unwise unless the family members were certain of what would be involved and how it might be useful to them. Instead, we offered simply to meet them and hear their own story about the situation in which they presently found themselves. We also agreed to try again to describe what a family evaluation was and to discuss questions they might have before determining a next step. On these terms, the two persons representing our family evaluation team were invited to the Millers' home at a mutually determined time. The first step in defining the relationship had been accomplished.

The initial visit to the home immediately provided a flood of data relevant to the evaluation effort. However, the task of developing a relationship with the family remained the highest priority at this stage, with other relational data filed for future reference. Face-to-face introductions and the occasion of being guests in the family's home gave the team members ample opportunities for acknowledging the family boundary with respect and affirmation. An attentive hearing of the family's distress over the teacher's actions and SRS's response further validated the family's right to its own view of their recent experience. The team's recognition of positive family values and strengths mentioned during the family's description further promoted an atmosphere of respect. The content for facilitating an inclusion process was abundant once the interaction began.

As the in-home visit progressed, the nature and purpose of the family evaluation was revisited. The family was noticeably less protective during this conversation, though still maintaining a measure of distance and caution. Its experience of being judged without benefit of its own testimony was recited again. With patient discussion, the family evaluation process was reviewed, its purpose of assisting the family in presenting a fair and accurate picture of itself to SRS described, and questions about the evaluation team members' roles discussed. By the session's end, the parents requested that the evaluation process proceed. Enough trust had been accomplished to join in the mutual goal of taking a snapshot of the family functioning and looking at the picture together. The foundation of a therapeutic relationship had been negotiated.

Stage 3: Facilitating Family Evaluation

Engaging family evaluation is obtained by utilizing a multimethod assessment model. Each of the methods of the model (self-report instruments, observation, and family interview) provides a distinct and important contribution to the overall evaluation of a family's functioning. The use of self-report instruments is by no means central to the evaluation of families, but it does provide supplemental information that "tempers" clinical judgment. These instruments give all age-appropriate members an additional means to individually express components of their family life experience. The "tempering" process for the evaluator is having to take account of these multiple descriptions by comparing and contrasting them amongst themselves and to the interviewer's own estimate of the family's functioning and then reaching a conclusion that gives regard to each perspective. Though not a simple task, it is one worth pursuing.

The observation (Olson, 1988) aspect of assessment is obtained by having an "outside" perspective (the evaluation team) and an "inside" perspective (the family itself). Both of these vantage points are important to the overall evaluation endeavor. Observation provides information that cannot realistically be obtained through the other two methods. For example, careful attention is paid to the neighborhood in which the family lives, the care and upkeep of the house, the level of organization and physical environment of the home, and, most importantly, the interactive behavior of the family members in their familiar surroundings. These areas and more provide additional information that more accurately reflect the immense complexity of family life.

It is important for the interviewers to be cognizant of the reality that they are and will always be on the outside of a family looking in. Though joining is an essential element of the assessment process, it nonetheless does not constitute family membership. Therefore, the only way to obtain a truly close-up view is through the lenses of family members. However, the importance of an outside perspective should not be minimized, for it is often the medium through which the family must present itself to child welfare service agencies, schools, and courts that are involved in its life. Therefore, it is crucial that evaluators take seriously the profound effect their viewpoint will have on the integral functioning of families. Additionally, because the nature of family life is dynamically complex, it is the outside perspective (theory) that gives form to the monumental amount of information available during the evaluation process.

The clinical interview is the focal point of the family evaluation. Our model does not contain a detailed query. Rather, the interview is broadly contained by the Family FIRO framework, which provides conceptual dimensions that channel the flow of information as it is being dynamically disclosed. This format permits flexibility by allowing communication to unfold in a more natural and less contrived fashion. However, it does necessitate that the interviewer possess sufficient knowledge of both family functioning and life span developmental theories.

The natural tendency of an evaluation is to go expeditiously looking for "something wrong." In medical settings this might be appropriate, but in assessing relationships it is important to not allow "something wrong" to become the totality of the focus. This is particularly so at the onset of a clinical interview. Understandably, it is awkward at best to initiate a discussion when the topic of concern is a family's own foibles. Therefore, it is important to not place a family in the difficult position of having to instigate a conversation based upon its shortcomings. Setting the occasion to converse about family life is done by giving each capable member an opportunity to express what he or she appreciates about the family. Once this has been accomplished, the interviewer then purposefully moves the conversation to focus on areas of relational functioning that the family voices to be problematic. This part of the conversation can be distressing, for in a real way the deficiencies are being brought into the open and relational accountability is confronted.

It seems that the interviewers' respectful curiosity activates the unfolding nature of self-disclosure. In other words, there is an attractive quality about experiencing someone who can be authentically interested in the inner workings of a family's life without being judgmental or demeaning. This creates a conversational momentum whereby the interviewer then listens for and organizes the information being provided by the family according to the Family FIRO dimensions. Although a structured protocol is not adhered to, there is still a steady pace of gathering family functioning information, albeit through a more informal and spontaneous style.

The final area in this stage is to hear what the family thinks it needs. Relational accountability results when the family formulates a plan that enables it to better attend to the needs of each family member. All of the preceding evaluation efforts have been training their intent toward this crucial province. It is here that the concern of each involved person, both outside and inside, is most prominent. And it is here that family members determine the direction and goals they will commit themselves to. This is the bottom line.

Case Example

At the conclusion of the previous visit, a second home-based meeting was scheduled in order to proceed with the next phase of the family evaluation. Given the number of individuals represented, with the family and the team, it proved to be somewhat of an obstacle. As a team we were interested in proceeding efficiently with the evaluation, yet we were careful to not send a wrong message that our scheduling convenience took precedence over their own full-time work (not to mention income). Eventually, an evening was selected that best assured the attendance of the entire family, including Tanya and the maternal grandmother.

The first component of this third stage involved each age-appropriate member of the Miller family (including the maternal grandmother) completing a selection of family functioning instruments. In order to lessen the sense of mystery that typically surrounds measurement devices, each of the instruments was explained at length. It was the team's hope that this effort would lessen the impression that something unknown was about to be done to them. We further explained that testing is but one of several ways whereby an individual can describe aspects of his or her family life. Once we received their agreement to participate in this segment of the evaluation, a selection of instruments was then distributed.

When each member had completed the testing, the clinical interview then proceeded with the Millers. The team remained cognizant from the beginning moments of working with this family that the last few weeks had been a time of emotional distress for the children and adults alike. Therefore, the team knew that protective responses could easily be drawn from this family and that we, too, could be tossed onto the compost heap, just like the other well-intentioned professionals who had preceded us.

Using the Family FIRO as a guide, we believed that the best way to proceed with the clinical interview was to engage the Millers in a conversation about the strengths of their family life. Because the Family FIRO suggests that there is a relational need to feel valued and appreciated, we set the occasion for this family's members to discuss important areas of their life that they take pride in and would like to express to us. It is important to note that this discussion was not a momentary distraction, only to be followed by questions of real import. Rather, we believed it was critical that the Miller family members give verbal expression to their strengths, that we to receive their story and then acknowledge their integrity as a distinct family. We understand this to be an effective way to further promote a sense of inclusion between the family and the evaluation team.

In this segment of the interview, the Millers described several areas they believed worked well for them, while the team again used the Family FIRO as a guide to shape the information being given. The family discussed at length the structural components of their home that served them well. As the executive leaders of the family, both Beverly and Jim voiced pride that they were able to live independently of social services for the financial needs of their family. Although this blue-collar family was experiencing significant financial pressure, they both expressed the mutual commitment to remain economically free from governmental aid. In fact, because of this couple's shared belief in their strength to stand emotionally and financially independent, they experienced the efforts of social services (ourselves included) as an intrusion upon the integrity of their family life. Additional aspects they deemed important were their parental efforts to raise compliant children and the nuclear and extended family connections they both enjoyed and benefited from. Multiple family members lived within the same neighborhood and were readily available as important resources of much needed emotional support and reassurance.

Because the site of the evaluation was the home, rather than a clinic, the team was able to observe firsthand the wider environmental context of the home. The African American neighborhood in which this family lived was plagued by high crime and significant gang activity. By observing the surroundings of the home and becoming better acquainted with the daily uncertainties this family lived with, the team was profoundly affected. Only then could the team appreciate the central priority placed by Jim and Beverly upon their parental authority and the extensive family network they often utilized. It was clear that the world outside their home was not a safe one. Therefore, in order to insure the safety of family members, they took definitive steps to organize their relationships in a hierarchical manner and to formulate rules that carefully governed the children's behavior and relationships both inside and outside the home.

Upon concluding the preceding segment, the interview then shifted its emphasis from one of soliciting descriptions of family strengths to the reported incident of abuse that eventually resulted in Tanya being placed in out-of-home care with Beverly's mother. Because the team had verbally acknowledged the strengths of this couple, and the obvious efforts they expended on behalf of their family, Beverly and Jim were better prepared to enter a discussion that focused specifically on the alleged abuse incident with Tanya. Engaging the topic of the abuse report was an uncomfortable process for the family and team alike. However, it was a subject needing to be breached in order to sufficiently assess the present functioning of the family as well as to eventually coordinate a reintegration plan for the Millers.

Given the stressful nature of the topic, the family was hesitant to discuss the abuse incident with clarity and not surprisingly took a defensive posture in relaying its story. Jim and Beverly, occasionally joined by the grandmother and the older two children, expressed outrage at all they had experienced over the last few weeks. Rather than be discouraged by the intensity of the discussion, the team understood the family's disclosures as indication that a relational connectedness had been established and that it was working. Once the family's distress was communicated to us, discussion of Tanya's injury proceeded with little distraction.

It was at this point in the conversation that the relational pattern of the family became more evident. The pileup effect (McCubbin & McCubbin, 1987) of chronic financial and family stress, Jim's alcohol abuse, and the recent removal of Tanya from their home was overwhelming the couple's capacity to manage their relationship. They were having difficulty negotiating their disagreements and consequently experienced escalating conflicts that were poising them on the edge of marital separation. The couple then described how it was during one of these ever more violent episodes that Tanya was hurt. Fearing the high-pitched verbal battle that had embroiled her parents, she entered the room where they were conflicting and was struck on the chest by a heavy glass object thrown by Beverly but meant for Jim. Both parents expressed grief over the incident and dismay at how their spousal conflicts had more recently become unmanageable.

Taking note from the Family FIRO, we decided it was important to continue in a collaborative effort in order to construct a reintegration plan that best fit the family's circumstances and needs. This relational model suggests that reactive control responses are most likely to occur when there is a disparity of influence. Therefore, in order to best assure the eventual success of the proposal, we believed that it was crucial to have the family actively construct the plan it would have to carry to completion. For us to proceed with making a plan separate from its influence would have established us as authorities over the Millers, while simultaneously eroding their competence to make decisions on their own behalf. It seemed to us that this would be a costly misjudgment and one the family had previously shown little tolerance for. During the remaining portion of the interview, a proposal was formulated that would allow Tanya to rejoin her family. The Millers were then informed that the next step involved having the team write the evaluation document, and upon its completion a final home-based appointment would be arranged so that the family could read the document if they so desired. This met with their approval.

Stage 4: Constructing a Relational View of the Family

The responsibility of constructing an evaluation document that is balanced, fair, and useful for both the family and the referring agency can be a daunting task. The evaluation team must be able to bring the many disparate pieces of information gathered over the course of the previous three stages into a coherent aggregate. This is no small task, for a comprehensive multi-method approach presents a monumental amount of data. However, the enormity of this endeavor is greatly reduced by the capacity of the Family FIRO to order the information into an organizational framework.

Even as the Family FIRO is useful in observing and interviewing families, it is also beneficial in constructing the evaluation document itself. The inclusion subdomains and the control dimension provide broad groupings to structure the information and arrange it in such a fashion as to make sense of the interrelatedness of these various matters. For example, the subcategory of inclusion–structure concerns the organization of the family. All of the relevant information to this aspect of family interaction, such as boundaries, rules, roles, and expectations are compared, contrasted, and, finally, synthesized. The summary description of this area of structural functioning should be congruent with each sectional summary that follows. In other words, the overarching relational view of the family should present a clear and understandable gestalt that expresses the distinct and yet interactive nature of the various family functioning domains.

Writing up the assessment results requires a balanced presentation. The document deliberately is fashioned to present a family's strengths as well as its shortcomings. The Friends University project intentionally does not use the language of psychological pathology to describe family members and their relational functioning. Undoubtedly, utilizing family functioning theories whose concepts emphasize normative rather than pathological functioning plays a significant role in this matter (Walsh, 1982). By describing familial strengths and difficulties, the focus remains on what is integral for adequate relational functioning and how the challenges of these dimensions are being met.

The final concern in this stage involves the recommendations for treatment. The effort here is to move beyond corrective prescriptions to propose ideas through which the family's own resilience can be accessed. In order to utilize this qualitative dimension, the integrity of the family as a natural and essential belonging group for its members must be respected and not compromised. The evaluation team must guard against the seduction to independently create a laundry list of recommended ideas that will help fix something "broken." To do so is to maintain the perspective that these families are inhabited by incapacitated people with limited ability to understand their own resourcefulness. The project is diligent not to place these individuals into such a dependent and potentially reactive position, for this would undermine their competence and sense of responsibility. Rather, by participating in a collaborative fashion with families to identify important goals for change, we work to better secure their emotional investment in these goals and thereby lessen the likelihood of activating their protective behavior.

Case Example

Constructing a relational view of the Miller family was facilitated by using the Family FIRO Model. We used the model's conceptual dimensions as a way to structure the information that we had gathered through the multimethod approach and as a way to effectively present the family in the document. The following is an outline of the document that we used to describe the Millers:

I. Case Data
   A. Demographic information (including addresses, race and/or ethnicity, family membership, date of births)
   B. Agencies currently involved with the family
   C. Purpose of the family evaluation referral
   D. Self-report instruments administered
   E. Interview location(s) and dates
II. Summary of Family Functioning
   A. Introduction
   B. Family structure
   C. Family cohesion
   D. Family stress
   E. Family functioning overview
III. Recommendations
IV. Family response to the evaluation summary (inserted after the Stage 5 visit)

We have found the Case Data section of the document to be more than just a collection of minutiae. Rather, this is a first-step presentation of the family to the readers of the document. Contained in this section are important fundamental items that briefly introduce the family and its context. Note that the item of family membership is important, for it is the Millers themselves (and not the team) who identify individuals recognized as inside members of their group. Additionally, it is important to understand who is involved on the outside of the family (current agency involvement), for this helps to define its context. (It has been our experience that the higher the level of outside agency involvement, the more distress reported by families.) Last, the purpose of the evaluation, based upon the referral request, briefly introduces the reader to the intent of the document. Each of these fundamental items provides a unique contribution to the overall family evaluation.

As stated earlier, a central role of the document is to provide an instrument whereby a family can more effectively introduce itself to a variety of service agencies that are or may be involved in its life. Therefore, we consider the second section to be the heart of the document, for it presents broad yet crucial areas of family life. As evidenced from the outline, summary sections (utilizing dimensions of the Family FIRO model) are used to discuss the strengths and areas of challenge for the family. The crucial areas of family structure and cohesion are addressed in detail. Both arenas allow for an informative discussion of key family functioning dimensions with practical application. Such discussion works to present a common language bridging the family's self-perception and the referral agency's immediate concern for therapeutic change. The following discussion on family structure will be used to present our efforts in this portion of the document.

The structure of a family is largely comprised of its rules, roles, and boundaries. A family must be adequately organized in order to sufficiently meet the emotional, physical, and social needs of its members. According to the testing results and the clinical interview, the Miller family emphasizes its familial structure more than its sense of cohesion. The role arrangements of this family are distributed in traditional fashion in that the locus of power and decision making is primarily held by the parents. Although the children have a voice in family discussions, their ability to influence decisions is significantly less than the parents.

It is evident that Jim and Beverly take a firm parental position with their children in that they expect strict behavioral compliance toward the rules governing the children's behavior. The home rules largely revolve around the themes of "safety" (strict curfew and scrutiny of peer group involvement) and "order" (obedience and domestic tasks). During the home-site visits, the team observed these rules in action through the compliant manner of the children and the direct fashion in which they attended to the tasks assigned them.

The themes of "safety" and "order" were also apparent in the efforts the parents took in the care and management of the home. Both adults expressed personal pride in owning their home and discussed how its upkeep, both inside and out, was important to them. It was clear that the physical environment of the home provided not only comfort but also a sense of security for its members. Jim and Beverly discussed at length the gang activity that frequented their neighborhood and why they were vigilant in their efforts to keep their children and home safe.

During the course of the interview, it became apparent that there was a great deal of unresolved conflict between Beverly and Jim on a variety of important issues, most notable being distribution of family responsibilities, financial decisions, and the disturbing effects of Jim's alcohol misuse on their family life. The absence of a shared perspective on these matters resulted in personal distress for the couple and an erosion of their relationship. Therefore, the nature of the unresolved conflict is better understood as a reflection of the couple's ongoing struggle to organize themselves in an equitable fashion and Beverly's efforts to protect the family against the disruptive influence of Jim's drinking.

Although the Family FIRO model is useful in organizing the text, additional subject summaries may be needed in order to highlight other areas of the family that lie outside the model's purview. An example of this issue is the summary on family stress. The team decided to discuss this topic at length because of the chronic and acute stress facing the Millers. In our estimate, the sustained nature of the stress confronting this family was affecting both the structure and the cohesion dimensions of family life in deleterious ways. Therefore, it provided a theme that brought together the various summaries that had preceded it in the outline. The following discussion will be used to present our efforts in this section of the document.

Although family life continually experiences stressful events and transitions, it is the pileup of stressors that threatens the stability of a family. Should a family face a chronic onslaught of stressful events, the capacity to adequately cope becomes overwhelmed. Both the self-report instruments and the clinical interviews indicate that the Miller family is currently experiencing extraordinary amounts of stress, eroding their capacity to adapt and maintain stable functioning.

To give a clearer indication of the present level of stress for the adult members of the Miller family, the averaged score obtained by Jim and Beverly on the "Family Inventory of Life Events and Changes" places them at the highest category of stress. The high-stress category indicates that the family unit is experiencing an unusual number of stressors, which are overwhelming its relational and emotional resources (such as hope and sense of morale).

While many components within the structural and cohesion dimensions of this family are currently functioning in a normal range, there is indication that the immensity of the couple's stress is taking its toll on their ability to adequately meet the emotional and physical demands of family life. Because the coping capacity of the Millers is being severely taxed, the structural and cohesive elements of the family are under increasing pressure and are beginning to unravel.

The recommendations section of the document should naturally emerge from the summaries that precede it. It bears repeating that the recommendations are collaboratively formed, in the effort to secure inter- and intrafamilial accountability and "corporate" ownership of the goals. This is not to suggest that the team passively participates in the formation of the goals. On the contrary, it is the team's responsibility to ensure that difficult topics are engaged and that the scope of the family's goals are sufficient for the tasks that lie ahead of them. The following discussion will highlight this section of the document.

Through a joint effort between the Miller family and the evaluation team, it is recommended that Tanya immediately rejoin her family. Both Beverly and Jim have mutually agreed to the following items to ensure the present and ongoing safety of their family members.

1. To enter family therapy with the following goals:
   - renegotiate family roles, power, and responsibilities between the spouses;
   - work on conflict management skills and establish a "no-violence agreement" between the couple;
   - facilitate communicating in a more negotiating fashion about their life stressors in order to increase their problem-solving capacity and significantly lessen the likelihood of their conflicts escalating out of control;
   - promote the establishment of regular routines whereby the couple can communicate to each other the issues they are facing daily; and
   - help the couple cultivate an increase of family cohesion by enacting more nurturing behaviors toward their children, thereby balancing out their present overreliance upon behavior control in order to obtain child compliance.
2. For Jim to enter alcohol abuse treatment in order to assist him in re-establishing his emotional and physical functioning.

Stage 5: Receiving the Family's Response to the Evaluation Document

The fifth stage represents an additional opportunity for the family to actively participate in its own evaluation. This is done in three ways. The first involves presenting the final document to the family in order to receive its response to it. Given the profoundly personal nature of assessments, it is crucial that the family be the recipient of the document's first presentation. To do so detours the pervasive practice of first acquainting a family with the evaluation's content in court settings. An often reported grievance is the humiliation of not having the opportunity to appraise the text before having it presented as public information. We believe this mismanagement is easily corrected by extending to the family the courtesy of being the first readers of the document.

The second way a family actively participates is in a roundtable discussion of the evaluation document itself. After each willing participant concludes the reading, the team engages in a conversation where all questions and concerns are addressed. The effort here is to be open and straightforward about the assessment information and to give the family an opportunity to address the evaluation team about any possible misgivings they may have. This collaborative approach keeps families in an active position by encouraging them to express their level of agreement with the assessment's contents and recommendations.

The third way a family participates is through the inclusion of a "family response" section in the document itself. The family's perspective is concretely acknowledged through a summary statement. The effort here is to visibly demonstrate to the family (and the referring agency) that their "inside" perspective has been considered essential by the evauation team and integrated throughout the entirety of the assessment process. Negotiated at the very beginning moments of contact, this task finalizes the collaborative effort between the team and the family.

Case Example

Upon completion of the evaluation document, the Miller family was contacted and another home-based meeting was scheduled. We requested that all members of the family be available, including the maternal grandmother, so that we could present the document and receive their responses. Because of the collaborative nature of the relationship between the Millers and the team, we believed it was respectful to allow them to be the first readers of the document.

While meeting with the family, it was explained that the evaluation would be read slowly and carefully and that any questions they might have would be addressed. The team further clarified that because the document reflected our own thinking (about all that we had previously discussed), the family members might take exception to some of our descriptions. Therefore, we were interested in receiving their feedback on whether it presented the family in a fair and balanced fashion. Last, we informed them that their response would be inserted at the conclusion of the document. This met with their approval. The following is an excerpt of the Millers' response.

The evaluation team met with Beverly, Jim, the maternal grandmother, and the children on June 5, 1993. On that date, the adult members, along with the eldest daughter, were given the opportunity to read the document in its entirety. When questioned specifically about their perception of the document's accuracy, Jim stated that he believed it was a fair representation of their family. Though slower to respond, Beverly eventually agreed that she, too, thought it was fair and took no exception to its content.

The family expressed surprise at the opportunity to read the evaluation prior to its being forwarded to the referring agency. Because of the collaborative relationship that was established during the evaluation process, the family was observably comfortable in asking for clarification of the documents. Their ability to hold it, read it, and comment on it took much of the mystery away from the document, and they voiced a great deal of relief at knowing its content before hearing it discussed in an upcoming court appearance. At the conclusion of this time, the family was asked to sign a form giving us permission to forward the document to the referring agency.

Stage 6: Receiving the Referring Agency's Response to the Evaluation Document

Because the family evaluation project represents a different type of assessment and a different way of doing assessments, we understood that our efforts would be received with some amount of hesitance. Anticipating this from the outset, we believed that the most efficient and effective path of gaining acceptance into this community would be through a collaborative approach. The final stage of the model again reflects this central theme of the project. Upon receiving the family's permission to forward the document, the team then writes a cover letter (attached to the text) to the referring agency, thanking its members for the referral and requesting their feedback about its strengths, weaknesses, and usefulness. We have found this stage to be particularly beneficial, for the information we have received has either directly supported our efforts or has given us invaluable information on the areas that have needed improvement. Additionally, it communicates to the legion of caseworkers, school counselors, teachers, and court personnel that we value their perspectives and that their ideas will be seriously considered. This sixth stage concludes the discussion of the model.

Case Example

Once the response section was completed and attached to the document, it was sent to the caseworker who had originally requested the service. The completed evaluation was accompanied by a cover letter wherein we solicited the feedback of the caseworker on the usefulness of the evaluation service. Sometime later she made contact with a team member and commented, "This put words to what I was seeing and hearing." Much to our relief, the caseworker liked the idea of having the family be the first readers of the document and including their response in a separate section. We received this feedback as a confirmation not only of our efforts to provide a different type of service but also of the importance of a collaborative approach to promote ourselves in the network of our community service providers.

To date we have served 15 families in this pilot project. The reception of the project by the court and child welfare agencies has been overwhelmingly supportive. Clearly, the court has found the comprehensive evaluations useful in matters of disposition and has adopted with little, if any, exception the recommendations to have children rejoin their families. Out of these 15 cases, there have been only 3 in which children did not rejoin their families. These exceptions were based upon the families' decision (rather than the Court's) not to have their children rejoin them due to extraordinary circumstances beyond their present control. In these cases, other intermediate plans were developed that would eventually have the displaced child returned to his or her family. The project is readying itself to move beyond the pilot stage and into a standardized service for our community. We envision the rapid expansion of this service, given its reception by the sources listed above.

ACKNOWLEDGMENTS

Special thanks to Judge James Burgess and Marcia Wasinger of the 18th Judicial District of the State of Kansas, Juvenile Department of the District Court, and to Mr. Joe Kuttler, Mr. John Sullivan, and Ms. Jean Hogan of Sedgwick County Social Rehabilitation Services, Wichita, Kansas, for their support of this pilot project. Also special thanks to Candyce S. Russell, Ph.D., Vera Mowery McAninch Professor of Human Development and Family Studies, Kansas State University, for reading and responding to portions of this chapter.

REFERENCES

Bray, J. H., Williamson, D. S., & Malone, P. E. (1984). Personal authority in the family system: Development of a questionnaire to measure personal authority in intergenerational processes. *Journal of Marital and Family Therapy, 10,* 167–178.

Doherty, W. J., Colangelo, N., & Hovander, D. (1991). Priority setting in family change and clinical practice: The Family FIRO model. *Family Process, 30,* 227–240.

Doherty, W. J., & Hovander, D. (1990). Why don't family measures of cohesion and control behave the way they're suppose to? *American Journal of Family Therapy, 18*(1), 5–18.

Epstein, N. B., Bishop, D. S., & Baldwin, L. M. (1982). McMaster Model of Family Functioning: A view of the normal family. In F. Walsh (Ed.), *Normal family processes* (pp. 115–141). New York: Guilford Press.

Gurman, A. S., & Kniskern, D. P. (Eds.). (1991). *Handbook of family therapy* (Vol. 2). New York: Brunner/Mazel.

McCubbin, M. A., & McCubbin, H. I. (1987). Family stress theory and assessment: The T-Double ABCX Model of family adjustment and adaptation. In H. McCubbin & A. Thompson (Eds.), *Family assessment inventories for research and practice* (pp. 3–32). Madison: The University of Wisconsin Press.

Olson, D. H. (1988). Capturing family change: Multi-system level of assessment. In L. C. Wynne (Ed.), *The state of the art in family therapy research: Controversies and recommendations* (pp. 75–80). New York: Family Process Press.

Olson, D. H., Russell, C. S., & Sprenkle, D. H. (1983). Circumplex model of marital and family systems: VI. Theoretical update. *Family Process, 22,* 69–83.

Schutz, W. C. (1958). *The interpersonal underworld.* Palo Alto, CA: Science & Behavior Books.

Walsh, F. (Ed.). (1982). *Normal family processes.* New York: Guilford Press.

White, M., & Epston, D. (1990). *Narrative means to therapeutic ends.* New York: W. W. Norton.

3

Psychiatric Emergencies and Family Preservation: Partnerships in an Array of Community-Based Services

Stephen Christian-Michaels

Institutions have long been seen as places to put away seemingly unsolvable problems ranging from mental illness and emotional disturbance to social disorders such as vagrancy, delinquency, and child abuse. From 1980 to 1984 there was a fourfold increase in the number of children and adolescents hospitalized in psychiatric units (Weithorn, 1988). Many have questioned whether or not these are unnecessary, costly and inefficient interventions (Friedman, 1984; Kiesler & Sibulkin, 1987; Winsberg, Bialer, Kupietz, Botti, & Balka, 1980). The dramatic increase in the hospitalization of children and adolescents followed an opportunistic proliferation in the number of private psychiatric inpatient beds. There has never been a benefits incentive to attempt outpatient treatment in difficult situations, and this situation supported a health care system that gives economic incentives to use inpatient and residential facilities rather than community-based outpatient services. Far from being helpful, this backward incentive system may have promoted a context that is harmful to children and families. There is also a tremendous financial cost to families, business, government, and, ultimately, taxpayers. Some of the negative outcomes include widespread inappropriate diagnosing, separation of a child from his or her family at stressful times, and parent-blaming. After experiencing these abuses, families frequently have then had to contend with the exhausting of their mental health insurance benefits, large outstanding debts to hospitals and professionals, and even financial ruin. Also contributing to the problem is the public sector of human services, which is a maze of unclear responsibility, fragmented services, and an inadequate amount of advocacy and leadership concerning children's services, which include child welfare, mental health, education, juvenile justice, and health services. These problems have contributed to the public agencies' over reliance on inpatient psychiatric care. All this has occurred despite the fact that for 25 years we have been familiar with methods that can substantially reduce the need for institutional care (Goodacre, Coles, McCurdy, Coates, & Kendall, 1975; Langsley, Pittman, Machotka, & Flomenhaft, 1968; Polak & Kirby, 1976). This technology evolved into what we now call a Family Preservation model. Employed in most states across the country, the Family Preservation model has been applied to youth with conduct disorders or delinquency problems (Tavantziz, Tavantziz, Brown, & Rohrabaugh, 1985) and serious emotional disturbance (SED; Seelig, Goldman-Hall, & Jerrell, 1992).

This chapter will describe the development of a program system in DuPage County, Illinois, that is based on the Family Preservation model and was conceived to provide a healthy alternative to a state-run system that revolved around the state psychiatric hospital and (usually out-of-state) residential treatment. The case example that follows describes the effectiveness of Family Preservation interventions.

Case Example: Brian

Brian, age 17, had been hospitalized many times in his life for mental illness. When Brian was 6 it is reported that he ate a glass after drinking out of it, talked to inanimate objects, and often endangered himself by running into walls and furniture and into the street. This bizarre behavior earned him the diagnosis of psychosis. When Brian was 17, his father abandoned the family, and Brian, his mother, and younger brother were emotionally and financially devastated. Brian's behavior got worse. He threatened young children, as well as adults, in the neighborhood. His mother was forced by the neighbors to resign from her job so that she could provide constant supervision of Brian. She was frightened of him because he was threatening to her and had damaged walls in the home. One night he spent several hours in the car in the garage, playing with the ignition, turning it on and off.

Brian's mother was referred by his school social worker. She reported that Brian had been last hospitalized 4 months previously and had not improved while there. In addition, his younger brother had been very upset about Brian's last hospitalization and, with the father having left so recently, the mother wanted to avoid another separation from the family. Following an assessment in the home, the assessor drew up a crisis treatment plan with the mother and authorized intensive in-home services: therapy, case management, and respite services. The Family Preservation team began providing these services to the family within 24 hours. Family therapy sessions were held every other day for the first 6 weeks to redirect Brian's anger over his father's departure, to assist the mother in alternative ways to calm Brian down when he became threatening, and to assist all the family members in supporting Brian. After the first 6 weeks, the frequency of sessions was reduced to twice per week.

The case manager met with the mother once a week to address family stress issues due to the pending divorce and financial strain. The case manager provided education regarding single parenting, education, and employment possibilities. At the same time, the school administration was changing; the new administration wanted to change Brian's school program. The case manager advocated for Brian to remain in his current school program and to graduate on time. Case management services also assisted the mother in the process of obtaining a state grant to fund a transitional adult group home program and other adult services for Brian.

The respite worker provided 6 to 8 hours of relief, supervision, and recreational activities each week. He provided Brian with the opportunity for a relationship with a stable male figure, introduced him to some new recreational, activities and taught him appropriate social skills.

Although Brian had been hospitalized nearly every year of his adolescence, he has now remained out of the hospital for 4 years. He continues to receive psychiatric services and is still on psychotropic medication, but he successfully completed high school and moved into a transitional living program when he became 18. The group home he lives in is only 8 miles from his family, and they visit him weekly. He spends vacations and holidays with them. He has a part-time job and attends the local community college.

THEORIES AND ASSUMPTIONS

The institutional approach to mental health focuses disproportionately on the individual patient, even when the patient is a child. To treat youth with serious emotional disturbance effectively, the child must be evaluated in the contexts of family, school setting, social structure, cultural background, and community of origin. The theories and practical experiences on which this mental health Family Preservation model is based include family systems, wraparound services, community systems of care, parents as partners, and collaboration among community agencies.

Family Systems

Structural Family Therapy provides the basic framework for our understanding of how the family functions (Minuchin, 1974). The emphasis on strengths, creation of new realities, and a focus on change are essential to a Family Preservation model. Frequently, families in crisis have many agencies involved in their lives, such as, school, probation, child welfare, police, and mental health. The coordination of services is usually minimal, with no one taking on a primary, convening role. Using the therapist or case manager to convene all the "players," including the family, is a crucial tool that helps to improve treatment, reduce duplication of service, and put the key mental health professional in a leadership role of the larger helping system. This concept of hierarchy is adapted from structural family therapy, speaking to the need for a leader in the larger helping system. Strategic Family Therapy, as articulated by Haley and the Mental Research Institute (MRI) group, offers an interactive-communication focus where repetition of family patterns, avoidance of past attempted solutions, and the importance of the family's style of language are all the focus of treatment (Haley, 1976; Watzlawick, Weakland, & Fisch, 1974). A solution-oriented approach seeks out the exceptions to the problem behavior enabling the therapist and the family to identify positive behaviors that drives the treatment rapidly toward change (Berg, 1992).

Given that seriously disturbed children and their families most frequently present in an emergency, treatment must be immediate. Crisis intervention strategies are used that focus on the family as well as the child. The focus of Crisis Family Therapy is to engage the family in stabilizing the crisis as an alternative to psychiatric hospitalization. Quite often a family appears to be extremely dysfunctional in the middle of a crisis, while the precrisis level of functioning is higher. Treatment, which is usually provided at the site of the crisis, focuses on basic needs, de-escalating the conflict between family members and reframing the problem (Pittman, DeYoung, Flomenhaft, Kaplan, & Langsley, 1966).

A Wraparound Philosophy

Wraparound is a term referring to devising services to fit a child and family. Wraparound services counter practices of placing children in existing, but possibly inappropriate, service systems, requiring the child and family to conform to what is already in place. Wraparound services provide ways to individualize treatment plans based on child and family needs in a collaborative process that includes the family and a network of community agencies, professionals, and self-help resources (Boyd, 1992; Clarke, Schaefer, Burchard, & Welkowitz, 1992; Knizter, 1993). In-home respite is a commonly used wraparound service that can provide relief to parents taking care of a child who requires constant supervision, helping to avert a hospitalization. Treatment integrated into the home or school is more natural for people and reduces barriers to treatment, such as the need for transportation or for day care. Too often professionals prescribe treatment with little input from the client and consumer as Traditional services are often delivered in a narrow, compartmentalized, and bureaucratic manner that does not address the needs of a given family.

A mechanism for funding wraparound services is a special fund, often an amount per family, that can be used at the discretion of the case manager. In some states, these funds are pooled by different governmental agencies and managed by a local case management entity. Discretionary wraparound funds might be used to purchase goods and services to support a family who might otherwise turn to the state and relinquish their parental rights. Examples may be purchasing a wheelchair, so that a child can be discharged from the hospital sooner; paying for an in-home behavior modification training program for the parents of a child with psychotic and developmental disabilities; or buying a lockbox for weapons to minimize the risk of harm to self and others.

Systems of Care

The term *systems of care* refers both to an adequate array of services and resources (accessible through wraparound) and the capacity to maintain continuity of care through different systems and different system levels. The mechanisms used to manage services in a system of care are gatekeeping and case management. Coordination of services is an essential component of a Family Preservation model, providing the seamless continuity of care. Many professionals were trained in community mental health centers where the continuum of care principle was a central organizing concept. However, this continuum assumes a linear ladder of services from most restrictive to least restrictive. The Community Mental Health Systems Act of 1979 described an array of services. This shifts the emphasis to a "menu of services" that is more responsive to the client's needs and ideal for creating individual treatment packages. The Child and Adolescent Service System Program (CASSP) principles expand this concept by involving all the child-serving agencies in a comprehensive, holistic array of services, not just mental health services (Stroul & Friedman, 1986). A recommended array of services across child serving agencies is shown in Figure 3.1.

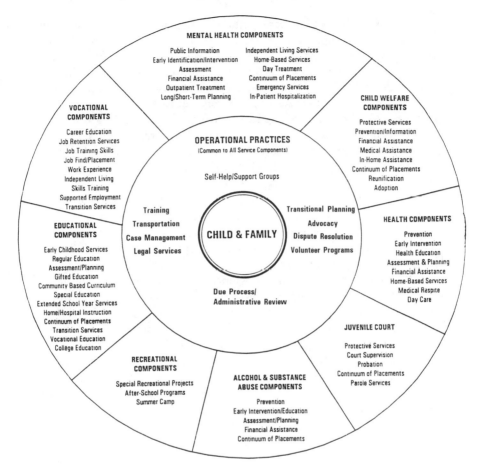

FIGURE 3.1. Components for building service partnerships for children and families. From Stroul & Friedman (1986). Copyright 1986 by CRSA. Reprinted by permission.

With the advent of managed care, the use of gatekeepers has become a more recognized method for controlling access to more restrictive or expensive services. The screener/assessor, who acts as a gatekeeper, works on controlling the access to the front door of many kinds of institutions (hospitals, residential treatment centers, and even foster care). The functions of a gatekeeper are (1) *screening*—frequently deciding over the phone about the need for an immediate emergency assessment (30 minutes to two hours), a assessment (1 to 3 days), or direct referral to less intense outpatient services; (2) *assessment,* a face-to-face comprehensive assessment to determine the level of care necessary; and (3) *author-*

ization of expenditures for therapy, case management, respite, restrictive care, and other wraparound services. The team's assessor evaluates all clients being referred for admission to the institution. In a small number of cases, after a face-to-face evaluation the child is sent to the hospital for medical stabilization or to foster care for protection. In most situations, the assessor authorizes immediately accessible home-based treatment services that could cost up to $6,000 per client for 3 months. With the gatekeeper function, families who need less intense outpatient services are given appropriate referrals. The authority of the gatekeeper to make clinical decisions involving hospitalization, deflection of hospitalization, home-based therapy, respite, and group-home alternatives is essential. This gatekeeper may also refer to private hospitals for brief stays at inpatient or partial hospital programs. These stays will then be reviewed and approved in increments of 5 days, with discretionary wraparound funds used. Length-of-stay extensions are typically approved by the assessor for both in-home services and brief hospital stays.

Case management is another essential activity for implementing the system of care. Case managers provide a myriad of functions that are defined by the needs of the child and family. Case management is a dynamic wraparound-service delivery mechanism. The functions could include but are not limited to outreach, advocacy, coordination, creation of new resources, convening a treatment team, linkage, and discharge planning. As part of delivering these services, the case manager incorporates an attitude that failures are due to problems in the system, not in the client, and the case manager endeavors "to do different, not more." Case management is the essential glue that holds the treatment plan together (Ronnau, Rutter, & Donner, 1988).

Parents as Partners

Traditionally parents, most notably mothers, have been blamed for their children's mental health problems. As parents of children and adults with disabilities have become more vocal about their children's needs, effective mental health systems have begun to include parents as partners (Donner et al., 1993). While a meaningful partnership provides a powerful tool to treating youth with serious emotional disturbances, it also requires new ways of thinking, diagnosing, and building treatment plans. The parents-as-partners philosophy means giving decision making power back to the parents. For the professionals this means learning how to share decision making, which also means learning how to bring parents in on gathering and evaluating the information needed to make educated decisions. The shared decision making then makes it possible to develop effective individualized treatment plans. The result is a client-driven delivery service with shared goals. These goals tend to be behavioral and outcome oriented. Parents will assume responsibility for making changes and thus will make the treatment plan work.

Collaboration, Not Just Cooperation or Coordination

Just as it is not enough to elicit merely the cooperation of the parents, coordination or cooperation between the "players" is not enough. The parents-as-partners philosophy requires a collaboration in diagnosis, planning, and treatment. Family Preservation services require all the players to collaborate, not just cooperate. Too often we refuse to take down the barriers between agencies, and the result is ineffective services that are fragmented. For example, until recently, Illinois children who are wards of the court often had difficulty accessing mental health services, due to a long-standing conflict between mental health and child welfare agencies. Vocational, recreational, and transitional services are frequently not incorporated in a holistic treatment plan. Those services which are being provided in a parallel fashion are often conducted with no joint planning or coordination.

The mental health Family Preservation team weaves the treatment considerations into these operational principles using developmental, behavioral, and genetic/biological perspectives. Interventions at home and school are frequently based on behavior therapy principles, while a psychoeducational approach is used to educate the youth and his or her family about the nature of a chronic mental disorder. Medication treatment is employed frequently as an adjunct. These additional interventions are essential as part of the team's treatment of the child in context with the family and community.

DESCRIPTION OF THE CLIENTS, AGENCIES, AND COMMUNITY

The children served in this Family Preservation program ranged from age 5 to 18. The average age was 14.5. The clients whom we have served have been referred to the state psychiatric hospital, state funded inpatient care at a private hospital, or residential treatment. While many clients were screened and found not to be appropriate for hospitalization, approximately 50 clients a year are treated in an intensive in-home treatment modality as an alternative to being hospitalized. The diagnoses include major depression, bipolar disorder, conduct disorder, pervasive developmental disorder, schizophrenia, post-traumatic stress disorder, and dual diagnoses of mental illness and developmental disability. The clients come from a

full range of socioeconomic levels. Many upper middle class families have
problems with the lifetime insurance benefit caps and end up seeking help
through the public mental health system. The clients are evenly distributed between male and female. The community is predominately White and
middle class, and the county has one of the highest per capita incomes
in Illinois. However, there are several minority populations, including
Hispanics and Asian Americans of Korean, Vietnamese, Cambodian, and
Laotian origins.

DuPage County as a Context for Change

The mental health Family Preservation program described in this chapter
is part of a large county health department. The DuPage County Health
Department's Mental Health Division serves a community of 800,000 people. There is a total of 155 full-time staff and 220 part-time staff in the
division. There are four programs: adult, substance abuse, child and
adolescent, and community consultation/education. The mental health
Family Preservation program is part of a home-based subunit of the children's program. Other home-based programs include a Family Preservation child welfare program and a less intense case management program
designed to prevent rehospitalization. The overall Mental Health Division funding comes from the county (60%), the State (38%), Medicaid
(1%) and client fees (1%). The Illinois Department of Mental Health is
the principal funding source for this in-home program.

DuPage is the second most populous county in Illinois, after Cook
County. There are 48 school districts, four special education cooperatives,
and 400 school buildings in the county. Other major players include the
circuit court probation department and local child welfare department field
office. There are five not-for-profit hospitals with psychiatric inpatient
units (with child and adolescent or adolescent units), two freestanding private psychiatric and/or chemical dependency hospitals and six hospitals
complete with psychiatric units in the contiguous counties, near the county
boundaries. There are six youth service agencies and at least ten family
service counseling centers. There are also many private practitioners,
providing both hospital inpatient services and outpatient services in the
county. The state hospital is 25 miles from the center of the county, approximately a 1 hour drive.

Situated 30 miles due west of downtown Chicago, DuPage has been
a rapidly growing suburban area that is slowly becoming more urban. It
is made up of 37 municipalities and 9 townships. The local human services tend to mirror the state departments of human services, which frag-
ment children's services. The legislative bodies have been largely
unresponsive to children's needs, thus promoting interagency competition

for scarce resources. In short, in 1988, when the mental health Family Preservation program began its development, DuPage County children's services suffered from all the same problems experienced by children's services nationwide.

DEVELOPMENT OF THE PARTNERSHIP FOR FAMILY PRESERVATION

Forming an Interagency Steering Committee

The DuPage Consortium, Inc., was formed as the beginning of a collaborative work in DuPage County, in 1973. It is a loose confederation of 60 agencies concerned with children and their families, providing advocacy, networking, and educational functions. The DuPage Consortium, Inc., is the place where many ideas are seeded and nurtured. It has helped break down the walls between agencies and has been the embryo of several multiagency ventures. The Consortium created a context of collaboration in a county occupied by fragmented services.

The Partnership for Family Preservation is a steering committee that was formed to develop home-based services and interagency joint ventures. The Partnership is made up of the special education cooperatives, child welfare department, juvenile probation department, health department, parents, youth service providers, state-level department of mental health, legislators, and a juvenile court judge. The state Department of Mental Health funded both a Family Preservation program and a joint-agency steering committee. The Partnership for Family Preservation has since received several other grants and is pursuing research, training, and treatment funds based on an interagency model of planning, intervention, and systems change. Barriers to collaborative treatment and planning are identified within the partnership and the proposed solutions are communicated to state level department directors and to local legislators with the goal of changing state policies and procedures.

Clinical Services

The clinical services of this program involve two general components: (1) screening and assessments, and (2) support services. The screening and assessment services function as gatekeeper to the state hospital and provide authorization for intensive in-home services as an alternative to hospitalization. Support services include whatever it takes to keep a child out of the hospital. Figure 3.2 describes the components of this mental health Family Preservation program.

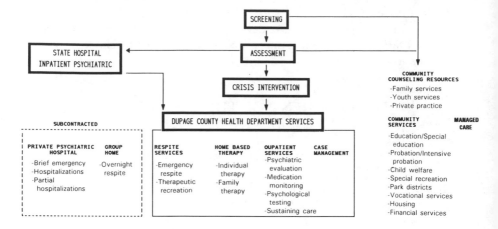

FIGURE 3.2. DuPage County Health Department mental health Family Preservation program.

The goals of the program are the following:

1. to decrease admissions to the state hospital,
2. to decrease the length of stay at the state hospital for those clients who are admitted, and
3. to decrease the number of assessments conducted at the state hospital and then deflected back to the community.

Screening Assessment Services

Screening and assessment services provide 24-hour immediate access to all clients who meet specific criteria of serious emotional disturbance and risk of psychiatric hospitalization in the public sector. Screening and assessment activities are separate from the treatment component. Given the move toward independent evaluations and concern about utilization review, the assessors focus exclusively on assessment and utilization review. Utilization review activities in managed care, insurance companies and larger agencies are concerned with how evaluators might benefit from their clinical recommendations: For example, a provider may refer someone for inpatient care and then get paid for providing treatment during the inpatient care. Having the assessors not provide ongoing treatment eliminates a conflict of interest and has made them more available for emergency evaluations. Establishing ability and willingness to make an assessment at the scene of a crisis (home, police station, emergency room) was the first step in defining this as a different type of intervention. It also allows us to see the family in crisis in its own context, not in our setting, where the family members may have mobilized their defenses. The context of the crisis assessment also makes it possible to see the real-world basic needs that must be addressed first and to obtain vast amounts of evaluation information very quickly. One of the problems this approach eliminated is the process wherein a family mobilizes to hospitalize one of its members; once started, this process begins to take on a life of its own. If the family member is turned away following an evaluation at the hospital, the family is then left feeling disappointed, frustrated, and angry, viewing any alternative services as less than the optimum. The client may be blamed by the family and may also be exposed to a very dysfunctional population at the state hospital intake/emergency room. At night, children and adult clients are often served out of the same waiting room, a potentially disturbing experience for a child or adolescent.

Crisis intervention often begins immediately via the assessor when it is determined that hospitalization is not necessary. The crisis intervention helps to develop a community-based treatment focus for the family.

The In-Home Intensive Services are delivered in the home because it is easier to flexibly serve clients in their own homes. In-home services can deal with behavior problems as they occur, *in vivo*, with modeling, coaching, and role plays after the event. Families report preferring home-based therapy. Therapy moves faster given the richness of the environment. The length of stay in the program is 90 days, and the intensity often begins at 20 hours per week and decreases down to 1 to 2 hours per week.

Clinical Team

The Family Preservation team in DuPage County, Illinois, is made up of 2 bachelor's-level case managers, any one of 40 respite workers, and 2 master's-level therapists, a team leader, and a consulting child psychiatrist. The individual team members carry caseloads varying between five and seven families. The families usually have a therapist, a case manager, and one or two respite workers assigned to them. The team is supervised by a team leader who is available 24 hours a day. The team also has consultation with a child psychiatrist once a week.

The therapist takes the lead in developing the treatment plan with the parents and the client. Therapists can provide family therapy and individual therapy daily if necessary, but twice a week is typical. The family therapy sessions often include the case manager as cotherapist. The case manager may work with the adolescent, providing supportive counseling and advocacy services. The functions of a case manager include coordination of services, linkage, leveraging flexible funds, and making sure basic needs are met. The client and/or parents might be transported by a case manager to a group, with the group being facilitated by the case manager. The case manager has access to an emergency checking account that is maintained to purchase supplies or services that the family is unable to obtain. Half of our clients are prescribed psychotropic medication and are seen by a child psychiatrist, usually within the Health Department. Emergency psychiatric evaluations can be obtained quickly to promote medical stabilization, thus avoiding hospitalization.

In-home respite services are provided to many of the clients, ranging from 3 to 25 hours per week, to help reduce the level of crisis. The respite care may be decreased over time, but it is a service that parents find invaluable. It is often respite services that immediately demonstrate that this program is different from the other programs the family has encountered. Respite staff members are part-time employees who are frequently in college or graduate school or work as aides in special education programs. The respite workers typically provide therapeutic recreation or vocational activities, with the goal being to give respite to the parents. Respite workers can be mobilized and put into an emergency situation within several hours. Occasionally, when the family needs time out from one another, a group home can provide overnight respite. These resources are authorized by the assessor either at the beginning of treatment or later, if it is required.

The Necessary "Can Do" Attitude

The staff members hired for this type of program have to be very optimistic and proactive. A "do whatever it takes" attitude is important. The families of SED children are often demoralized, exhausted, and pessimistic. The staff over time shows them that there is hope. Staff members have to be persistent and willing to reach out even when the door is closed in their face. The wraparound approach emphasizes changing the plan as the needs change and creating new services where none exist. The staff needs to be able to tolerate ambiguity, to be constantly flexible, and to avoid thinking in confining terms such as "slots," "placements," and "standard protocols." The supervisor has to be able to view every mistake as an opportunity to improve and model that to the staff. The messages that supervisors send should be "If you are not making mistakes, you're not trying very hard. You need to admit your errors, correct them, and learn from them. Problems or failures are opportunities to fine-tune therapy skills and our system of care." The supervisor must engage the staff members in a continual review of problems encountered and help them develop a solution, should a similar client or situation be re-encountered. Staff is encouraged to look for systems problems and gaps, modeling that can-do attitude at every level of intervention, all the way to the directors of state departments and legislators. Staff also helps convene self-help groups which, in addition to being a support resource, also become part of a the legislative advocacy process.

The supervisory staff is constantly informing staff, management, board, community and state-level policymakers of our innovations and the remaining barriers that need to be addressed. The 24-hour access for support by the team leader and upper management is critical in order to maintain the can-do attitude. Support within the team via frequent staffings, planning prior to sessions, and collaborative phone calls throughout are critical to the creation of the proactive attitude at the team level.

PERSUADING STAKEHOLDERS TO ACTIVELY BECOME PARTNERS

Overall, as with other Family Preservation implementation plans, the rationale for reforming a delivery system is often primarily the saving of financial resources and reduced institutional placements. The demonstration of better treatment outcomes is used, but tends to be more subjective than other measures, given the lack of solid outcome research in this area. How the stakeholders have been engaged in our program and have become partners is an interesting story. Generally our approach was to develop a common self-interest and then demonstrate success, making all the partners appear in the best light to their constituents or customers.

Parents

Parents are our first and foremost partners. By seeing the family and identified patient when they need services and by going to them wherever they are, we have become more user friendly. Families report that it is much easier to be involved in an intense 20-hour-a-week treatment modality when services are provided in the home. Parents report being happy with the intense manner in which they are involved in the treatment as opposed to a once-a-week family therapy session, a group therapy session, and a family group session that families typically receive in most hospital settings. The treatment is more individualized and focuses on basic needs as well as the mental health needs. In-home respite services are used to provide therapeutic recreation to the children and, for the parents, some relief from the constant demands of a caring for a youth with severe emotional disturbance.

Another way parents are involved as partners is by teaching them how to advocate for their children's needs. Too often parents have been uninvolved in the treatment and seen as the problem. The most important way of engaging parents as partners is to treat parents-as-partners. Parents quickly respond when they are shown respect.

State Psychiatric Hospital, State Department of Mental Health

With the general trend toward community-based services, state hospital employees could have been opposed to our program initiative, given the perceived threat to their future employment. In other states, state employee unions have objected to a shift to a community-based priority. In the state hospitals, attrition is being used to slowly reduce the number of units while building a higher staff: patient ratio for those units that remain. The collaborative relationship with the state hospital staff developed as the screener/assessors showed that they would not make inappropriate referrals to the state psychiatric hospital. As we demonstrated to the hospital staff that our criteria of admission were more stringent than hospital standards, the trust increased. Similarly, as the treatment teams showed how effective they were with very disturbed youth, the partnership grew that allowed for shorter lengths of stays. Currently, for those few youths who are admitted, the Family Preservation team now begins the treatment in the hospital, with the goal being to reduce the length of time in the hospital. This has been persuasive to the hospital staff that this collaboration is valuable. Finally, the state hospital staff members had often reflected that their work is for naught. Clients in the old system of care frequently did not follow through on outpatient referrals and were often readmitted. Now, for those few clients who are admitted, the follow through back in the community is 100%. The average readmission rate per year for the years 1985 to 1988 was 3.25, while for the years after the implementation of Family Preservation, 1989 to 1993, the average was 1. For state hospital staff this contributes to their own sense of effectiveness, thus enhancing their role as a partner.

Mental Health Policymakers, State Department of Mental Health

The Department of Mental Health/Developmental Disabilities (DMH/DD) is both a customer and partner. DMH/DD provides the primary funding stream for this program and yet is a codeveloper. We have explored together how to best implement the Family Preservation initiative. The success of reducing hospital-bed days and admissions has been attributed to the DMH-funded initiative. For the first time in quite a while, dramatic success is being attributed to this state department. The reduction of admissions both from this program and similar programs made it possible to consolidate three metropolitan inpatient programs into one, with a reduction of 140 beds, or a 70% reduction. Similar consolidation is being planned for the future. Involving the state-level mental health policymakers in the steering committee planning sessions, public relations events, and state association meetings has all contributed to this sense of partnership.

Private Psychiatric Hospitals

Initially, tensions ran very high between private psychiatric hospitals and the Family Preservation program, as psychiatrists, unit staff, and hospital administrators resented our role as a gatekeeper to the state hospital. Psychiatrists were angry that the gatekeeper was not a physician, and they had little respect for the screener/assessors. There was already friction between the state hospital and the private psychiatric hospitals. Now the doctors could no longer transfer clients without going through a local gatekeeper. Even with all of these challenges, good relations developed as the screener/assessor's ability to access immediate services as an alternative to hospitalization became evident. The challenge was for the screener/assessor to be seen as a resource, not as an obstacle to the state mental health system. Those clients who required long-term institutional care were expedited more quickly than in the past. Other clients who were deflected from hospitalization received less restrictive and more appropriate levels of care more quickly. The follow-through on these referrals was perceived as highly effective. Hospital staff reported that they saw clients getting services, where previously they tended to fall through the cracks. Private psychiatric hospitals were also given the opportunity to provide brief inpatient care with the families immediately linked to intensive home-based services as an alternative to state hospital care. Hospitals are given a guaranteed reimbursement, and the screener/assessor authorizes inpatient days in private hospitals in increments of 5 days. Partial hospitalization with guaranteed funding also has been used as an alternative. This expansion of the array of services has involved the hospitals and physicians in a much more collaborative manner than in the past.

Schools

Schools are frequently frustrated with the unwillingness of community mental health centers (CMHC) to work with students and their families who are hard to engage, the slow response to requests for help, and the unwillingness to engage 17- to 21-year-old clients and the dually diagnosed mentally ill and developmentally disabled. Mental health centers have been perceived as isolated prima donnas who have used the cloak of confidentiality to avoid collaborative relationships.

The speed with which emergency assessments and treatment has been provided began to change these old perceptions in DuPage County. The willingness of the Family Preservation team to meet basic needs and collaborate with the schools, and the development of the steering committee to plan joint ventures has helped to change the relationships. The schools have also been concerned about the increase of psychiatric hospitalizations, as discharge recommendations frequently include expensive residential treatment with the direct cost to the local school district/special education cooperative. Several joint community development projects involved the schools and the CMHC banding together to educate the professional community to alternatives to residential treatment and other restrictive care.

The development of a joint 10-hour day-treatment program for severe conduct disordered youth is another example of collaboration. Education, mental health, and probation staff planned and now fund this unique program, which provides an alternative to residential treatment. Other examples of an improved relationship include (1) a special education cooperative purchasing benefit coordinating services from the mental health center and (2) the mental health agency purchasing psychiatric time for special education evaluations. Currently, representatives from mental health and education cochair a steering committee, with the major discretionary funds coming from mental health and education. Federal grants are being jointly pursued to further reform the system of care. The special education cooperatives are now advocating for expansion of home-based services and are very strong partners.

State Department of Child Welfare

The different missions of child welfare and mental health have traditionally placed them at odds. Similarly, the lack of cross training has contributed to little understanding of the other's context or basis of intervention. The home-based unit had the opportunity to move into the same office building as the local child welfare agency. This has helped by providing easy access, quicker ability to clarify misunderstandings, and the opportunity to educate each other. Child welfare workers have not been trained to identify major forms of mental illness. With easier access to mental health professionals, there have been more referrals for services from the child welfare agency. The state wide success of mental health Family Preservation programs has prompted the Department of Children and Family Services to develop a similar program for wards of the state. As a result of a recent consent decree, the Department is mandated to provide mental health services to wards. Mental health Family Preservation programs provide a method of meeting the mandate. The steering committee of the Partnership for Family Preservation has had steady participation from the child welfare agency. The relationship has grown slowly but steadily, now to the point where a federal grant is being pursued involving a substantial matching of state child welfare funds for a systems change initiative. Collaborative planning has begun as child welfare and mental health staff have learned to work together.

Juvenile Probation

The friction between juvenile probation and mental health has evolved for a number of reasons. These include the inability of the outpatient clinic to serve clients who are hard to engage, an unwillingness to serve youth with conduct disorders, the slow response to requests for services, and the isolated manner in which outpatient staff seemed to operate. Juvenile staff at the detention center have been known to try to admit clients to the state hospital after hours so as to improve their client's chances of being admitted. The attempts to build bridges to the court and probation system predated the mental health Family Preservation program. The number of residential treatment placements funded by probation were going up as the per diem rates were also going up. A joint committee to establish a 12-hour day-treatment program for conduct disordered youth demonstrated how collaborative relationships serve our clients better. The probation, special education, mental health and child welfare organizations cofunded clients as an alternative to residential treatment. This collaborative planning process and the relationships established there are used in the current steering committee. A juvenile court judge has been attending the steering committee, and his presence has helped build more trust and commitment to the process. The willingness of the screener/assessor to assess youth in detention and even to contribute staff to aid in a suicide watch in the detention facility has helped build that collaborative relationship.

Managed Care Entities

With the dramatic demonstration of decreases in bed days and admissions at the state hospitals, insurance companies, managed care entities, and self-insured pools are beginning to explore ways to apply this program to private sector clients. Currently, clients are admitted to hospitals at the behest of a psychiatrist who benefits from the decision to hospitalize. The managed care response has most frequently been to insert a telephone authorization process. This authorization process is difficult in that the gatekeeper is totally dependent on the conclusions of the admitting physicians. The gatekeeping function allows for an independent evaluation, many times a second opinion. The gatekeeper function together with

Family Preservation services provide managed care with an alternative to hospitalization. This relationship is just in the beginning stage. Community mental health centers provide comprehensive services and a level of collaborative trust with other human service providers not currently available in the private sector.

Case Example: Mike

Nine-year-old Mike was referred by his psychiatrist when insurance no longer reimbursed for his hospitalization. He had been diagnosed since the age of 6 with pervasive developmental disorder, autism, attention-deficit/hyperactivity disorder, obsessive–compulsive disorder, and Tourette's disorder. Since age 6, Mike had been prescribed antipsychotic drugs, stimulants, and other medications. While he had been stable periodically, it appeared now that the current medication regime was not working. He had become quite distant, impulsive, obsessive, and ritualistic. He was unable to dress himself due to the rituals. The school reported that he was so distractible that he could not attend to any assignment or activity, and in their opinion he was not learning. At home, the family reported incidents of aggression, such as when he hit his the mother in the head from behind in a surprise attack and had pushed and shoved his younger sisters, ages 6 and 18 months. They reported that he had attacked each family member on different occasions, in unprovoked situations.

The attending psychiatrist felt that Mike needed a drug-free period to assess the best method of treatment. In addition, the psychiatrist also stated he felt that family stress was contributing to Mike's behavior. It was reported that there were marital and financial stresses: There were two new infants in the past few years, the mother's health had deteriorated during the two pregnancies and she had uncontrolled diabetes, and the stepfather's daughter, age 15, had moved into the home within the last 2 months because she had been sexually abused by her mother's boyfriend.

The Family Preservation team provided therapy, case management, and respite services. Therapy was provided twice per week during the 90-day period to address all the family stress issues, the sexual abuse issue, and assist in evaluating Mike while he became medication-free.

Case management services provided parenting education for step-parenting the 15-year-old, as well as general parenting education for Mike and his younger sisters. The case manager linked with the psychiatrist, making phone calls every other day, relaying observations about Mike's behavior off medication. The case manager also coordinated services with school staff regarding Mike's special needs during this medication free period.

The respite worker took Mike out of the home three afternoons each week to provide some relief for the family during this period. The respite worker encouraged Mike to relax, play games, and talk.

Ninety days after the initiation of Family Preservation services, Mike was at home, on new medication, continuing with his psychiatrist, focusing better in school and at home. Two years later, he remains at home and in his school program with no out-of-home institutional care. The family continues to be supported by twice monthly therapy sessions and medication monitoring.

OUTCOME RESULTS

Family Preservation is expected to reduce the costs of providing care by reducing the reliance on expensive institutions. The program as it has been implemented in DuPage County has demonstrated these expectations can be realized. In Figure 3.3, the reduction in the number of admissions is displayed, showing a 90% reduction of admissions since 1989.

In Figure 3.4, similar findings are seen with the annual cumulative bed days. The decrease in bed days from 1989 to 1994 is a reduction of 96%. The annual savings, based on an estimated cost of $500 per day, can be estimated at $1,440,000 in savings per year.

There was a fear that with fewer admissions, the length of stay for those admitted would increase, as those who were hospitalized would be more dysfunctional. This has not been borne out in the data. The aver-

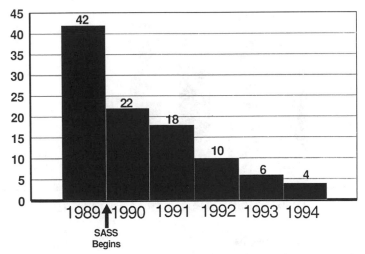

FIGURE 3.3. Child admissions to public psychiatric hospitals in DuPage County, 1989–1994.

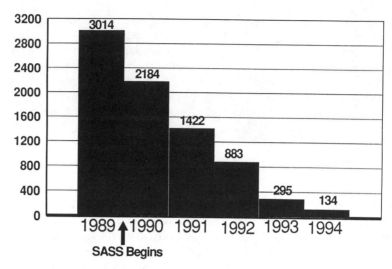

FIGURE 3.4. Child bed days at public psychiatric hospitals in DuPage County, 1989–1994.

age length of stay is listed in Figure 3.5 for each of the 5 years and declined after efforts were taken to shorten stays.

And finally, the number of children and adolescents actually assessed at the state hospital and then deflected has been almost reduced to zero. The reduction of these numbers means that many families are not having

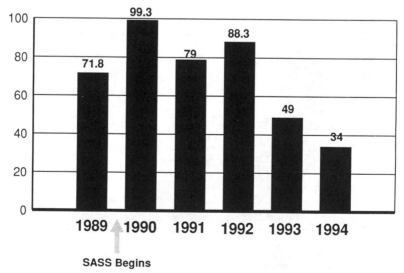

FIGURE 3.5. Average child bed days at public psychiatric hospitals in DuPage County, 1989–1994.

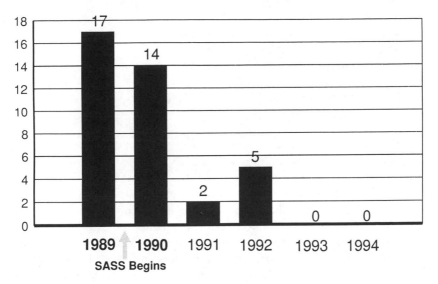

FIGURE 3.6. DuPage child deflections at public psychiatric hospitals.

to travel 25 miles by car or ambulance with an acutely distressed youth, sit in a waiting room with ambulatory chronic mentally ill adults, and then be sent home because the youth was not dysfunctional enough to receive services. When this did occur, it made it that much harder to engage the family, given that trauma of the refusal of the state hospital to meet the family's perceived immediate needs. In Figure 3.6, the number of state hospital deflections are displayed.

CONCLUSION

We have the technology now to serve severely disturbed and mentally ill children and adolescents and their families without relying on expensive and perhaps ineffective institutional care. For a Family Preservation program to work, the parents must be involved as partners, as must be all the human service providers. The current liaison relationships between professionals must be replaced by collaboration. The service delivery system must provide services that are relevant to families and are based on a comprehensive assessment of all domains of family life. Treatment must then be provided through an individualized treatment plan developed in collaboration with parents and other human service providers.

The curative factors of this program that have been reported by parents include the following:

- instillation of hope,
- rapid reduction of crisis via intense service delivery,
- shared decision making — parents as partners,
- self–reliance promoted — be our own case manger,
- realistic focus,
- coordinated care, and
- learning new skills.

With these kinds of successes, we need to expand the use of mental health Family Preservation. Outcome research needs to be conducted to determine which youth are better served by different in-home treatment strategies. Funding streams need to be developed that make it possible to serve families before there is a need for imminent hospitalization by today's standard. Finally, we need to recognize that the addition of Family Preservation services into a system of care will affect the whole system, by including youth with more severe disorders and lower levels of functioning to the caseload of all the agencies. This will increase the cost of all community-based programs. The additional costs can be more than made up for with the savings of inpatient and residential care costs, if policymakers invest the savings back into the community.

REFERENCES

Berg, I. K. (1992). *Family based service: Solution focused approach*. Milwaukee: Brief Family Treatment Center.

Boyd, A. (1992). *Integrating systems of care for children and families: An overview of values, methods, and characteristics of developing models with examples and recommendations*. Tampa: University of South Florida, Florida Mental Health Institute, Department of Children and Family Studies.

Clarke, R., Schaefer, M., Burchard, J., & Welkowitz, J. (1992). Wrapping community based mental health services around children with a severe behavioral disorder: An evaluation of Project Wrap. *Journal of Child and Family Studies, 1*(3), 241–261.

Donner, R., Huff, B., Gentry, M., McKenney, D., Duncan, J., Thompson, S., & Silver, P. (1993). Expectations of case management for children with emotional problems: A parent's perspective. *Focal Point, 7*(1), 5–6.

Friedman, R. M. (1984). *Seriously emotionally disturbed children: An underserved and ineffectively served population*. Tampa: University of South Florida, Florida Mental Health Institute, Department of Children and Family Studies.

Goodacre, R. H., Coles, E. M., McCurdy, E. A., Coates, D. B., & Kendall, L. M. (1975). Hospitalization and hospital bed replacement. *Canadian Psychiatric Association Journal, 20*, 7–14.

Haley, J. (1976). *Problem solving therapy: New strategies for effective family therapy*. San Francisco: Jossey-Bass.

Kiesler, C. A., & Sibulkin, A. E. (1987). *Mental hospitalization: Myths and facts about a national crisis.* Newbury Park, CA: Sage Publications.

Knizter, J. (1993). Children's mental health policy: Challenging the future. *Journal of Emotional and Behavioral Disorders, 1*(1), pp. 8–16.

Langsley, D. G., Pittman, F. S., Machotka, P., & Flomenhaft, K. (1968). Family crisis therapy: Results and implications. *Family Process, 7,* 145–158.

Minuchin, S. (1974). *Families and family therapy.* Cambridge, MA: Harvard University Press.

Pittman, F. S., DeYoung, C. D., Flomenhaft, K., Kaplan, D. M., & Langsley, D. G. (1966). Techniques of crisis family therapy. In J. Masserman (Ed.), *Current psychiatric therapies* (pp. 187–196). New York: Grune & Stratton.

Polak, P. R., & Kirby, M. W. (1976). A model to replace psychiatric hospitals. *Journal of Nervous and Mental Disorders, 162*(1), 13–27.

Ronnau, J., Rutter, J., & Donner, R. (1988). *Resource training manual for family advocacy case management with adolescents with emotional disabilities.* Lawrence: University of Kansas, School of Social Work.

Seelig, W. R., Goldman-Hall, B. J., & Jerrell, J. M. (1992). In-home treatment of families with seriously emotionally disturbed adolescents in crisis. *Family Process, 31*(2), 135–150.

Stroul, B. A., & Friedman, R. M. (1986). *A system of care for severely emotionally disturbed children and youth.* Washington, DC: Children and Adolescent Service System Program Technical Assistance Center.

Tavantziz, T. N., Tavantziz, M., Brown, L. G., & Rohrabaugh, M. (1985). Home-based structural family therapy with delinquents at risk of placement. In M. P. Mirkin & S. L. Koman (Eds.), *Handbook of adolescent and family therapy.* New York: Gardner Press.

Watzlawick, P., Weakland, J., & Fisch, R. (1974). *Change: Principles of problem formation and problem resolution.* New York: W. W. Norton.

Weithorn, L. A. (1988). Mental hospitalization of troublesome youth: An analysis of skyrocketing admission rates. *Stanford Law Review, 40,* 773–838.

Winsberg, B. G., Bialer, I., Kupietz, S., Botti, E.,& Balka, E. (1980). Home versus hospital care of children with behavior disorders. *Archives of General Psychiatry, 37*(3), 413–418.

II

FAMILY PRESERVATION

Family preservation became popular only in the mid- to late 1980s when public consciousness about the plight of emotionally disturbed children and adolescents was raised by the federal Child and Adolescent Service System Program (CASSP) initiative and further provoked by the Mental Health Association study of children placed out of their communities. Since the first family preservation programs were developed for families whose children were at risk of being placed out of the home because of abuse and neglect, these programs were sponsored by child welfare agencies. The programs described here are intended for families in which the children are emotionally and behaviorally disturbed, these are children who would otherwise be placed in a treatment setting out of the home.

Laura Fraser's chapter presents a program developed at Eastfield Ming Quong, a comprehensive mental health agency that serves children and families through outpatient, school-based day treatment; residential, wraparound programs; and in-home services. The multiple impact model was created in response to the overwhelming demand and need for an alternative to traditional practices of placing children of families in crisis into shelter or foster care. Their program utilizes a multiple impact model which addresses families at multiple levels: individual and dyadic relationships as well as the whole family system and the intergenerational context.

Cynthia Stone's chapter on family preservation in the mental health system in Pennsylvania represents another program developed from a family systems approach—this one from the structural family therapy approach of the Philadelphia Child Guidance Center.

While Raymond De Maio's chapter describes an approach that does not call itself "family preservation," the effect of his work with children who have been victims of incest is to preserve family relationships in the face of a tradition that has dismantled these families. Please note the sensitive handling even of the relationships with the perpetrators, who are, after all, also family members.

The work of these authors and family preservation programs in general affirm that, properly supported, many beleaguered families can take care of their children—a fact that could save a lot of the money currently being spent on out-of-home care and on the chronic problems that often follow out-of-home placement, if professionals and policymakers would take note of it.

4

Eastfield Ming Quong: Multiple-Impact In-Home Treatment Model

Laura H. Fraser

Seven-year-old Jason Patterson was referred to the Child/Adolescent In-Home Program (CAIHP) by the therapist of the residential unit where he had been placed for 6 months. He was described as severely oppositional, engaged in extreme tantrums, and possibly suffering from Posttraumatic Stress Disorder (PTSD). His mother, Kathy, was 26 years old and had four children; Jason was the oldest. Kathy and her children were living in a transitional shelter designed to help women leave violent spousal relationships. Her ex-husband was extremely physically abusive to Kathy, was a drug addict, and had raped Kathy in front of the children on several occasions; he was also severely punitive to his young children. Kathy was motivated to have Jason home with her, but she was also working on her individual issues stemming from growing up with two alcoholic adoptive parents and was in the midst of trying to locate her birth parents. Jason's next youngest sibling, Cassandra, 5 years old, was engaging in self-mutilating behavior and was alleged to have been involved in precocious sexual behavior with Jason. The referral source feared that the level of difficulty with which the family had to grapple, as well as their limited resources, would preclude Jason from being able to remain at home.

The Tapahonsos, a Navajo family, were referred to the CAIHP by the Department of Children and Family Services (DFCS) following reports of physical abuse by the mother. Lisa, the 16-year-old, was reported to be oppositional at home and school, had intermittent suicidal ideation, and her school grades were rapidly declining. Angie, her 14-year-old sister, was alleged to have been involved in some neighborhood petty crimes and was beginning to be truant from school on a regular basis. The parents reported themselves as being chronic alcoholics with 2 months of sobriety. The father had recently lost his job as a city mechanic as a result of driver's license suspension from numerous episodes of driving under the influence (DUIs) and was likely to have to serve jail time for those offenses. The referral source felt the girls were at high risk of being placed outside of their home if family patterns of abuse and acting out remained unchanged.

Kathleen Spencer, 16 years old, was referred by DFCS and her current family therapist. Kathleen had been in the county shelter for a month following a brief inpatient psychiatric hospitalization for suicidal ideation and reports of harsh punishments by her parents. Kathleen was demanding a foster care placement, threatening to kill herself if denied, since she felt "there is no other way out of my parents' house." The referring therapist was frustrated and felt the family members "stalemated" each time they came to his office. Kathleen agreed to make a trial move home for the 90 days of in-home treatment.

Families such as these, who present with complex needs on multiple levels, and families with children who are exhibiting dangerous and provocative behaviors are deeply troubling to those practitioners who attempt to provide intervention. Often, such families cannot be "contained" long enough to effect change that enables their children to remain at home. When abuse and neglect are an aspect of a family problem, "policeman" types of intervention are often employed by the larger system (e.g., child protection services, juvenile probation, etc.) to "remediate" the problem(s). Adhering to legislative mandates, those approaches are not necessarily structured to promote the activation of naturally occurring family system strengths. Moreover, when larger system agencies make an exploration of underlying emotional and structural issues, the findings are often used as evidence to remove children from their families, rather than an opportunity to further understand and remediate the factors that have generated the crisis in the first place. Finally, these are often families that are not self-referred; rather, they are brought to the attention of the "authorities" as a result of perpetual crisis (Kagan & Schlosberg, 1989). Such intervention strategies inevitably elicit feelings of incompetence, defensiveness, and secretiveness on the part of the client family. This, coupled with the feelings generated by the nature and complexity of the family trauma and the threat of losing a child, makes the work of the intervening practitioner difficult indeed. This is especially true when therapists are constrained by traditional models of treatment (such as a 50-minute "hour," one time per week, in the clinic). They soon experience the same hopeless feelings as their client families.

The philosophy of CAIHP is that traditional treatment approaches do not provide the clinical intensity that is required when a child (or children) is at risk of being removed from the family. The staff at CAIHP adheres to the belief that families have inherent strength and healing power which, when accessed and shaped, allows families to transcend their dilemmas. The CAIHP model is structured to provide treatment from a variety of entry points. Often in multiproblem, chaotic families, there is significant impairment in a number of subsystems and dyads.

Therapy is a process of challenging how things are done. A major target of the challenge is family subsystems, as they are the context for development of complexity and competence (Minuchin, 1981, p. 143). We utilize a blend of therapeutic approaches at CAIHP, including Structural and Strategic family systems approaches, as well as marital, individual, and play modalities. Our approach is designed to "hold" a family long enough to reach below the presenting problem (or series of crises) and create change that will last across time. In addition, the CAIHP operates on the premise that interventions must be provided expediently and intensely to divert an out-of-home placement.

The "larger" CAIHP team consists of three clinical social workers, a bachelor's-level child/adolescent specialist, the clinical program manager, and the consulting psychiatrist. We are a tight and cohesive team with specific tasks for each member. The clinical program manager handles administrative responsibilities, operates as liaison to the greater agency, provides individual supervision, and sometimes provides direct treatment. The consulting psychiatrist oversees clinical functions and adherence to psychiatry protocol. The clinical social workers and child/adolescent specialist provide direct treatment to families.

The success of our intervention rests largely on the productive functioning of the larger CAIHP team. The client families with whom we work have powerful inductive qualities. If the clinical team falls prey to an extended induction, we will serve only to perpetuate harmful, non-productive patterns. To counterbalance this potential process, team members provide each other with consultation, emotional support, and a good dose of humor. Although each family is assigned three therapists from the larger team, the larger team is always actively involved in treatment from behind the scenes. Each member of the team takes turns carrying the beeper and may be called upon to help a family that is not on their caseload to manage a crisis.

We have weekly 3-hour clinical meetings where the bulk of treatment planning occurs. During clinical meetings, therapists bring in their client families for live mirror consultations with the larger team. In this way, each team member "meets" the family, is able to observe it during treatment, and can provide valuable feedback to the primary therapist. In addition, team meetings are used to address the inevitable countertransference issues that arise throughout the 90-day period. It is here that differences between therapists and consultants must be "hashed out." Our team would not be able to carry out these sometimes threatening functions without an established method of team process, cohesiveness, and a strong belief that diversity of ideas is positive. Otherwise, our team would become "stuck" in much the same way that our clients are when they enter treatment.

From the larger team, varying configurations of two clinical social workers and the child/adolescent specialist are assigned to work with a given family. Each therapist has a specific role to play with a particular subsystem of the family. The primary therapist heads up the clinical team and provides family and parent sessions on a weekly basis (and more frequently if indicated). The secondary, or backup, therapist has a more flexible role. He or she may serve as co–family therapist and/or work with sibling groups or other integral extended family members. The secondary therapist's role is shaped by the specific needs of a given family. The third therapist is a child/adolescent specialist who has weekly individual sessions with the identified patient (IP) and, on occasion, joins family sessions to help the IP to have a voice within the family.

With the exception of one live consultation session at the clinic, treatment takes place in the family's home. Meeting in the family's home is advantageous on a number of levels. Most importantly, it allows families to feel a greater degree of comfort and control because they are in their own surroundings. Thus, the process of engaging families in treatment can be expedited. Diagnostically, working in the family's home is of great value to the treatment team because such things as how often the phone rings, the frequency of neighbors dropping by, whether bedrooms have doors, and so forth can be observed firsthand. Therapists need to be on-site in the families' environments to realistically assess what tools are available to their clients. Perhaps most importantly, in many non-White cultures, it is often far more appropriate to discuss painful and shameladen issues in the family home, rather than in a public place such as the clinic setting.

We are a short-term program; we have only 90 days to assist families to effect change that is dramatic and enduring so children will not have to be placed away from their natural families. When families are referred to the CAIHP they are in a crisis; our intervention capitalizes on the system energy being generated by the crisis to mobilize the family to work toward change. Our intervention model matches treatment intensity to family crisis intensity.

The CAIHP treatment model was designed in 1985 in an effort to provide a creative (and more effective) treatment alternative for seriously disturbed children and adolescents and their families. In a conjoint effort, the Mental Health Department of Santa Clara County and Eastfield Ming Quong, the large comprehensive mental health agency, which "houses" the CAIHP program, designed the intensive 90-day model as an alternative to costly, and often ineffective, out-of-home treatment options. The original creators of the program recognized that the level of need for families in crisis could not be addressed in a weekly, 50-minute outpatient session, nor were the needs of the clients being met in out-of-home care settings. Furthermore, they recognized that family system issues could not be effectively addressed when children are not living with their families. Thus, the 90-day, frequent weekly contact, clinical team approach was designed. At the CAIHP, we sometimes feel frustration that we cannot continue treatment beyond 90 days. Such an intensive entrance into the lives of families reveals a multitude of issues that are compelling to address. However, we must make an extensive assessment and then carefully deliberate on which point of entry into the family system will yield the greatest opportunity to create change that will last across time and generations of children.

The program is funded primarily by Short–Doyle funds channeled to Eastfield Ming Quong via the local mental health bureau. Referrals to the program come largely from the mental health system (community mental health clinics), inpatient psychiatric units, the Department of Children and Family Services, juvenile probation, the local schools, and private practitioners. Since the program's inception, we have been successful in thwarting the out-of-home placement of hundreds of children.

BEGINNING PHASE OF TREATMENT

The first phase of treatment includes the orientation, multiple-impact, and initial weekly sessions. This stage lasts approximately 4 weeks. During this phase the team is attempting to accomplish many things: engaging the family in treatment, gathering intergenerational family history, developing an initial hypothesis of family system operation, assessing alliances and hierarchical structure, and testing the hypotheses. Therapeutic work is commenced and is aimed at transforming nonproductive (or destructive) family functioning, de-escalating presenting problem behavior, and establishing cohesion as a clinical team. These treatment tasks are accomplished through a number of structured sessions, each with a specific goal.

The Orientation Session

The first contact with the family is the orientation session. This is not a therapeutic session, although this meeting yields much family system information that is essential for the development of an initial hypothesis.

In the case of the Tapahonso family, Mr. Tapahonso was nearly silent throughout the orientation. However, when questioned, he stated that his primary concern was to maintain his sobriety and he was unsure about the amount of emotional energy he could expend on the therapeutic process. It was clear that this angered his wife, as she felt the responsibility of management of their daughters rested solely upon her. She was also angry because she was now the family's only wage earner. Lisa was extremely articulate and seemed to be attempting to create enthusiasm within her family to participate in treatment. Lisa tearfully expressed her fear that her parents would return to drinking and the accompanying violence. Angie listened, but spoke less than her father. She did respond affirmatively that she was willing to participate in treatment, if that was what her family chose to do. When the referral source attempted to highlight concern for the younger sister's recent brushes with the law, the father downplayed the seriousness by stating that her "antics" were typical of 14-year-olds on the reservation (where he grew up). The family was asked to take 24 hours to decide whether they were willing to commit to treatment.

The orientation yielded much important information about the coming work with the Tapahonso family. Perhaps most prominent was the lack of a working alliance between husband and wife. As a result, Mrs. Tapahonso, and particularly Lisa, appeared to carry a disproportionate share of responsibility for the family, which contrasted with the more passive positions of the father and Angie. Lisa, more so than any other family member, demonstrated an overburdening in her role as she alone stated the "family problem" and was attempting to persuade her family to participate in confronting those issues. There seemed to be strong alliances between the mother and Lisa and between the father and Angie. However, despite the fact that the mother and Lisa were similarly overfunctioning in their roles, their anger and frustration about their status was expressed between them. The orientation also revealed that the team would need to assume the role of student to learn about the Navajo culture and family structure and to assist the family to negotiate cultural conflict between mainstream American practices and traditional Navajo practices.

Not all orientations yield as much information about family functioning as did the orientation with the Tapahonso family. However, generally the team will have gathered information via the referral source as well as the orientation, and thus is able to enter the multiple-impact session with an initial hypothesis that can be tested and refined.

The Multiple-Impact Session

The multiple-impact session is a daylong (6 to 8 hours) session that is actually a compilation of a number of sessions, each with a specific purpose designed to gradually build an in-depth understanding of the family system operation as a whole and in its subcontexts. It is also an opportunity to introduce the family to the therapeutic process that will occur over the next 90 days.

By the close of the multiple-impact, the team will have completed work in the following areas: engaging the family, assessment, gathering a full intergenerational history (through use of a genogram), and developing a working hypothesis upon which the treatment plan will be generated.

First Phase: Introductions

The goal of the first hour is to give the family members a chance to introduce themselves and to become acquainted with the team. During this time, we attempt to discourage family members from delving into the presenting family issues, saving that piece until later, when we will lead them to tackling the "problem" in a structured manner. Often our clients are families that have experienced repeated frustration and been labeled "failures" or "resistant" in their previous contacts with helping professionals. This is not because of some inherent deficiency on the part of the family, but instead on the part of the treatment modality. The needs of our families are complex and their defensive structure may be highly developed. Placing blame on the IP for the entirety of the family problems is many times a powerful protective device used to keep the focus away from painful underlying issues. It is our intent that the multiple-impact format will assist the family to begin to view the problem(s) as a greater family system issue, rather then simply the IP's presenting problem.

In the case of Kathleen Spencer, when the team arrived, Kathleen sat sullen and uncommunicative, while her mother fluttered about nervously. Mr. Spencer greeted the team as if we had arrived for a social tea. When the team asked the family to introduce themselves, Kathleen and Mrs. Spencer immediately engaged in struggle; nary a sentence could pass from one without the other perceiving it as an invitation to do battle. The team members had to continually prompt the mother–daughter dyad to return to the task rather than delve into the problem. While the constant verbal battle raged, Dad was quietly fingering a photo of an emaciated and sickly young boy. After repeated redirection from the team, the Spencers were finally able to introduce themselves. Shortly thereafter, Mrs. Spencer "introduced" their son, pictured in the photo. He died from a birth defect of the liver, 3 months prior to Kathleen's adoption.

The above account serves many important functions with our families, especially those families that are volatile, like the Spencer family. There was a great deal of family "investment" in keeping Kathleen in the role of IP. However, when the team established treatment structure and worked to divert the Spencer family from their stalemate of focusing on the overt issue of Kathleen's behavior, the Spencers quickly revealed the issue that was going to be central to treatment. There was a great deal of unresolved grief regarding the death of the parents' natural son; their grief was activated by Kathleen's need to establish her autonomy and to individuate from her family.

Second Phase: Rules

The next phase in the multiple-impact is the "rule" phase. To continue with the joining process, the family is asked if they have any rules they would like us to observe while we are guests in their home. This is done to acknowledge the "control" they have in the treatment process and to acknowledge that we are "guests" in their journey through their important family issues.

Next, the family is asked to tell us about rules they have for one another. This offers us an opportunity to assess family boundaries, hierarchical structure, and "loyalty" to the family.

Kathleen told us tearfully that she was not allowed to have her bedroom door closed unless she was dressing. She was not allowed to take phone calls unless her parents had first screened the call. Kathleen could not listen to the radio stations her peers were allowed to hear, but instead her parents permitted her to listen only to an approved Christian radio station. As Kathleen became more animated in her description of the tight rein her parents maintained, Mr. and Mrs. Spencer became very activated and another battle ensued, with parents arguing the need for more stringent controls upon their daughter and Kathleen feeling more and more like a "caged animal, with no way out." Kathleen told the team that her parents forbade her to talk with family and church friends about her problems, because it was a great embarrassment to them. Kathleen stated that she felt "cut off."

The family rules segment of the multiple-impact revealed a demand for loyalty to an impermeable boundary around the family system as well as a series of deadlocked transactional patterns between family members. Thus, patterns remained fixed and unchanged until Kathleen created a crisis by running away and thereby involving external members in the family system. Kathleen was not allowed the usual freedom of other children her age and, at the outset of treatment, the family was unable to negotiate any changes in those rules. The team's initial hypothesis, based on Kathleen's statement about her reasons for running away and her suicidal ideation, was that the Spencer family was rigidly entrenched in family transactions aimed at diverting Kathleen from engaging in the necessary adolescent task of preparing to leave home (and her parents). The earlier "introduction" of the Spencer's deceased son lent credence to this hypothesis; the emotional loss of the Spencer's "little girl" appeared to be activating the unresolved grief of their son's death.

The team also uses the rules segment to lay the foundation for treatment guidelines. It is at this time that families are forewarned about mandated reporting laws, confidentiality, and the like. The family is also given the CAIHP crisis beeper number; they are able to reach at least one member of the larger clinical team 24 hours a day, 7 days a week.

In our model, the rule that is perhaps most integral to treatment is "the no family secrets" rule. It is explained to families that we believe secrets are harmful to families and because of that belief we will not honor any requests to keep information secret from other family members. This is critical as much of treatment occurs within subsystems of the family unit. Therefore the team is in a prime position to be triangulated, inducted into dysfunctional alliances or covert family rules organized to maintain powerful family secrets. Clinicians working with each subsystem will offer assistance when a family member needs to reveal (or challenge the presence of) a secret to the larger system, but will not participate in maintaining a secret from other family or team members. The treatment team models open communication via sharing the content of individual sessions among clinicians so pertinent information may be used during family sessions or as relevant to work within other subsystems.

It is important to note here, that the multiple-impact follows a planned progression of gathering information and working toward discussion of the issues that brought the family into treatment with the CAIHP. Unlike a traditional visit to the clinic office, where the presenting problem is often discussed first, the family is introduced to the process of therapy and has an extended opportunity to engage with the treatment team before the discussion of highly volatile issues begins. In this way the family is not immediately re-enacting contacts with other helping professionals from the larger system. However, this is still the first treatment session, and, thus, families must be left with a sense that the "real" problem has been addressed and that the clinician(s) is not horrified by the depth of the family's problems. A primary goal of working with this format is to generate "buy-in" from the family and to activate the hope that family life, despite firmly entrenched patterns, can be different.

Third Phase: The Problems

The next phase of the multiple-impact is the problem session. It is the task of this part of the session to have each family member, down to the youngest person, tell the team what he or she feels the family needs to be helped with, and how they would like to see the family change. This is an opportunity for the team to begin to put their initial hypotheses through the first intensive round of testing. Through the structured multiple-impact method of slowly building to the presenting problem, the team lays the groundwork for treating the issues in a new manner. Thus, the goal of helping the family move toward viewing the issues as a family problem rather than one that is generated exclusively by one member, is further accomplished. It is here that the team is able to join with the IP and help him or her to move out of the role of scapegoat. If the team is successful in assisting the family to have glimpses of the larger family issues, we are able to reframe the function of the IP as positive because it has called attention to painful family struggles that are in need of attention.

Returning to the Tapahonso family: Mr. Tapahonso was not present for the multiple-impact session because he had returned to the reservation to visit his ailing mother who had just suffered a debilitating stroke. In his absence, he was described as the "problem" by Mrs. Tapahonso and Lisa. The mother revealed a long history of battery by her own father, but made no mention of her physical abuse of Lisa. Both the mother and Lisa expressed their concerns about Mr. Tapahonso and talked about how much Angie was becoming like her father. Angie remained quiet throughout the multiple-impact, but did talk about feeling close to her father and boasted about his ability to speak the Navajo tongue fluently. When each member concluded her viewpoint of the problem, the team reminded the family that they were originally brought to the attention of the "authorities" as a result of allegations of physical abuse of Lisa by Mrs. Tapahonso.

With the help of the adolescent specialist, Lisa was able to share that she would often intervene in the spousal violence and subsequently be hit by her mother. Lisa had difficulty maintaining a position that was in opposition to her mother and slipped into a less direct position of describing the parental role she often assumed with her mother and father. On numerous occasions, she would wait until the wee hours of the morning for her parents to return from outings where drinking was involved. Lisa described waiting and worrying that her parents would be killed in a drunk-driving accident or be arrested in a barroom brawl. Lisa also described various undesirables whom her parents would invite home from the bar, whom Lisa would have to send away. At that time, a marked and dramatic shift in alliances took place: Lisa and Angie moved physically closer together and began to tell many stories of chaotic and violent events that occurred when their parents were drinking. During such events, Lisa physically intervened to protect her sister and, as a result, was often beaten by her mother. Mrs. Tapahonso became increasingly angry and began to interrupt her daughters to tell of Lisa's oppositional behavior at school and home.

The problem section of the multiple-impact demonstrated the rapid shift in alliances and coalitions that occurred within the Tapahonso family. The team began to surmise that the family of these adolescent girls had little stability from which they could individuate. This might explain why they sometimes dabbled in dangerous behavior and peer groups outside the home and at other times showed remarkable responsibility in managing their lives. Because the hierarchical structure of the family was impaired, there was little internal stability. This hypothesis was supported by our observation of rapid and dramatic shifts in coalitions.

Fourth Phase: Genograms

The next stage of the multiple-impact is the genogram session. At this point, the team has established the ground rules for treatment, has heard each member's view of the problem, and has begun to invite their clients into seeing the problem as a larger family issue. Moreover, the genogram continues the process of moving responsibility beyond the IP, and the immediate family, to the intergenerational context and provides the team with additional assessment information. The genogram often reveals tacit family rules that dictate interactions between members and how emotions are handled. Finally, the genogram provides the team with yet another opportunity to test the efficacy of their initial hypothesis.

The Campbell family was referred by 14-year-old Allen's probation officer. Allen was becoming increasingly delinquent and had recently been hospitalized as a result of suicidal ideation. In addition to the issues presented by Allen, his 15-year-old sister was briefly hospitalized after she intentionally ingested an overdose of Allen's Ritalin. When the team entered the family's home and began to move through the stages of the multiple-impact, they were struck by the lack of affect in this family of three teenagers, a mother, and father. No one initiated any interactions with each other or the team. When the team pressed the family to explore the recent suicidal behavior of two of its members, the family was compliant in describing the concrete events of the incident, but they were unable to explore the emotional implications. On a break, the team almost simultaneously described the family as being emotionally "dead." The team returned to the family with a large piece of paper and began to draw out the family genogram. When it came to the mother's family of origin, she surprisingly revealed to the team that she had been extensively molested by her father until 17 years of age.

The molestation stopped because she moved out of her family home to marry the children's father. The mother disclosed this without affect and used language that was concrete and void of emotional descriptors. The family looked on in shock, but didn't speak. No one in the family, including her husband, had ever known of her trauma. The team probed deeper; eventually some of the children followed the lead of the therapists and timidly questioned their mother about her trauma. To them, the mother replied, "It's over and I'm still alive, so there's nothing to talk about." The family fell silent again.

In a sentence, the mother described the tacit family rule about dealing with painful emotional issues. "It's over, so there is nothing to talk about." This explained the family's method of mechanically recounting the events of the recent suicide attempts with such striking lack of affect. The coming work with the Campbell family was going to center on how to help the family find its heart, so the children would not be so emotionally isolated and cut off as to feel suicide was their only option.

Fifth Phase: Individuals

When the genogram sequence is completed, the multiple-impact moves to individual sessions. It is at this time that the primary therapist meets with the parents, the adolescent specialist with the IP, and the secondary therapist with remaining family members (or different groupings of the remaining family members). The purpose of these sessions is to further join with each subsystem and to assess how the subsystems function when they are separate from the whole.

The individual sessions allow an opportunity to assess for risk factors, to complete a mental status exam, and so forth. Often, at this time the adolescent specialist makes a no-suicide contract with the IP and makes an agreement that the IP will call the team if the need arises. It is a final opportunity to test the efficacy of the hypothesis as well as to test the "strength" of tacit family rules for transactions and methods of handling emotion at the subsystem level.

During individual sessions with the Campbell family, Carol, Allen's sister, who had made a recent suicide attempt, described her family as "lines on a paper that never touch." Her affect was flat and depressed, and the secondary therapist noted that her description of her family, although more laden with sadness, was congruent with the team's impression of the whole family system: lifeless. For the daughters, however, it was hopeless rather than mechanical. More clinically hopeful was Allen, who was able to be far more animated in his session with the adolescent specialist. He made a quick and genuine emotional connection to the therapist and articulated his wish to be attached to others. He also expressed a hopefulness and an interest in trying to have a deeper relationship with his father.

It was from information gleaned from the individual sessions that the primary therapist was able to commence work on helping this family to find its "heart." The challenge for the middle phase of treatment lay in working with the spousal system to test whether the mother in particular could tolerate a more affective relationship with her family.

Individual sessions lay the groundwork for future treatment. It is in this context that different subsystem members can experiment with new methods of transactions, receive reinforcement from clinicians, and gain an increasing sense of mastery, armed with new tools for challenging the entire family system. The primary therapist must orchestrate the overall process to thwart powerful family processes that perpetuate existing nonproductive patterns of interaction.

The subsystem configurations pose a challenge to the clinical team, as powerful family mechanisms are at work to induct therapists into operating as yet another participant in the nonproductive family dance. Families with rigid alliances and patterns of transactions are especially challenging, as was the case in the Spencer family.

When the adolescent specialist met with Kathleen during the multiple-impact session, Kathleen's first question was, "Are you on my side or my parents' side?" She then listed all the helping professionals who had been involved with the family thus far, and what "side" they had chosen. Kathleen attempted to structure the relationship into the same rigid patterns that she had experienced in her family: There are only two options for our family—either submit and give complete loyalty at individual expense, or meet one's own needs and be cut off, entirely, from the family.

This proved to be a challenge throughout treatment. In their individual session with the primary therapist, the Spencer parents asked the same question as their daughter, "Whose side are you on?" Throughout treatment, the primary therapist and adolescent specialist had to pay close attention to their own clinical relationship. On several occasions they found themselves "arguing" with each other about treatment with the family, particularly when a crisis arose. With help from the larger team, they found that each time they were at odds, they were inducted into the rigid family coalitions and the belief that there are only two options to resolve a crisis. Through consultation with the larger clinical team, the Spencer's therapists were able to extricate themselves from powerful inductive forces and re-enter the family "centered" once again.

Final Phase: Wrap-Up

The final phase of the multiple-impact session is the wrap-up. The purpose is always the same: to report to the family what major issues can be addressed in treatment, to underscore family system and individual strengths, and to give predictions about the "emotional rollercoaster" the family will ride on its journey through treatment. The method of providing "wrap-up" is spontaneously designed on the multiple-impact day so as to best access the particular family's listening powers.

When the team assembled the Spencer family for the final stage of the multiple-impact (to give feedback), they chose to use the "fishbowl" technique. They directed the family to remain quiet and observe the clinical team discussing their family in the same manner as a team meeting would be conducted at the agency. The team chose this method because of the family's increasing anxiety that they would "break apart" again following the team's departure for that day. Furthermore, the team did not want to provide the family an with an opportunity to "undo" the work the Spencers had accomplished thus far by having an interactive discussion that could lead the way back to stalemated communication patterns. The team began by each clinician stating a strength he or she had observed in the family (e.g., love, a wish to have a "happy family," and a reframing of the mother and daughter's emotional tenacity as a demonstration of their ability to endure the emotional intensity that would be elicited by change). Next, the team discussed the constant impasse between mother and daughter and the challenge that both would have to undertake to achieve compromise. The team predicted that moving away from power struggles was going to open old wounds of loss for the Spencer parents and therefore "leave room" for Kathleen to work on issues about her personal identity, particularly with regard to her adoption. The team predicted that the family might find themselves at a point in treatment when it seemed as if things had become "worse" instead of better, but the Spencers would need to persevere to achieve the sort of family life they wished to have. Finally, the family was given the homework assignment to refrain from attempting to negotiate major rules until the next session.

MIDDLE PHASE

In the middle phase, the therapeutic work is focused upon effecting change that is fundamental and structural in nature. With family preservation as a primary goal of treatment, the team continually ponders the question, "What skills, abilities, and changes does the family need to develop to enable them to stay together?" As the middle phase of treatment progresses, families are challenged to assume responsibility for answering those questions as well. Therapeutic pressure is applied to different subsystems, and family members begin to experiment with new role functions and transactions. Utilizing the support of their individual therapists, family members grapple with identifying what they need from each other and how to enact those changes. One method is what Minuchin (1981) refers to as "unbalancing" and is something the CAIHP is well suited to employ.

> The therapist joins and supports one individual or one subsystem at the expense of the others. She affiliates with a family member low in the hierarchy, empowering him instead of undercutting him. . . . She joins a family member in a coalition that attacks another family member. These operations handicap the recognition of the signals by which family members commonly indicate to each other the appropriateness of their interpersonal behavior. . . . These changes may produce new realities for the family members . . . alternatives within all subsystems may therefore be uncovered and become possible. (Minuchin, 1981, pp. 161–162)

The team must work to understand how things have been done in the past and weave change into the existing fabric of family patterns of interaction. This is especially important when working with families who culturally and ethnically differ from their therapist(s).

In the case of the Tapahonso family, the primary therapist spent a large part of earlier parent sessions comparing and contrasting life on the reservation to life in suburban California. It was clear that many values of the two cultures were in conflict. The biggest difference the parents identified was with regard to the father's role in parenting children. It was the couple's experience, in their families of origin on the reservation, that a father was not centrally involved in the day-to-day tasks of child rearing. Instead, it is the mother who has primary responsibility; however, she has constant and regular access to support from an extended network of kin. The Tapahonsos moved to suburban California shortly after they were married. When the children were born, Mrs. Tapahonso did not have the support of her Navajo community. Thus, she grew to feel overwhelmed and harbored intense resentment for her burden. Her resentment was often directed at Lisa, who attempted to thwart it by taking on parenting responsibilities. Consequently, mother and daughter frequently battled; their role responsibilities were blurred and unclear. In the middle phase of treatment, the primary therapist repeatedly challenged the parents to develop strategies for responding to the needs of their adolescent daughters and therefore to establish a more productive parental hierarchy. Initially, Mr. Tapahonso was passive and silent; however, as he began to develop an alliance with the therapist and felt that she respected his opinion and ideas, he spontaneously began to take a more active role in disciplining, and talking with, his daughters. Concurrently, the mother began to reach out to her daughters and spend "fun" time with them.

During an individual session with her adolescent specialist, Lisa revealed an important family secret around which many tacit rules had developed. The couple's first child was a son. The child died from SIDS while under the father's care. When the death occurred, Mr. Tapahonso was drunk. The couple had not spoken about their son's death in many years. As the pain and anguish surfaced, the spousal subsystem was challenged to grapple with their grief as a couple and together answer the questions that their daughters asked about the death.

It was here that the family was able to make some fundamental changes in their interactions with each other. The father was able to take a more active role in parenting as the "myth" about his incompetence surfaced (via discussion of the death). This freed the mother to build a more emotionally appropriate relationship with her daughters and for the family to experience greater intimacy. At the same time, the parents were adopting parenting styles that were more congruent with their present resources. As the primary therapist underscored the changes in parental functioning, she also encouraged the Tapahonsos to evaluate what aspects of their Navajo culture they wanted to preserve for their daughters and how they might actively pursue that goal.

As the Tapahonso family spousal system altered and worked to become more of a team, their interactions with their daughters changed. All family members and the team agreed that a real shift had occurred when Lisa had a date and came home to find both her parents sitting on the couch waiting for her to return home safely.

Another integral piece to work with families with adolescent children is of a psychoeducational nature. Many of the parents in our families left home abruptly during their own adolescence or in other cases were unable to leave their families of origin until much later stages in life. Through our earlier work with the genogram, the team is able to identify where parents may need information about the developmental tasks their adolescent children are compelled to master. Assuring parents that it is normal for teenagers to experiment with leaving home and becoming autonomous adults often alleviates much of the resistance that parents present to their teenagers when their adolescents seem to be suddenly "rejecting" them. In addition, as this family life stage is understood from a more "universal" perspective, parents may be able to separate from the present "wounds" of rejection inflicted by an individuating adolescent.

Many of the families with whom we work have developed rigidly entrenched transactional patterns as a method of maintaining a homeostasis that protects them from dealing with painful underlying issues. The middle phase is integral to the successful treatment of chaotic families. As the IP's symptomatology decreases, the family, and particularly, the therapists, are often lulled into a false sense of "cure." This is especially inviting for the clinical team that has spent 4 to 5 weeks battling through chaos and blowups and sometimes outright hostility to the treatment process. However, this is a key juncture when clinical intervention must intensify, as family members will often become frightened by this new found family quiet. It is at this time that the underlying problems are most accessible to therapists and most frightening to clients. If the clinical work slows down, chaotic families will often experience another crisis, apparently to protect themselves from experiencing the underlying pain. This form of "resistance" can be so intense and the family may generate a conflict so large that a child might have to be removed from the home and all treatment efforts and family work may be lost. This is why the CAIHP team must be in the family's home frequently and always available by beeper.

After 5 weeks of intensive work with Kathy and Jason, as well as play therapy sessions for Cassandra, the Patterson family seemed to be doing very well. In her individual sessions, Kathy began to touch upon the extreme loneliness and abandonment she experienced while growing up in her adoptive home. Furthermore, Kathy described fears that her natural parents, when she located them, would reject her and find her inadequate as a daughter. As Kathy's personal struggles came to the surface, so, too, did her feelings of self-doubt when it came to disciplining Jason. Simultaneously, Jason grew more and more anxious and outrageous in his behavior. His acting out seemed to be a challenge to his mother, as if he were saying, "Can you take control of our family? When you are scared and anxious, Mom, I'm not so sure you can keep things safe for us, so I don't think the world is safe." After two incidents in which Jason climbed to the roof of the two-story apartment building and pelted people with rocks, Kathy wondered whether he should return to residential treatment. The team reminded Kathy that she could use the CAIHP beeper system when a crisis arose. Kathy did; when the next two incidents occurred, the team coached Kathy through the events and the intervention while interpreting the meaning of Jason's behavior. Kathy was encouraged and reinforced for her strength and ability to parent Jason (and her other children). Simultaneously, in individual sessions, Kathy was helped to identify the link between her personal recall of her feelings of abandonment, Jason's awareness of her precarious emotional state, and the return to passivity in disciplining Jason.

Another powerful form of resistance is when there is a pseudocalm and treatment becomes diffuse. Families that begin treatment with such an intensity of crisis that they may have a child placed outside their home require a great deal of clinical intensity and emotional energy from the involved therapists. Thus, when there is pseudocalm, therapists may unconsciously respond to family messages to refrain from the process of making deeper clinical "incisions."

In the CAIHP we often utilize the larger team to help restore the clinical focus. This may take the form of a clinical consultation, a live mirror session, or the inclusion of the secondary therapist in family sessions. Work with families such as these, and particularly families where the parents are needy and dependent, takes a tremendous toll on the therapist. At the CAIHP program we do not believe it is healthy nor indicated for therapists to treat crisis-oriented families without the assistance of their team partners. These are powerful family systems that can easily and swiftly induct the clinical team. When this occurs, the clinician can become an unwitting participant in destructive family patterns whose eventual result is the breakup of a family.

Resistance in the middle stage may take a psychodynamic form (as illustrated in Kathy's case history), or other sorts of resistance may occur. One common form is the emergence of a new "IP." Families are likely to present resistance to truly establishing second-order change in their systemic structure. In other words, once the IP's presenting problem(s) have abated, the family may unwittingly signal other family members to reestablish familiar (yet nonproductive) homeostatic mechanisms. Thus, a second child may begin to act out and become the "new IP." When this happens, the family and team can easily be invited into feeling hopeless about the future of the family. However, when recognized as yet another form of family resistance, the "symptoms" are often more quickly remediated by helping the family to enact the new skills and transactional patterns they have learned to use with the initial IP. Moreover, the middle phase is often a time when the family needs to repeat transactions that utilize newly discovered (productive) methods of interaction.

The Tapahonso family was initially pleased that Lisa, the IP, was responding to the rules of the household and had begun to do exceptionally well at school. Angie, however, was getting into increasing amounts of trouble on the street. A neighbor reported that she believed Angie stole a bicycle from her garage, and the police implicated Angie in an incident of vandalism but did not have definitive proof of her involvement. When her father learned of this, he became enraged and hit Angie. He was immediately remorseful and called the primary therapist. The primary therapist met with Mr. and Mrs. Tapahonso. She actively pushed the Tapahonsos to work as a parenting unit to resolve this latest crisis. Together, the couple decided that Mr. Tapahonso would call Child Protective Services and report the incident (it was not considered by the authorities to be child abuse), and together the Tapahonsos resolved to give Angie an appropriate consequence for her behavior. The therapist worked closely with the parents, getting them to acknowledge their fears of parenting as a team. They used this as a starting point for discussing the lack of intimacy that had so long existed in their relationship and their respective individual panic and fear of being close to one another.

Finally, during a pivotal family session, Angie became enraged when her parents jointly responded to her inappropriate behavior. She ran out of the room and out of the house. With minimal prompting from the therapist, the parents quickly devised a plan to bring Angie back to the house and to continue to work on the issue at hand. They brought her back and as a unit expressed frustration at her behavior while also providing her with emotional support for her feelings of shame and frustration at being confronted for her misdeeds.

The preceding example highlights another typical form of resistance encountered during the middle phase. Once the children's behavior has stopped consuming the parents' emotional energy and time, the spouses are left to face one another. This is of particular importance when we are working with families that are in the family life cycle stage of adolescence. When the last teen leaves home, a couple must learn how to be alone with each other once again. If there are many unresolved spousal issues, fears of intimacy, or a poorly established spousal boundary, a couple may become terrified at the notion of being alone again and may therefore unwittingly signal children to act out, which creates a pseudoalliance between parents. This is a time when the CAIHP model is very efficacious for treating families, as we have built marital therapy into the treatment structure. We assume from the outset that the spousal system will need assistance to face its own life cycle challenges. This is addressed throughout treatment.

TERMINATION PHASE

During the final phase of treatment (the last 3 to 4 weeks), many tasks must be accomplished. Termination is a delicate and difficult process in any intense therapeutic relationship, but it is especially difficult for families who have been in turmoil and have multigenerational patterns of loss, abandonment, and incomplete life cycle transitions. In some senses, the CAIHP team has been saying "good-bye" since the outset of treatment as we are continually reminding the family (and ourselves) that we have only 90 days in which to effect change that is long lasting and will preclude the need to place a child outside the family's home.

In some cases, as the termination phase approaches, the clinical team has recognized that the family is not, at that point in time, able to make all the changes that the treatment plan originally incorporated. There are families (and individuals within those families) that do not have the internal resources to enact those shifts that would ultimately most benefit future family functioning. Thus, the clinical team must always be poised to redirect the course of treatment to incorporate an impasse. When this occurs, the team must refocus treatment to alternative areas where the most substantial gains can be made.

During the middle stages of treatment, the Campbell adolescents had made significant progress with their respective therapists. The Campell children were able to state clearly that they wanted a more affective relationship within their family. In their individual sessions, the kids articulated the things they would like their parents to know about their lives and their wishes for how their parents might provide nurturing to them. The primary therapist spent many sessions providing an opportunity for the children to address their mother and to articulate to her directly those needs they had identified in their individual sessions. The primary therapist attempted to coach Mrs. Campbell in how to begin to respond to the emotional needs of her children. However, it soon became clear that Mrs. Campbell did not have the emotional resources to give to the children what they so clearly stated that they needed. In parent sessions, she stated that having an affective relationship with her children made her feel as if she would have to open "Pandora's box" and begin the difficult process of confronting her own family-of-origin issues. She was unequivocal in stating that she could not, at this time in her life, make the changes that were being asked of her. Thus treatment focus had to be redirected to other family resources.

Simultaneous to the work focused on the mother, Mr. Campbell began to build a positive relationship with Allen. Allen initiated a connection with his father by entering his father's garage and "hanging out" with his dad. Prior to the start of treatment, Dad would spend the bulk of his time at home, alone, out in the garage. Allen and his Dad started work on a car that had been waiting for years to be rebuilt. Soon after that project commenced, the father spontaneously arrived at his son's basketball game. The next time Dad attended a game, he brought Allen's sisters with him. During a very poignant live session at the clinic, Dad lead the way in expressing emotion about a painful family event. He began to cry when the primary therapist asked him to talk about how he felt when one of his daughters made a suicide attempt. He described going up to her bedroom, and the deep well of sadness and fear he experienced when he looked into her room and saw her teddy bears so carefully arranged on her bed. He talked about the extreme loss he knew he would experience if his daughter was no longer alive to attend to the "teddy bear task" that he had watched her do almost every day of her life. All the children were crying as father spoke, but mother sat stony-faced, neither sad nor disapproving. In that session, Dad gave the family tacit permission to break the family rule of "it's over, so there's nothing to talk about."

During the termination phase, the primary therapist worked with the family to recognize the impasse and to strengthen their alternative resources for change. Mrs. Campbell was able to say to the children that she recognized their needs and found them to be valid, but she was unable to make the changes they were requesting of her. In parent sessions, the couple acknowledged that their marriage was void of emotional connection, but both partners felt that they worked well as a team to provide for the concrete needs of their family. They did not feel they needed to make any changes in their relationship at that point in time. They agreed that they would call the CAIHP if they ever chose to pursue a different sort of relationship with one another.

For the termination session, Mrs. Campbell made an elaborate spread of food for the departing clinical team. The children and their father were able to articulate, with great affect, their gratitude for the changes that the CAIHP helped them to make in their family life.

As is evident in the case example cited above, the CAIHP is not always able to effect change according to the original intervention strategy. However, the model allows for intensive work to occur at many subsystem levels within the greater family system operation. Thus, if one entry point does not allow for the desired result, alternative routes may be accessed to create the closest approximation to the original treatment goal.

One of the concrete tasks that must be completed is linkage to other resources. This may include a referral to continued family therapy in a more traditional setting. If this is the case, the CAIHP team works with the new therapist to bring them into treatment and to the work the family has achieved thus far. In addition, the CAIHP works with the family and new therapist to identify those issues that will need to be addressed in future treatment. When possible, collateral sessions are held to help the family make the transition to the new therapist.

More often, families are not financially able to continue in treatment particularly in the present economic climate of shrinking services. Thus, throughout the 90 days, therapists work with families to facilitate more regular "use" of naturally occurring supports (extended family, neighbors, etc.) and community organizations (e.g., church, 12-step programs, sports teams, parent organizations, etc.). For many families, this is a more natural transition, as CAIHP treatment may have been their first experience in therapy. Further, work throughout the 90 days offers families, particularly those that have been involved with the court systems, a corrective experience. In other words, families learn that you can ask for help, reveal yourself, and not be punished for doing so. It is our aim to increase the likelihood that families will reach out for support when the familiar signs of stress and "stuckness" present themselves.

Termination is discussed for the last 3 to 4 weeks of treatment and is "used" to further access underlying loss and abandonment issues that have contributed to the presenting problem. Family members are encouraged to share their sadness as well as anger at the departing therapists. Therapists model acceptance of anger and responsiveness to those feelings. With the clinical team, the family plans for the termination session. Families are asked how they would like to say good-bye to the team, and sometimes together the team and family plan a good-bye party to acknowledge the work and the change that the family has completed.

Frequently with CAIHP families, feelings of loss and fear of backsliding may cause families to create a crisis and thereby make the symbolic statement, "We're not ready for you to leave; we still have many problems we want you to help us with." CAIHP therapists help clients to recognize those final phase crises for what they are and use them to help clients to look toward utilizing newly acquired skills and to access other existing community resources.

During the very last session, clients are asked to give the team feedback about treatment, both positive and negative, and they are asked to predict what the next crisis will be. Finally, the team gives the family feedback on their clinical achievements as well as personal feedback on the therapists' feelings about leaving the family with whom they have journeyed through the struggle and beauty of change.

Work with the Spencer family was long and arduous; both the IP and her mother battled fiercely throughout. The father was assisted to take a more active role in family life. He was often the pivotal member in this very small family. At the close of treatment, the Spencer parents had begun to allow Kathleen far more freedom (relative to the start of treatment) than she had ever before experienced. At the termination session, the family stated proudly that they knew there would be a lot more battles ahead of them, but they felt they would be able to remain together while struggling through those battles. Laughingly, Kathleen showed the team one of the ways the family had learned to tolerate her individuation. Kathleen flipped up her beautiful long black hair (which was always worn in a girlish, Rebecca of Sunny Brook Farm style of which her parents approved), and revealed that she had it shaved underneath to have "lines," just like many of her peers wore their hair. Her parents rolled their eyes, but felt they could tolerate Kathleen's coiffure choice as long as they didn't have to stare at it constantly. The Spencers showed the team their appointment card for their first session with a therapist who was going to assist them not only with navigating further parenting struggles, but to undertake the long overdue grief work that had never been completed.

The treatment team was pleased when they left the Spencer home for the last time. They had worked long and hard and were able to maintain a strong clinical focus despite the powerful inductive forces that this small family presented. They felt a certain degree of frustration, however, that they could not continue on with the Spencers as they traveled through their grief work and Kathleen's later adolescent stages.

Work with Kathy and her children, Jason and Cassandra, came to a surprising conclusion. As termination was approaching, so, too, was the prison release date of Kathy's abusive ex-husband (the children's father). Although many clinical advances had been made with the children, they were still unable to talk about their father in any way that acknowledged the fear and anger they felt for him. In the last weeks of treatment, Cassandra, through her play sessions, revealed the opportunity to complete the treatment goals.

For weeks Cassandra had been playing out scenes that included a ferocious bulldog attacking children, ruining "safe" play houses she had created, and gobbling up "nice people." The team, who sat behind the mirror weekly to watch the play sessions, interpreted the "bulldog" to be a symbol of the fear Cassandra felt for the outside world and the chaotic, internal world of her family in earlier stages. However, when the play therapist met with Kathy to discuss treatment in that subsystem arena, Mom revealed that Cassandra's abusive father had a large tattoo of a bulldog on his chest. Indeed, "Bulldog" was his nickname. The secondary therapist brought this new information into the play therapy room. Cassandra then began to talk about all the "rules" and threats that her father had imposed about never saying anything "bad" about him to anyone. Cassandra "practiced" stating her "bad" feelings out loud and found that those feelings were accepted. With that newly experienced confidence, Cassandra was able to reveal many terrifying events that had occurred at the hands of her father. Kathy's new found emotional strength and invigorated parental tenacity allowed all the children to explore their memories. With their mother, away from treatment sessions, the kids began to release their memories. Kathy called the beeper and worked with the team to manage the deep sadness and guilt she felt for not having been able to protect her children from the trauma they had experienced. Jason and Cassandra told their mother of several incidents of sexual molestation that were perpetrated by their father and his "drug" friends. With that evidence, she was able to get a no-contact order between the father and the children.

Work in the final stages of treatment was swift and intense. When the team and the family met for the final termination session, it was to eat pizza and then wave good-bye to the kids as they piled into the car, with all their belongings. They were moving away from the transitional battered women's shelter to a distant town where Kathy was going to re-establish herself with the help of her birth family.

Work with the Tapahonso family terminated at a point when the family was truly ready to make it on its own. Lisa managed to become enrolled in a very special alternative school program in which the students were working on many community activities to raise money to travel to South Africa. Both Mr. and Mrs. Tapahonso became actively involved in assisting the the school program to achieve its goals. Angie was placed on probation, and both of her parents accompanied her to meetings with her probation officer. Accompanied by the primary therapist, the parents met with the school to establish a more comprehensive educational program to meet Angie's needs.

At the final session, the girls told the team of a social event that they attended together and all the gossip they had gathered from that event. As the team prepared to leave, the family members became tearful and expressed their gratitude for the help they received and their sense of readiness to tackle family life alone, with their newly developed skills. As the team departed the Tapahonsos said, "We're like baby birds who are ready to leave the nest and fly on our own; we're scared, just a bit sad, but ready to fly alone."

REFERENCES

Kagan, R., & Schlosberg, S. (1989). *Families in perpetual crisis.* New York: W. W. Norton

Minuchin, S. (1981). *Family therapy techniques.* Cambridge, MA: Harvard University Press.

5

Family-Based Mental Health Services

Cynthia Archacki-Stone

People never cease to amaze me.
— PATTI R. LESH

THE ADVENTURE BEGINS . . .

Providing mental health services to children and families in their homes is a new initiative in the mental health field. This movement is growing in strength across the country. There are significant attempts to design individualized services to meet the special needs of children and their families. Family-Based Mental Health Services in Pennsylvania began in the mid-1980s. Ten pilot projects were funded by the Commonwealth of Pennsylvania, Office of Mental Health, by 1988. The purpose behind this movement is to strengthen the family unit in an effort to prevent the out-of-home placement of children. The future goal is for every catchment area in Pennsylvania to establish Family-Based Mental Health Services. In 1994, there were 52 programs in existence across the state.

The Pennsylvania services are designed to provide intensive support and therapeutic intervention to families in crisis. There are three criteria for referral: a child with a history of unsuccessful treatment, involvement of at least one adult or parent, and the willingness of other involved agencies to participate. Since these services are the most restrictive (most costly and most intensive) outpatient services, it is necessary to establish that traditional services provided in therapists' offices have not been effective, that the child's behavior and emotional difficulties persist and the risk of out-of-home placement is a probable outcome unless effective treatment can be provided. The voluntary participation of at least one adult who fulfills the parental role for the child is required. But despite the voluntary nature of Family-Based Services, families rarely enter treatment feeling as though they have a choice. By the time referral is directed to our services, numerous agencies have attempted to provide assistance without success. The threat of placement looms and the family is desperately trying to stay together. The child and family's involvement with other child care agencies, such as child welfare, juvenile justice, drug and alcohol, the mental health system, and the school districts is important. Because treatment planning with the child, family, and other involved agencies is critical to continuity of care, this partnership approach is required at the time of referral (Kaplan, 1986).

To further complicate the referral process, there are additional requirements to meet before the services can begin. These are generated by the ever-present funding issues. In 1990, the Pennsylvania Office of Mental Health, Department of Public Welfare, worked to assure the existence of the services in Pennsylvania. Prior to this time, all programs were limited to grant funding from the state budget for mental health. The funding stream of medical assistance (MA) dollars was investigated. By 1992, Family-Based Mental Health Services began to be able to draw down these monies. Billing for services was initiated as each county negotiated reimbursement rates with the Pennsylvania Office of Mental Health in its region. Because Pennsylvania is such a large state with diverse populations in rural and urban areas, rates vary considerably. Some insurance companies have approved payment for Family-Based Mental Health treatment. Categorical state funds are still available to each program and are utilized to pay for services that are not reimbursed by MA or insurance monies. In 1994, the services survived with a creative blending of these monies, reflecting the reality that good clinical programs must be provided within fiscal constraints. It is never enjoyable to ponder the financial realities of providing service.

Because of limited funds, each child referred to our program must be evaluated by a child psychiatrist and/or a licensed child psychologist to insure the appropriateness of the referral prior to the initiation of service. The County Office of Mental Health/Mental Retardation must then authorize services.

If this sounds like a lot of hoops to jump through—well, it is! Acceptance of referrals from the general public is very difficult. Referrals from the child-serving agencies previously mentioned are more commonly considered, since these child care professionals have been working with the child and the family. Usually, we rely on their assessment for referral, coordination of agency agreement, and introduction of our program as a possible treatment option to the family. Continual development of our professional relationships within the community is necessary if our program is to continue to get appropriate referrals. Fortunately, these activities to coordinate a child and family's treatment are considered necessary and are reimbursable services.

The philosophy of Pennsylvania Family-Based Mental Health Services is anchored in the belief in the family's strength (Kaplan, 1986). Unfortunately, all too often the child and family's problems dominate the treatment process. Families ask for help out of despair; parents have a deep sense of guilt, blame, and failure. Often, the family and its members are convinced their situation is hopeless and beyond their control (Kagen & Schlosberg, 1989). As we think of those who are faced with such circumstances, we must remember an old saying: "Do not remind me of my failures, I have not forgotten them." We have found that to dwell on what is wrong only further intensifies the desperation felt by the family.

The child and family have no sense of control over their situation when we first enter their home. However, there is a desire to believe that we can somehow "fix" the problem. Often the family members have given up on their own abilities to make things better. They are overwhelmed, exhausted, and just trying to get through another day. Family-Based Services emphasize the child and family members' resources and attributes. It is continuously emphasized that the family is the key to a child's improved functioning. The family knows what has been tried, what has worked, and what has not worked. There is a foundation of rules, limits, and relationships that have been established long before the family-based therapist entered this household (Satir, 1988). Our goal is to build on what is not broken. Therefore, services include the entire family whenever possible. Each family member holds a valuable perception of how the family functions. As we attempt to gain the full picture of how the family works, our focus must remain on empowering family members to help one another to resolve problematic issues in the direction that they choose. It is not our job to remake families or insist that the family function as our values might dictate. To maintain this focus, we have to remind ourselves that each family makes unique choices about how the members live their lives. Our role is to present alternatives so that that they can hear them and make responsible choices as they attempt to put an end to their chaos.

The theoretical framework selected by the Pennsylvania Office of Mental Health in their design of the program is that of Structural Family Therapy (Minuchin, 1974). Given the lack of available education and training programs for family therapy in America, there has been a limited number of therapists available to do this work. This is particularly true in the rural county in which we operate. To address this deficit, the Pennsylvania Office of Mental Health implemented a mandatory training requirement for all therapists and program directors who provide family-based treatment. Over a 3½-year period (17 days per year) the Philadelphia Child Guidance Clinic at the Family Training Center in Philadelphia and the Western Psychiatric Institute and Clinic in Pittsburgh have provided a wide range of didactic presentations and clinical skill development sessions specifically oriented to the family-based setting. There are five training sites throughout the state. Each month an in-service day is presented from a comprehensive curriculum. Topics have included remarriage, single parenthood, substance abuse, death and dying, child abuse, school-related problems, attention deficit disorders, agency collaboration, and professional fatigue, among others.

In addition, a clinical skill development day is held monthly. During the course of this day, therapists present written assessments outlining aspects of structural family therapy such as hierarchy, family rules and boundaries, enmeshed and disengaged relationships, triads, and coalitions, and videotaped vignettes of families currently in treatment. It is during the clinical days that theories are applied and practiced. Role playing is frequently used to focus on such interventions as enactments, unbalancing, punctuating, challenging, and others. Treatment strategies and planning are primary activities.

Training offers a unified and consistent theoretical map for the programs and a strong emphasis on the competence and quality of clinical skill development. The training program also provides therapists with an opportunity to interact with their peers. Thus, a network of professional support is created. Sharing the struggles of the work, knowing others are coping with the same demands, and having a safe environment to learn and develop offers a much needed respite to recharge a therapist's batteries.

In addition, a summer practicum (1 month long) is offered to program directors. This is held at the Philadelphia Child Guidance Clinic, and attendance is strongly encouraged by the Pennsylvania Office of Mental Health. Also on the training menu is participation in a supervision course for program directors. It goes without saying that Family-Based Services are dedicated to continuous improvement, as seen through its commitment to training.

Family-Based Mental Health Services involve extremely intensive work. The staff is required to be on-call 24 hours a day, always available to families in times of crisis. The staff consists of a program director with a master's-level education in a mental-health-related field and experience with direct service to children and families, as well as supervisory experience. The program director does not carry a caseload, but is able to provide direct service in the absence of a family-based therapist. The director is permitted to supervise a maximum of three treatment teams (six therapists). The Pennsylvania program usually operates with a team of two therapists who provide the majority of the direct and case management services. Individual interaction also occurs, but the ideal is for the team to work together modeling how parents might work together. Beyond "two heads are better than one," the motto is that the more heads you have working together, the more comprehensive and coordinated your treatment will be.

On paper, the treatment team is composed of a therapist with a master's-level education in a mental-health-related field, whose team function is to facilitate the treatment planning process, and a therapist with a bachelor's-level education in a mental-health-related field, whose team function is to facilitate the case management coordination. In reality, the team members must function on an equal basis. This is a challenge given the differences in education and experience. (It should be noted that there is allowable equivalency of experience for educational requirements. The specific regulations of the program have been published in the *Pennsylvania Bulletin,* May 1993.)

The maximum team caseload is eight families. In order to spread the extensive demands for documentation, four families are assigned to each therapist. In treatment, the team combines its forces and jointly "dances" to form a partnership with the family. Each family is eligible for 32 consecutive weeks of treatment. The length of service may be extended if approved by the child psychiatrist. The frequency of treatment sessions is determined by the family and the therapists (the minimum being once a week). Generally, sessions are held in the home, but families have the option of meeting in the office as well.

A great deal of time is spent developing the team relationship. Direct communication is essential. After 7 years of being a program director with two teams, I have found no painless means of getting this to happen. Many challenges occur in creating a cotherapy team, such as differing stages of personal and professional development, conflicting values, issues of trust, and questioning of competence. But, through it all, a mutual respect and rapport develops. Team dynamics play a significant role in the treatment of families. When the team is in disarray, so is the treatment, usually. The power of the family, as well as the team, combines to create the treatment experience. When the team is "out of step" and their "dance" is not synchronized, the treatment suffers. We must pay close attention to this dynamic.

In our program structure, the staff meets together a minimum of 4 hours a week to review cases and air concerns. Supervision with an individual therapist or team occurs a minimum of 3 hours per week. More time can always be scheduled at the program director's, therapist's, or team's discretion. To further our commitment to the team concept, the majority of program operational procedures and decisions are made with group consensus. Planning meetings are held quarterly (away from the office) to brainstorm, plan, and problem solve all issues that affect the program; be they administrative or clinical.

Simply put, the program director has one primary responsibility: to promote, facilitate, and provide the staff with therapeutic expertise to function in a professional and conscientious manner. Through these efforts each and every child and family will be assured the best treatment possible. The treatment team's goal is to join with the child and family members in a partnership, identify and employ their strengths, and struggle with them to find solutions to their difficulties. The team is responsible to be ever mindful of protecting the children from all forms of abuse and promoting safety within the home.

Although our goal is to prevent out-of-home placement, realistically this is not always possible. But placement does not reflect failure. At times, placement must occur in order for a child in the family to be safe. We attempt to establish a means for the family to maintain relationships and work toward resolution and reunification. Our program is not specifically designed to provide reunification intervention when a child is returning home from a long-term placement. For the most part, we work with children who have experienced psychiatric hospitalizations, brief foster care placements, or who have spent time with relatives and are now home again.

Our program is housed in a community mental health center located in a hospital. Prior to the family-based program being established, the center provided traditional individual-focused psychotherapy on an outpatient basis. Seventy-five percent of the clientele is adult, and most of the service was oriented to this population. Family therapy occurred only in times of crisis—it was not a treatment of choice. Everyone in the center worked autonomously, concentrating on the demands of his or her everincreasing caseload. To say that the creation of the family-based program caused a commotion would be an understatement. It was more like a revolution. Family-Based Services had start-up money to purchase a comprehensive library of training films, journals, and books, and office furniture and equipment, vehicles, therapeutic games, handouts, and other materials. It is easy to imagine how luxurious this looked to the overworked and undersupported therapists in the old mental health center.

Family-based treatment is time-limited. Many disagree with this restriction. Our caseloads are small—8 families, compared to 90 or more identified patients on an outpatient therapist's caseload. Our focus is children and families together, not just one identified patient. We videotape treatment sessions and expose our work for supervision and critique. We collaborate with all community agencies, breaking down the isolation of the mental health center. Controversy seems to be everywhere. To top it off, we are rarely in the office, so "do you really work?" is a frequent question. As Jay Haley (1975) wrote that "if a mental health center introduces family therapy as a treatment procedure, the consequences are likely to be disorientation of the staff, radically changed administrative procedures, less harmony among the professionals, and confusion in the administrative hierarchy" (p. 12). We can personally attest to the accuracy of his statement.

We were definitely outcasts. We were placed in a position of proving our worth—the very same position families are in when they enter treatment. We were working very hard to be accepted and to join the center, but our efforts never seemed enough. Unfortunately, this continues to some degree today.

The family-based staff, like families, turned inward and relied on one another. Enmeshed relationships were important to our survival. Training was also helpful in providing much-needed support. However, that, too, was a sore spot for the Center. The consensus of our fellow professionals was that "family-based staff needs training because they do not know what they are doing, and how is it that they get such a privilege and we do not?"

Through this conflict, we somehow managed to empower families to improve their lives. We were experiencing exactly what they were. We focused our energies on our clientele and avoided the organization as much as possible. We became labeled as the "oppositional children," and for the most part this still holds true today, after 7 years. But, like the "acting-out" child who is trying to alert others to the problems of the family system, we continued. The progress is slow, but changes have occurred. There are child and adolescent psychiatrists on staff now who have a family focus, and two family therapists on staff who are pursuing an American Association for Marriage and Family Therapy (AAMFT) membership. Live supervision is being accepted as a regular activity. Service requested by families is on the increase. We have a ways to go, but a systemic orientation is starting to emerge.

Crawford County, Pennsylvania, is rural, with a population of 85,000 in approximately 1000 square miles. There are many small communities of between 500 to 2000 residents scattered throughout the county. This is an agricultural county with some emphasis on tourism. The major industry is tool and die manufacturing. The unemployment rate is extremely high, generally between 8% and 9%. Much of the population is ethnic Italian, Polish, and German, predominately White, with African Americans comprising only 2% of the total population. Most family members have been born and raised in the county and have extended family nearby. It is common for our work to include three generations of family members. Many grandparents are involved in treatment. It is important to respect and utilize their impact within the families which are referred for services.

Family-based programming focuses on change, specifically, on change among the relationships within the family systems, which is facilitated by adding complexity and alternatives to family members' way of dealing with each other and the world around them. Their degree of freedom and control over their lives increases. This process has reached everyone that the family-based program has been associated with; the community mental health center, the other child care agencies, the community, the family-based staff, and, most importantly, the families. The families involved with Family-Based Services are often termed "chronic." These families have been attempting to help their emotionally disturbed children for many years by participating in traditional mental health services, and they have found little sustaining relief for the struggles they have encountered. Their problems have been called chronic, a label that has a negative connotation — of hopelessness, no possible cure. But haven't these families been labeled by a service approach that is itself chronic?

It has been our experience that by the time the mental health system has labeled the family "chronic" there is usually a belief among professionals that the family is "hopeless." Furthermore, the family is often called "resistant" because they do not keep their in-office appointments, or the family may not carry out the suggestions of the therapist. So, in addition to the sins of being chronic and hopeless, the family may also be called "uncooperative" and resistant.

The family-based program prides itself on addressing both family and individual child issues from the family's point of view. What do *family members* see as the problem? What are *they* willing to work toward? What are *their* goals (not the therapist's goals)? Initially, families have a difficult time with this type of approach because they have all too often experienced the humiliation and embarrassment of being told what to do. Their thinking has been neither encouraged nor nurtured by a mental health system that has been child centered and places emphasizes primarily on the individual. The family-based initiative in Pennsylvania follows a systemic point of view. This means we believe that everyone in the family system is important. We believe they have the capacity to survive; they are resilient.

The families who come to be labeled as "chronic" are frequently seen from a pathological point of view. This stance is commonly accepted by the medical profession, mental health professionals, and the public, as reflected on the 6 o'clock news. As a society, we very rarely see what is good, but we certainly know when things are wrong. Modifying and restructuring this way of thinking is very difficult. It is much easier to be critical than it is to be positive. Many of us do not know how to take compliments because we are so used to being criticized. Yet, when we take an honest look at the families who have suffered years of devastation, we must remember they have survived these perils. They have incredible defense mechanisms and coping skills. They may not look traditional, or like anything we have seen before. These families are survivors, and "but for the grace of God" our family may have traveled the same path as theirs has. Would we be anymore successful than they have been? So within a framework of unconditional respect for the family, and the knowledge that these dignified individuals have much to teach us, the family-based professionals start their work.

CASE EXAMPLE

Throughout this chapter reference will be made to the Band family. This is a family who participated in 5 months of family-based therapy. The mother, twice divorced, was attempting to raise her two youngest children, who were 16 and 14 years old, respectively, as a single parent. The case was originally referred because the 16-year-old was at serious risk of being placed outside of her home. This youngster, May, was involved in a simple assault charge, and the juvenile court had placed her on probation. She also had many problems at school, both with fighting and with her failing academic status. The 14-year-old, April, was not displaying any behavioral problems at school, but she was doing very poorly academically. She was also truant.

May had been receiving outpatient therapy. Her attendance for these appointments was sporadic because she had problems with transportation. In addition, the juvenile probation officer and the outpatient mental health therapist had concerns with May's drug and/or alcohol abuse and her association with other teenagers who were known to be in trouble with the law. The impression the mother had given to both the probation officer and the mental health therapist was that she, too, was concerned about what was happening with May, as well as April, but she could not control their behavior any longer. These professionals labeled the mother an "ineffective parent." Therefore, the family-based program was recommended by the professionals. Mrs. Band felt as though she had no choice. The program was introduced as "the last alternative" to prevent May's placement out of the home. This mother was full of fear—fear of losing her daughter, fear of hopelessness, and fear of the unknown strangers who would be coming to her home.

Grudgingly, the mother and her two children agreed to allow the family-based program strangers to enter into their home. This highlights the first dilemma of family-based therapist. The pivotal step to gaining entry into their home and being allowed to work with this reluctant family was the process of joining in their pain, in their crisis. As this mother would tell us, "I don't know about you, but the privacy of my home is very important for me and my family. I am not in the practice of inviting strangers into my home!" Resistance to joining is a normal reaction. It is not a purposeful act to reject treatment. Mrs. Band and her children were doing the best they knew how to do. Their defensiveness was natural. Therefore, the therapists had to be acutely aware of the strain placed upon the family when they agreed to have someone come into their home. Even though service is time limited (32 weeks), for many families this seems like an eternity, especially when they feel forced to participate. The family's introduction to the service was laden with intimidation: "If this does not work, May will be placed." Many unrealistic expectations were set into motion. The mother believed the family-based therapists had the power to place her girls. Naturally, she wanted to please us to avoid such a horrible outcome. She was also angry that such power was in the hands of people she did not know nor want to know.

Our first goal was to present the program clearly, defining how we could work together and explaining that we could not place her children. The focus of our initial contact was to begin the construction of a partnership with this family. Mrs. Band was not convinced, and we encouraged her not to trust us until she was sure we had merited her trust.

Like many others, this mother was extremely concerned about the appearance of her home, and embarrassed by what she deemed "meager furnishings." She was very apologetic because she did not have the things that she wanted. This family was strapped financially. The mother was working part-time at a retail outlet store, but she was making only minimum wage and receiving no benefits. The family had to rely on the welfare system for cash supplements, food stamps, and medical assistance. There was some financial support from the children's father, but he, too, was in financial straits. He lived out of state and was raising the couple's oldest child who was, at that time, 18 and pregnant. The oldest sister had also had a serious involvement with drug abuse and was receiving rehabilitation counseling. Those expenses were weighing heavily on the father.

In addition, the mother had two children from her first marriage, a son, age 22, who had been raised by his father (the mother rarely had contact with him) and a daughter, age 20, who was separated from her husband and raising an infant child. This daughter was raised for a time by her mother, but spent the majority of her childhood with her father. Nevertheless, the mother attempted to assist this daughter financially.

The first task of the family-based therapist is to be inducted into the family system. To "be inducted" simply means to experience what the family has experienced—to communicate to the family that you are willing to take a journey with them on their road, and they are the tour guides

(McColderrick & Gerson, 1985). Mrs. Band and her two children, May and April, guided us as we began this powerful journey with them.

Treatment issues surfaced within the first week when both girls refused to go to school, and the mother felt helpless because she could not get them to attend (Hoffman, 1981). The girls were bigger than she was, and she felt as though the days of "manhandling" them were over. What could she do? In the past she allowed them to stay home while she went off to work. She was fully confident the children were capable of caring for themselves. Her assessment of the children was that they were very responsible. Mrs. Band was quite right. The children were very responsible in many ways, but they were supposed to be in school.

Using the emergency 24-hour on-call system, Mrs. Band contacted us at 7:30 A.M. We went to her house that morning and helped her to escort both of the girls to school. This worked once, but the second time was not as successful. The older daughter, May, had no problem with us being supportive of her mother. However, April resented our involvement. She went to school the next day, but she immediately went to the nurse's office, lay down on the cot, and refused to talk to anyone. The school notified Mrs. Band. She directly used the on-call system at 9:00 A.M. We went to the school with the mother. April showed blatant resistance to the treatment team. She also refused to talk to her mother. Since we had known the family only for 1 week, we were not sure what we were seeing. Mrs. Band had been totally alone raising these girls. She may not have wanted us in her home, but she had accepted that we were there to help. She was committed to keep her family together and decided to give this service a try. The girls were testing our intentions—were we honest? Would we say what we mean and mean what we say? May and April had been their mother's only support, but now home-based treatment was in the picture. We hypothesized that April was afraid of losing what she perceived to be her job within the family—to protect and keep people away from her family, almost as if she was the gatekeeper. Even though she was finally able to say she did not like the way her life was, that life was familiar. Change was too frightening for her. The mother agreed. April needed some time away from her in a safe place, because at this point in time, she did not know what to do or say to this child. Mrs. Band was afraid April might run away as she had threatened to do.

The family-based program has the capacity to provide safe respite care for children when the situation becomes too volatile in the home. This occurs frequently at the onset of treatment. Respite care is a form of family support that is incorporated in the program's design. Frequently, crises escalate, creating an unsafe environment within the family. It is at these times that child-serving agencies like child welfare and juvenile justice become involved. Placement outside of the home becomes the only available resource to insure the child's protection. This process always necessitates the involvement of the court system. A critical amount of time lapses. The crisis passes, and the opportunity to intervene in a therapeutic way is lost, given the separation of child and family. It is also common, at least in Crawford County, that it is more difficult to reunify the family than it is to initiate placement. The longer the child is away from his or her home, the harder it is to resolve the conflict that led to the placement.

Facilities for respite were created for the family-based continuum for this reason. We have the capacity to provide specialized foster care or emergency shelter care for a child for a maximum of 72 working hours, without requiring a court order. This use of respite is initiated by the parent and is strictly voluntary. At the end of the 72 hours, respite is terminated and the child returns home. During the respite time, therapeutic intervention possibilities increase with all family members, as well as the family unit. It is during these times that the office setting is utilized as neutral grounds for family sessions.

To provide respite care, we have entered into a contract with a local provider, Bethesda Children's Home in Meadville, Pennsylvania. We meet on a regular basis to preplan all possibilities for each child we are serving. Coordination is essential, especially since the use of respite is generally unplanned and after working hours. Cross training between the foster parents, emergency shelter staff, and family-based therapists occurs regularly as we coordinate as a treatment team. Upon initiation of respite, the foster care parents, the emergency shelter staff, and their supervisors are briefed on the family–child situation. A treatment course is agreed upon and coordination among this team occurs daily. It is our experience that respite is invaluable, especially in the first few months of treatment when the family system shifts to accommodate restructuring changes.

April's respite was for 72 hours, the maximum allowable time. While she was away, May was a perfect angel. There were no problems. She attended school every day and did not act out or fight. Mrs. Band continued to go to work. The therapists were at the home, at the foster home, and in contact with the school every day. Family sessions were held in the office. Patterns of the family materialized. May was the facilitator of all communications. She spoke for April as though she were her parent, and for mother as though she were her coparent. The mother and April had great difficulty talking to one another when May was not present.

When April returned home, May began to act out. To further add to the turmoil, Mrs. Band was laid off.

During the initial involvement of the family-based therapists, Mrs. Band showed a remarkable increase in enthusiasm. She clearly defined her goal—to make sure her girls attended school daily and improved their grades. With the increased acting out of April, and then May, we noted a marked decline in mother's enthusiasm. She was once again feeling extremely overwhelmed and stated a desire to give up. Giving up to this woman meant relinquishing the custody of her children to a placement agency such as juvenile probation, which would raise her children over an undetermined period of time. She had already faced such a loss with her other three children (their care had been relinquished to their fathers). Losing April and May would mean total defeat for Mrs. Band.

The children's father was pressuring Mrs. Band to give him custody of the children, and she was easily intimidated by his demands. It seemed that the girls had become very successful at generating conflict between their parents. This mother saw this situation as hopeless, but she did agree to allow the therapists to contact Mr. Band, who lived out of state. He agreed to participate in one joint treatment session with Mrs. Band, as well as a family meeting. The result of this intervention (a 3-hour session) was that the parents were able to establish coparenting responsibilities for these girls. The parents successfully communicated their "orders" to April and May. They established basic rules for visits, phone calls, and school attendance, and jointly conveyed them to the girls. This marked a major change within this family, but once the father returned to his home, the girls' acting out resumed.

Family-based programs cannot function without the ongoing input of other professionals, family members, and coworkers. In this family we collaborated with a child psychiatrist, child psychologist, outpatient mental health therapist, school guidance counselor, juvenile probation officer, respite care foster parents, teachers, and a neighbor who served as surrogate mother to these girls a great deal of the time. Despite these efforts, we still remained stumped. It appeared that the family was having a very hard time doing something different. Each time Mrs. Band took the initiative to assert her parental role, the girls took measures to stop it. The therapists had developed relationships with each family member and the family unit. The family members said they wanted to stay together, but the girls' acting out behaviors continued to escalate. There was no indication as to what might be hiding in the family's history that was so horrifying they would not risk looking at it. The more we talked with this mother and her children, the more we came to appreciate their deep loyalty to one another and their behaviors that maintained things as they were. The relationships were closely enmeshed. Each family member appeared to have a deep responsibility and need to protect one another. Behaving differently seemed to threaten their very existence. The roller coaster continued with many crisis calls and a total of three episodes of respites for these children. What were we missing?

We had been with this family for over 3 months, and we were feeling overwhelmed and frustrated, just like this mother and her children. The roller coaster ride was exciting, but very tiring. We turned to the family and asked for their help. The family-based therapists tried to establish partnerships with the family. The program is not designed to dictate or "fix" the problems for which referrals are made. The family therapist's purpose is to be with this family and struggle with them through their difficulties. Because the family did not appear to feel safe with change, we did not feel safe either. Therefore, we disclosed to the family our thinking of how risky we thought change might be. We gave them the choice as to whether or not they would be able to weather change, or if it was something they should not consider at this point in time.

This is the critical place where therapists get stuck. It is not the therapist's right to determine what or when an individual or family will change or if they are even ready for that step. Our responsibility as family therapists is to reinforce the competence of an individual or family that will help them persist with changes. But before we can do anything different, we must know we are safe.

We soon discovered that April felt she was unsafe. In a riveting session upon her return from the third respite stay, she was asked what she was so afraid of. She disclosed she was afraid that her mother would seriously harm herself "if she unlocked the closet door" (April's metaphor). She did not know why her mother would do this, but she had a sense that her mother was carrying so many painful memories that if she had time on her hands, with nothing to do, she might have no reason for living. The mother did not know what to do with this information. She denied there were any problems, and she had not displayed openly to us any indication of serious depression or anxiety. Yet her daughter was fearful that if anyone got close to her mother, they would unleash the horrors she was trying so desperately to conceal. April then disclosed that she and her sister slept with their mother, despite the fact that everyone had their own bedroom. This had been a tightly guarded secret, but, somehow, April had come to trust that the therapists might help her with her mother. This was a remarkable achievement for her and her family.

It is important in work with families to recognize and acknowledge when they give you permission to be a part of their system. At this point, we needed the additional permission of these children to speak with their mother about what may be in her "closet." The children agreed to this, but they stipulated that we must be very careful. Treatment then focused on their mother. She had suffered enormous abuse (sexual, emotional, and physical) at the hands of family members whom she had trusted. These people remained in her life. Mrs. Band had convinced herself she was a good actress and could hide her pain from everyone. She gradually began to recognize that her daughters had seen through the facade. In addition to continued therapeutic intervention with the whole family, we encouraged individual sessions for the mother. Mrs. Band was offered several treatment options to help with her issues. These included referral to a women's center specializing in abuse and its recovery or referral to mental health services, with an outpatient therapist. She declined these options. She stated that she trusted the family-based team and preferred that we treat her issues. Because individual treatment of adults is not our primary treatment focus, we in turn sought the supervision of more expert clinicians to help us provide service to Mrs. Band (Figley, 1989).

Through our work together she began to know her competence and strength at managing her "demons." She began the process of healing. She was faced with a decision of whether or not to expose the details of her pain. She struggled and accomplished this with the therapists. However, she adamantly chose not to tell her daughters the details of her abuse. Again, the pace of the client must be respected. Mrs. Band was not ready to disclose her shame and humiliation to her daughters. She chose to continue to protect them from these secrets. Mrs. Band wanted to direct family treatment toward present-day concerns of her girls. This entailed her assertively informing her children, in a family session, that she no longer required their protection. She was attending to her needs, and she "fired" them from this job (Sherman, 1986). Her daughters were faced with finding new jobs within the family. They did not know quite what to do with this. Treatment focused on helping the family members talk to one another about what they needed and how these needs could be met. Mrs. Band and her girls began to individuate (Falicov, 1988). They were now sleeping in their own rooms.

After 5 months of treatment, the family decided that they wanted to get on with their lives without any additional therapeutic assistance. Mrs. Band had been introduced to other surviving abuse victims and a parent support group within the community. She became an active participant in these groups. She had experienced a positive involvement with Family-Based Services and agreed to reconnect with outpatient mental health treatment for herself or her children if, and when, they felt the need.

During family-based treatment, May's school placement was questioned by Mrs. Band. She had had concerns for years, but her requests for an evaluation were bypassed. The school attributed May's academic problems to her behavioral outbursts. Referral was made to a psychologist at the mental health center to complete a testing evaluation. It was discovered that May had learning disabilities. Through a coordinated meeting with the mother, the psychologist, the family-based team, and the school, specialized classes were arranged. At the end of our treatment, she had successfully passed the 10th grade. The younger girl was also achieving better academic scores and had become a cheerleader.

At 1 year follow-up, this family was still together. The mother was working full-time. She had had a boyfriend, but terminated the relationship when he did not meet her "expectations." Visits and phone contacts with the children's father had become more regular, and he had become much more supportive of Mrs. Band's parental decisions.

May had become pregnant and miscarried. As a result of the pregnancy, she quit school. However, after the miscarriage, she re-enrolled in school, had intentions of graduating, and had briefly reinvolved herself in outpatient therapy.

The younger daughter was no longer a truancy problem. Mrs. Band described her as a "normal" teenager who "did not like to do dishes or clean her room." April's grades were A's and B's and her cheerleading activity continued.

The premise of Family-Based Mental Health Services is really quite simple—to work within the family in the context of the community. However, the way in which this goal is carried out is complex and requires creativity and ingenuity. Staff in these programs are bombarded with everything from families living in isolated areas that are difficult to find, to families whose lives have been seriously altered by every kind of abuse and neglect imaginable. Yet therapists are asked to maintain a sense of objectivity while being in the middle of the "eye of the hurricane."

Certainly not every family we work with has the kind of outcome that this one did. There are times where we must recommend that the child be placed outside of the home because the family environment and members are not able to provide a safe haven for the child to grow. In these situations, our goal is to help facilitate the placement with the parents and the family and to help them so that relationships can continue with their children during and beyond placement.

Families have an incredible influence on home-based professionals. Families have much to teach us about flexibility and change. As therapists we have much to learn. We must listen to their needs, their wants, their desires, their struggles, their pain, and their triumphs. We must clear the way for them to be able to live their lives to the best of their abilities.

Work with families cannot be productive unless we can maintain our humility. We cannot learn from families until we can admit how little we really know. We are trained to restructure and unbalance, reframe and punctuate, assess the system, and add complexity. But the how and when of change rests with the family. The family and the therapist mutually impact on one another; both are necessary for therapy to exist.

CONCLUSION

Our basic mission is to believe in people's competence as opposed to focusing on their incompetence. If we are to do something and do it well, we must be able to believe it is possible. Most parents truly want what is best for their children. Most families are doing the best they can. When a family has a child who is at serious risk of being placed, they usually know that. The majority of families do not want that kind of separation to occur. They are working desperately to prevent it, but many times their solutions are ineffective and instead may make the problems worse. Do they want help from the outside? Certainly they do! Do they know how to accept it? Do we know how to deliver it? We must recognize that in order to be useful helpers, we must also be able to participate fully in the family's effectiveness. This is what is meant by a partnership. Families will not open their arms, and say, "Wow, we have wonderful family therapists here and they are going to solve the problem!" The family must decide what and when they will change; we, as therapists, must help instill the hope that change is possible. In order for home-based services to have the opportunity to do this work, we must follow the simple rule, "When in Rome, do as the Romans do": When you are in someone else's home, you follow their guidelines, not yours. This is the prerequisite of humility in family-based work. Unlike outpatient services, home-based services have an intimate sense of the client and family. It is important to know how they live, to see Uncle John's picture on the wall and know what influence he had. There is no substitute to seeing the pride on their faces when they tell you where they got this piece of furniture or that picture, or when they show you the photo album and talk to you about their memories. The richness of the family is abundant and we must focus on it.

Thus, the adventure entailed taking risks to be simply human. Risks of accommodating and challenging, trusting and being trustworthy, as well as of openness and honesty, fairness and vulnerability were all motivated by the common goal of change. Thus, growth has occurred for the clients and families as well as for the therapists. Choices have been made, competence has been realized, and resilience persisted as we learned new ways in a partnership of mutual respect.

REFERENCES

Department of Public Welfare. (1993). Family-Based Mental Health Services for children and adolescents. *Pennsylvania Bulletin, 23*(18), 2127–2136.

Falicov, C. J. (Ed.). (1988). *Family transitions: Continuity and change over the life cycle.* New York: Guilford Press.

Figley, C. R. (1989). *Helping traumatized families.* San Francisco: Jossey-Bass.

Hayley, J. (1975). Why a mental health clinic should avoid family therapy. *Journal of Marriage and Family Counseling, 1,* 3–13.

Hoffman, L. (1981). *The foundations of family therapy.* New York: Basic Books.

Kagen, R., & Schlosberg, S. (1989). *Families in perpetual crisis.* New York: W. W. Norton.

Kaplan, L. (1986). *Working with multi problem families.* Lexington, MA: D. C. Heath.

McGolderick, M., & Gerson, R. (1985). *Genograms in family assessment.* New York: W. W. Norton.

Minuchin, S. (1974). *Families and family therapy.* Cambridge, MA: Harvard University Press.

Satir, V. (1988). *The new peoplemaking.* Mountain View, CA: Science and Behavior Books.

Sherman, R., & Fredman, N. (1986). *Handbook of structured techniques in marriage and family therapy.* New York: Brunner/Mazel.

6

Helping Families Become Places of Healing: Systemic Treatment of Intrafamilial Sexual Abuse

Raymond X. De Maio

The problem of intrafamilial sexual abuse challenges therapists to work in exceedingly difficult contexts — contexts of broken connections, competing and emerging systems, conflicting cultural ideas, and hidden coalitions. Often there are multigenerational histories of abuse that support the abusive patterns. The family therapist who is trained to understand and work with multiple embedded systems, to reconnect relatives who have been cut off, and to appreciate and use multigenerational histories has the necessary skills to help these families. To illustrate, let's begin with a story.

Cindy Smith was 9 years old when her stepfather, John Walsh, first sexually abused her. Afterwards, whenever her mother Alice was not home, Cindy was terrified. The abuse left her feeling guilty, ashamed, and confused; she was dazed. On one occasion John held a knife to her throat and said he would kill her if she told her mother. Cindy couldn't bear to tell her mother anyway. It would devastate Alice, who seemed to love

John so much. Alice did not have much say in the household as John controlled the finances, and he knew just how to manipulate her.

When Cindy was 11, she confided in a friend about the sexual abuse. Her friend did not keep the secret, and eventually Cindy was interviewed by the child protective services. Her account of the incest was confusing, ambiguous, and contradictory. This was understandable given the way John had set things up, mixing tenderness with terror.

During the investigation, John convinced Alice that Cindy was lying. He pointed out the contradictions in her story. He claimed Cindy was jealous of his relationship with Alice. He acted as if he were betrayed, and he appeared righteously enraged when he was confronted by the authorities. The family stood behind him and decided that Cindy was crazy. It is easy to understand why Cindy recanted her story of sexual abuse.

Many ideas and assumptions of family therapists are problematic when dealing with a context marked by secrets, denial, betrayal, and violence. To base one's evaluation and therapeutic interventions solely on information gathered from seeing Alice, John, and Cindy together could put Cindy at a continued risk. For professionals to remain neutral when they know how denial and secrets work often covertly aligns them with the offender's perspective. To use positive connotation or positive reframing in the context of incest seems absurd. To view the family as a systemic unit in simple cybernetic terms that gives equal weight and responsibility to each participant reduces John's responsibility for his acts against his stepdaughter. This has been a major criticism of family systems therapy made by feminists (James & MacKinnon, 1990).

Yet therapists from any treatment modality dealing with incest have problems with treatment assumptions. Many models emphasize assessment. Because of the responsibility to protect children, the child welfare systems and courts need to know what happened in order to establish proof of the abuse. Thus, with a family like the Smith-Walshes, which is full of denial and secrets, "treatment" becomes investigation, and healing for family members is determined by the context of the investigation. Alice described her initial therapy as intrusive. She experienced the social workers who interviewed the family as condescending. This atmosphere contributed to Alice becoming more attached to John. Their denial became more impenetrable in the face of their common enemy. Further, John's and Alice's anger and frustration were often taken out on Cindy. Individual therapy for Cindy had its problems: It did not increase her connection with her siblings, and it may have contributed to a greater disconnection from her mother, who was angry that her daughter was being cared for by the female therapist. John was recommended for group therapy for offenders, but he refused to go, stating that he was not an offender.

CONDUCTING THE THERAPY: FUNDAMENTAL ASSUMPTIONS

This chapter is intended to give family therapists working with families where intrafamilial sexual abuse has occurred an introduction as to how to conduct therapy in such a way that the family is not decimated by the process of acknowledging, confronting, and working through the effects of the incest. It outlines my ideas in working with these families—ideas that have evolved from my participation in an incest project at the Ackerman Institute of Family Therapy called Making Families Safe for Children (Sheinberg, 1992). The ideas represent a multilevel perspective in working with a family where incest has occurred (see Trepper & Barrett, 1989; Wheeler, 1990). The therapy is systemic.

The act of incest greatly influences how the family is organized both prior to and after the disclosure. Each family member and each system involved with the family experiences the problem differently. The clash of these differences defines interactions among people around the problem.

One goal of therapy is to help families understand the contexts and interconnections of people and problems. All families and their members have multiple stories and multiple descriptions. Thus, a family where incest is occurring is not only described by this fact, it is also a family with stories of pride, connection, and disconnection. Likewise, the offending father is more than an offender, the hurt child more than a victim.

In addition to being part of a system, people are individuals. Each is responsible for his or her acts. Each must deal with denial, shame, and guilt. In the therapy each is encouraged to learn empathy and to relate in more intimate and constructive ways. Thus, in this framing the therapy is structured to help clients assess their responsibility for their own acts. It is particularly important to see the *children* in these families as individuals. Often as family therapists we help children by treating their parents; thus, we are less in tune with their special developmental needs. The treatment I am proposing focuses on the areas of their development that have been interrupted by the abuse.

The work is also feminist informed. Incest occurs in a cultural and historical context in which men have been allowed to dominate women. Moreover, incest is an act involving attitudes and beliefs about gender that is reinforced by the notion of male entitlement in the culture, the family, and the individuals' histories around themes of men and women. Understanding how family members operate according to their constructs of their femininity or masculinity is another important part of the therapy, for the acts of incest are related to the offenders' gender identification, and the incest experience is translated into the betrayed child's gender identification. Helping men and women relate empathically, mutually, and in connection are ideas advocated by feminist family therapists. These are major antidotes to ideas of male entitlement. Encouraging empathy, mutuality, and connection is a major part of this therapy.

This therapeutic approach recognizes that therapeutic choices are influences by the preconceived biases of therapy. The preceding ideas are my biases. Our biases are influenced by the cacophony of competing ideas in the culture.

WORKING WITH LARGER SYSTEMS

In order to create a safe therapeutic environment, the therapist must help the family cope with the complicated and often demoralizing social context that evolves after disclosure. Not addressing the larger system issues may lead to a major block of facilitating treatment. It is not unusual in these families to be involved with as many as 10 new systems—all playing a role around the problem of incest.

When I first met Alice Walsh 2 years after the disclosure of John's violation of Cindy, her involvement with outside systems related to the problem of incest could at best be described as adversarial and unproductive. As Alice interacted with the social welfare agency and court system a symmetrical conflict of blame evolved. The more Alice felt blamed as a "bad" mother, the more she failed to cooperate with the system. The more she failed to cooperate with the system, the more she was labeled a "bad" mother.

She did not trust any outside system. And with her daughter hospitalized for a suicide attempt while in foster placement, Alice entered therapy wanting to get her daughter back. Despite her staying attached to John, Alice had to be viewed as an important ally in her daughter's healing, so that Alice's interactions with both her daughter and with other agencies could change. Imber-Black (1988) speaks of the importance of changing labels and stigma to establish positive interactions with outside agencies. Working with the hospital social worker, who also adopted the idea of Alice as a potential partner in Cindy's recovery, enabled Alice to remove herself from her normal one-down position with social agencies.

The work of dealing with the larger systems is neither fancy nor brief. A therapist coaches the family to approach the systems in a collaborative spirit. Families learn their rights and share their frustrations. With the therapist the clients develop plans to facilitate the process of interagency involvement.

In consulting with other professionals, the therapist must be direct and forthcoming. These professionals are invited to become allies to the therapy in helping families overcome denial. The therapist explains that this work is best done in a positive and respectful context. Because the family needs time to understand the complexities of the incestuous acts, the therapist remains in contact with the other professionals throughout this initial period. The professional "stands between the family and larger systems, serving as mediator, translator, and shuttle diplomat" (Imber-Black, 1990, p. 183).

DEALING WITH DENIAL

Another area that will often block successful treatment is denial. The silence of the act of incest does not disappear with disclosure but evolves into the silence of denial. A family like the Smith-Walshes, which is tightly organized around the protection of the offender, will be in the greatest denial. Helping family members organize around other ideas is often the first step in the family's acceptance of the acts. It is like the first drops of rain in a desert, in which all types of life emerge from a lifeless, arid terrain. For Alice Smith, her raindrops were in beginning to help her daughter at the hospital.

Lifting the denial is a fragile process, however. As in the desert, if the rain stops—particularly early on—what has begun will die, and life becomes even more fragile with the first efforts of the rain wasted. Helping Alice look at her own childhood and the sexual abuse that she experienced and connecting her healing to the healing of her daughter were new organizing principles in her life.

For John this period was fraught with anxiety, and his efforts to protect himself from accepting the reality of his actions seemed insurmountable. As Alice made progress in changing her reality, he would double his efforts to extract her loyalty. Yet in working with John, a part of him began acknowledging the possibility that something may have happened. The real movement in John's accepting responsibility for his actions came when he was confronted by Alice's belief in her daughter and her willingness to press charges.

The key to dealing successfully with denial is managing the complex feelings generated in breaking the incest taboo. These feelings are generally embedded in a deep shame. When fully experienced, this shame can be obliterating. In order to help manage the deep feelings of shame, the therapist must set up a holding context.

CREATING THE APPROPRIATE
THERAPEUTIC CONTEXT

Winnicott (1965) first described a holding environment as the necessary environment for the child to develop his or her true personhood. He called this environment "good enough mothering." Trained as a pediatrician, Winnicott's observations of the early mother–child relationship became his metaphor for the therapeutic environment. Initially, holding consisted of the mother's intuitive behavior of making a totally dependent infant safe. According to Winnicott, her ability to empathize with the feelings of the infant and provide the appropriate environment were the conditions needed to develop the child's innate potential. The holding environment begins with the actual holding of the child and then extends to broader tasks in the child's environment. It eventually "include[s] the function of the family" (Winnicott, 1986, p. 27). Winnicott also extends it to society, to the tasks of social work, and to the therapeutic relationship. Thus, the holding environment provides safety based on the developmental needs of the person or persons being "held."

Establishing the family as the holding environment for the child who has been violated is the goal of family therapy. To accomplish this task the therapy should become a holding environment for the family, so that the family can feel that they are in safe hands. Luepnitz (1988) describes how the therapist "contains" or "holds onto the individual's or family's pain," just as the mother contains the distress of the infant—nondefensively, nonpunitively, reassuringly—thus sending the message that the feelings being experienced by family members can be tolerated by the therapist, and, therefore, are valid and meaningful. It is in this holding context that the family is able to understand the full extent of the incest. Alice was able finally to fully hear her daughter's painful story after having her own painful story heard and accepted. She acknowledged the shame of her denial in the safety of the therapeutic context.

Two major attitudes that facilitate holding contexts are mutuality and empathy, which enhance family connections. "In a mutual exchange one is both affecting the other and being affected by the other; one extends oneself out to the other and is also receptive to impact of the other" (Jordan, 1991a, p. 81). Empathy occurs within what the authors from the Stone Center call "mutual relationship processes" (Jordan, Kaplan, Miller, Stiver, & Surrey, 1991). "Optimally, it is a quality of relational flow, a mutual exchange in which each shares, absorbs, reflects upon, and enhances her own and the other's experience, and the relationship itself" (Jordan, 1991b, p. 6).

For the therapy to encourage mutuality and empathy, the therapist must model these behaviors. Setting up a positive holding environment for the family members is done with those fundamental counseling skills of genuineness, positive regard, caring, reflective listening, and the ability to hear feelings and support them. These are not techniques but ways of relating that are communicated through body language, eye contact, voice, and the demonstration of understanding. This way of relating parallels the feminist description of the self in connection (Jordan et al., 1991; Gilligan, 1982).

By asking questions to point out common experiences for women and men, using a language of connection, punctuating mutual support and empathy among family members, and understanding and addressing disconnection, a therapist builds a context of safety and connection in family relationships.

Using Mutual Enhancing Questions to Deepen Connections

As the therapy room evolves into a safe place for the family and as connections grow, family members will be encouraged to relate in more mutual and empathic ways. Thus, in Alice's therapy, when her mother and her sister participated, the women shared stories of their histories. Therapeutic questions are used to facilitate mutuality and empathy between family members. As each told their stories I would ask questions that would elicit responses of support from other family members. In one session after their mother spoke of her own abusive childhood, I asked Alice and her sister, "What is it like for you hearing about your mother's past?" And then when Alice stated she wished she had heard this earlier, I asked her mother, "What do you think of your daughter's idea that she should have heard this before?" Other questions are asked to increase mutual support and sharing: For example, "How do you feel about what happened to your daughter?" "Do you need anything else from you mother in regard to what has happened?" "Did you feel support from your daughters? These questions are aimed at creating a back and forth understanding between mother and daughter to enhance the experience of each.

Questions are also asked in a way that reflects the therapist's empathetic understanding and are framed to encourage positive and supportive comments from family members. Prior to Alice's participation in Cindy's therapy at the hospital, Alice described some of her painful encounters in the past in conversations about Cindy's abuse.

ALICE: I really want to go, but I'm not looking forward to it.

THERAPIST: What do you mean?

ALICE: I just begin feeling it's all my fault. I have a lot of guilt about it. It's like what the prosecutor told me. I'm as guilty as John. He said

I should be charged with endangering Cindy's life. I just get paralyzed when I think that way. I am afraid, so afraid to hear that.

THERAPIST (*to Alice's mother, Eve*): What do you think of the amount of pain your daughter is willing to experience now to help Cindy?

EVE: First of all, Alice, it's not your fault what John did to her. I am real proud how willing you are to go into the hospital. I don't know if I would have the courage to do this. They're going to judge you. But nobody else can help Cindy like you will be able to.

THERAPIST: What is it like for you to hear your mother saying these things?

ALICE: I appreciate my mom standing with me. I'm glad she's on my side.

The question: "What do you think of the amount of pain your daughter is willing to experience now to help Cindy?" empathically acknowledges what Alice is experiencing, and it asks of her mother not only to feel for Alice's reality but provide both the praise and support that Alice needs.

Sessions such as these help families build connections that have been eroded by acts of incest and the accompanying secrecy and denial. These connections are necessary for healing. In addition, feelings of pride are antidotes to disconnection in families. Questions eliciting what people are proud of, questions evoking individual and family strengths, and questions emphasizing surviving a difficult experience build pride. In turn, the feeling of pride enhances the bonds between people. Pride acts as an antidote to feelings of shame.

The family genogram is also a source to build both pride and connection. Doing a genogram on a large pad or blackboard gives a family a chance to recapture the picture of past connections. Children in these families often do not know about the connections (lines) between people in their parents or grandparents' lives.

HEALING CHILDREN, HEALING FAMILIES

The holding context, thus, is a therapeutic environment in which connection grows through empathy and mutuality. In this environment families that have been dangerous for women and children become places for healing. The process begins with a therapist's empathy for the predicament of each family member in the drama of incest. The ideal therapeutic context is set up for all family members to heal from the trauma of incest. The context, however, begins with an understanding of the child's hurt. Healing for the child is the driving force behind the organization of the therapy. We begin with a systemic understanding of the child caught in the incest drama.

UNDERSTANDING INCEST SYSTEMICALLY

In order to understand the full impact of incest on a child, one must appreciate what it is like for a child to be caught in a family when he or she is being sexually abused. Many theories of family therapy rest on what has been called the pathological triad (Hoffman, 1981). The most common pathological triad in families occurs when one parent forms a coalition with a child against the other parent. "The problem is most severe when the coalition . . . is denied or concealed" (Haley, 1987, p. 116). Therapy is conducted to break the cross-generational coalition and thus free the child. After this is accomplished, family therapy often ends and the couple begins working on the marital relationship.

Seeing the child's difficulties as coming from being caught in a triangle and helping the child out of this position as scapegoat has been one of the most significant contributions of family therapy. Clearly, the female child who is a victim of incest is part of the most destructive pathological triangle. Not only is the child betrayed and cheated of her role as child, she has played wife to her father, and by not telling her mother, she has protected her, thus playing mother to her own mother (Everstine & Everstine, 1989). The secret tends to isolate her from her siblings. Ending the abuse, of course, does not end her therapy. These children have been hurt by their untenable position in the family. The child has often been told by the father that the family's preservation is maintained by her keeping the secret; conversely, the family is threatened by her betrayal. From a systemic perspective, one can only imagine the child's pain. And thus, the systemic framing of the child saving the family at her expense is both explicit and implicit to the child. Although she may be convinced otherwise, her place in the system is not her choice. The following case example illustrates this point.

In a family where a 15-year-old girl was abused, the offending father, Tom, told me how he would get in a flirting mood with his stepdaughter Ana by being very playful. He would be an active listener and compliment Ana. They watched movies together, had long talks. Ana enjoyed the attention and saw her stepfather as a cool man. Then, one night when Tom came home in what he called a sexy mood, he pushed Ana down on her bed, kissing and groping at her. This was totally out of the realm of her thinking.

Although Tom went back to being "his cool self" with no mention of his behavior, Ana described herself as feeling as if she were going to explode. Her biggest worry was that if she told her mother, her mother would have a nervous breakdown. In the 2 weeks prior to disclosure, she was intensely trying to read her mother. How strong was she? Would the secret cause her mother to become sad and depressed? Would this break up the family? What would happen to her three younger siblings? She worried that she was at fault. She enjoyed being with Tom. Did she lead him on? Two weeks went by, and though she decided that her mother could not handle the situation, she blurted out the incident.

Ana was an extremely verbal adolescent who, because of her age and level of intellectual functioning, was able to tell what happened to her in a way that jived with both our theoretical expectations and an adult understanding of events. In this case her offending stepfather never denied the act and fully explored in a year and a half of therapy how he set up his sexual misconduct. His attention to his stepdaughter and his interest in her was the way he set up his "seduction." Thus, his active listening was on one level a tool to get closer, motivated by his needs. She clearly became his sexual object. This is not to deny other descriptions of his relationship with Ana, though I framed the objectifying as the dominant one.

In addition to being set up in the coalition and carrying the secret, the child has to deal with his or her own terror of the act. Recently, one of my adult clients described a panic experience to me. While she was sleeping, her husband came into the room and was taking off his pants, and at the sound of his unzipping his zipper she woke up in terror. The memory evoked the early terror that she first experienced at 6 years old and then forgot. As we tried to understand the fear that this would create for a child, it was incomprehensible. In the session, she began rocking. When her father first approached her, she thought he was going to kill her. With subsequent visits unpredictable, nights became terrifying. She could not sleep. Afterwards, she felt dirty, not there, depersonalized.

Thus, the impact of incest on a child in the family is multifaceted. There is the dance prior to the act—setting up of the incest. There is the act itself—the traumatic event. And then there is the carrying of the secret—the hidden coalition. Each facet, alone, impacts painfully on the child involved. Since these states are continuous and often contradictory, they have a cumulative and a recursive effect. Thus, for example, in setting up the act, "good daddy" will shape the way the child views the incest act. How does she explain his coming in the night doing these things? It must be her fault. He's so good to her. Maybe it's not him; maybe she's dreaming. Often in telling their story of incest, children will say that some stranger attacked them. This distortion may be very real to the child. In fact, they may have been told this by the offender.

It is easy to understand how the symptoms and behavioral problems of incest survivors emerge from this context of contradictory interpersonal demands.

DIFFERENTIATING "NOW" FROM "THEN"

In identifying symptoms and problems, it is important to determine the meaning of the behavior. Thus, we need to know what is informing the behavior and how the family is interacting around it. In order to construct the "meaning" of the problem behavior, questions are asked that are designed to ferret out temporal difference of the problem. Noting how events and experiences in the present are different from those at the time of the incest is an important distinction in helping family members move beyond the incest.

The following segment of an interview with Alice and Cindy occurred after Cindy was reunited with her mother. In the session we saw how the memory of the incest structures and influences the relationship between Cindy and Alice. During the session Cindy also began to work through her pain by a discussion of the past and present.

THERAPIST: Thinking back now, what changes do you remember in Cindy when the abuse began?

ALICE: I think she became quieter, sadder. . . . (*She begins to cry.*)

THERAPIST: It's real sad for you to think about this.

ALICE: I feel bad for her and I start feeling guilty.

THERAPIST: Cindy, what's it like for you when you think about the abuse?

CINDY: I try not to think about it, but sometimes I just start getting sad.

THERAPIST: Is the sadness now that you are safe different from the sadness when you weren't safe?

CINDY: It must be. I guess I'm not so alone and I'm not as afraid. Its not like it was.

THERAPIST: What's Mom do when you get sad?

CINDY: I'm not sure.

ALICE: I guess I get sad?

THERAPIST: Does being sad make you closer?

ALICE: Probably the opposite.

In this dialogue it appeared that Alice's sadness and guilt about her daughter did not allow her to fully participate in her daughter's recovery. Cindy's sadness and Alice's sadness and guilt tended to make each other sadder. And this effect promoted greater distance between Alice and Cindy at a time when Alice's support was crucial for Cindy. In a later session we co-constructed a ritual to interrupt and reorganize the pattern. Whenever Cindy was sad about the incest or when Alice was sad or guilty about it, they would light a candle together and they would watch the sadness and guilt go up in smoke. This activity became a way for daughter and mother to be close when remembering the incest.

Developing descriptions of the past and present and asking for differences and similarities is a systemic way to "work through the past." When Alice was present with Cindy we would often go back to past and compare it to the present. In this process, Cindy developed a way to own the past without ruining the present.

Present negative behaviors that are being influenced by the past traumatic events are contextualized in a way that allows the participants to see that the behaviors make sense because they are being informed by past trauma. These clients are not just crazy. Problem behaviors for children who have been abused include dissociation, compulsive sexual acting out, self-blame, and revictimization.

Dissociative States

Dissociative symptoms develop from the child's need to get away from the horror, the confusion, and betrayal of the sexual attack. Understandably, the child is unable to accept the reality of his or her situation. In a way, the child's body is there to absorb the violation, and her mind is elsewhere to survive it. Dissociation becomes problematic after the abuse is over because it is no longer adaptive, and it may even be dangerous. It is particularly important to elicit help from the child's family to understand if and how a child is blanking out. Children who are described as daydreamers or lazy or having trouble focusing may very well be blanking out or dissociating.

When working with children I usually go back to the original context of their dissociation and compare it to the present symptoms. The process is another way of working through the past, which was described above.

Often framing dissociation as a positive skill of self-hypnosis and survival of intolerably confounding experience makes the symptom much friendlier. Helping the child learn how to control his or her blanking out and saving it for times of stress may become a positive family task. This further differentiates the present dissociative symptoms from the past dissociation, which had been a necessary step for survival.

Compulsive Sexual Acting Out

Children who are sexually abused are often confused about the sexual meaning of the incest. Finklehor and Browne (1988) refer to the "traumatic sexualization of the child," which "is shaped in developmentally inappropriate and interpersonally dysfunctional ways" (p. 63). First, the child who is sexually approached does not necessarily associate the word abuse to the act. The child will construct meaning based on her previous knowledge of sex and her own shame about her body. In addition, she may receive from the offender explanations about her experiences that will influence her view of the abuse. Moreover, certain feelings and memories will get mixed up with the traumatic act.

Janet was 5 years old when she was sexually abused by an uncle. At 14 she began using a vibrator compulsively, and her mother, Eloise, discovered her masturbating in the living room on several occasions. She told her mother she felt compelled do it. "I had a feeling down there which felt good but also felt bad," and with the vibrator she explained, "I was able to forget the feelings when I was doing it." I underscored the positive aspect in the compulsive masturbation—her need to experience control of her own body as she was becoming a young woman.

Eloise admitted her own discomfort with sex. She wished she had shared a different view of sexuality with Janet. Building on that idea, we created a task that each evening Eloise would give Janet sex education. In the ritual Janet would pick an age, and her mother would give her appropriate information. For the assignment Eloise found books on teaching sexuality to children. In addition to this we deconstructed her experience of being sexually abused, viewing it as an act of violence of a man over a child. Janet regained the power of her sexuality.

Self-Blame

The context of sexual abuse—the secrets, the shame, the objectification, and the manipulation by the offender—infuses the child with self-blame. After the disclosure of sexual abuse, we tell children they are not at fault. If we ask children if they feel it is their fault, they will often answer no. In working with adult survivors, I have found that verbal denials of self-blame over traumatic events are not always accurate. I first discovered this when I used the Beck Inventory (Beck, Rush, Shaw, & Emery, 1979) in order to justify treatment to an insurance company. Despite previous claims of not blaming themselves for the trauma, survivors, on the question of blame, often check "I blame myself for everything bad that happens." Several authors (Everstine & Everstine, 1993; Mollica, 1988) have had similar experiences with a paper-and-pencil questionnaire. Everstine and Everstine suggest that "victims have a tendency to deny symptoms, not because they don't have them, but because they would rather not talk about them or are ashamed of having them" (p. 25).

It is important to figure out how a child is blaming himself or herself. If the blame has a global impact on the client, the survivor is walking around with the feeling of blame covering him or her like a shroud. This will be generalized to other situations and will have a strong negative impact on the survivor's life. On the other hand, when a child blames himself or herself for letting the act occur, this blame is somewhat specific and may have a preventive impact in the future. Because the blame implies some sense of control, it should not be explained away completely and should be explored. The following questions may be helpful in exploring the meaning of the blame. "How could you have told?" "What would have happened if you told your mother earlier?" "What stopped you from telling immediately?" "What do you mean you won't let it happen again?" Although the idea that the abuse could have been prevented is false on one level, on another level it adds to control, and I believe should be received more positively than it often is.

Global blaming occurs in a more passive and defeated feeling state. The following activities address global blaming. Taking a daily newspaper, I have read some of the headlines, suggesting to the clients they must have been at fault. (Often there are many very violent and heinous events in the newspaper. These should not be used.) "Airplane hijacked to Kennedy Airport. Yep, Jane caused that. IBM Big Layoff. You must have had a hand in that. Storm causes havoc. Come on, explain how you brought that about."

Another helpful idea is using a ritual to give the blame back to the offender. For example, in one case a mother and daughter made a card for the offending father, which included the gift of responsibility for the act. In this case the child made a drawing of her stepfather wearing a crown of guilt, shame, and blame.

Revictimization

One of the most important reasons to develop an early intervention program for children who are sexually abused is the phenomenon called revictimization. There is evidence that a child who is abused will be a likely candidate for future abuse. Since the steps of the dance of being abused may be strongly imprinted on him or her, interrupting this pattern is important. The following case is an example of stopping revictimization.

At the time of therapy, Cheryl was 16 years old. She lived with her mother Joyce, a single parent whose husband died 8 years prior. Joyce explained that she was very worried about her daughter. Cheryl would get extremely angry at her mother. She accused Joyce of being weak. In the fights during therapy, both in language and in tone, Cheryl was very attacking. Her mother described these attacks by saying, "It was like being jabbed with a stick." On another occasion she said, "It was like an arrow piercing through me." This theme of attack often appears indirectly in therapy when an attack has occurred.

In addition to this verbal abusive behavior, Joyce felt that Cheryl was in a bad relationship with an abusive boyfriend. The more Joyce tried to protect Cheryl, the angrier her daughter became.

Cheryl claimed that her mother was not strong enough to help her. Cheryl believed her boyfriend, Bob, protected her. I arranged for a session with Cheryl and Bob. During the session, Bob proceeded to tell me about an incident that occurred at a party on Memorial Day weekend. Cheryl got drunk that evening, and a group of boys began swinging her around. What followed was a description of a brutal sexual attack on Cheryl, with the boys using broom handles and their fists while jabbing her in the vaginal area. During Bob's telling of the story Cheryl held herself and cried.

Clearly, Cheryl and Bob came together over this story of the abuse, and Cheryl overlooked abusive aspects of Bob. In Bob she found someone with whom to share the story. It is not unusual for children and adolescents to first tell an abusive experience to another peer. Bringing in the trusted friend to therapy is often a safe way to help the child introduce the story of abuse to adults. Also, it utilizes the healing context that the child has already begun. Later in the session I asked Cheryl questions about her experience, and she told me her story through Bob.

Joyce seemed to represent to Cheryl that part of her she hated most — the part that was victimized. Her verbal attacks further immobilized Joyce. In the session the following week, I redid the family genogram with an emphasis on the roles women and men played in the family. Joyce talked about the way her mother was mistreated by her father. She described how he would beat her.

Ending the silence on how women were treated in this patriarchically informed family led to an expression of anger and resentment. The response of anger to a history of violence and abuse is an important step in empowering a victim. "Never again" is an appropriate theme for women who suffer violence: "Anger stirs and wakes in her; it opens its mouth, and like a hot-mouthed puppy, laps up the dredges of her shame. Anger is better. There is a sense of being in anger. A reality and presence. An awareness of worth" (Morrison, 1970, p. 43).

Joyce was aware that something happened to her daughter on that frightful May weekend. Yet whenever Joyce approached her, Cheryl would not talk about it. During a session after Joyce told Cheryl some of the stories of her mother's oppression and Joyce's anger about it, she asked Cheryl to tell her the story of her abuse. She promised she would not be weak, but she would be angry for her. Cheryl broke her silence about the rape. The context of the session was set up for Joyce to help Cheryl with the many feelings she had about the rape.

Particularly during the end of this session, questions were used as interventions to mobilize their anger over the heinous act. For example, to Joyce I asked, "What would you have done if you walked into the room and saw this happening to your daughter?" "What would you like to do to those boys now?" And to Cheryl, "What would you do if you saw this happening to your younger sister?" and "How would you feel if your mother ripped their heads off?"

Child molesters (on TV talk shows) often talk about their ability to single out a vulnerable child. They see a shyness, a body language that they observe in the child. In doing Cheryl's history, there was a pattern of vulnerability. An incident had occurred in the 8th grade, when she was hanging out on a dark corner and a stranger came up to her and began touching her. In another series of incidents, her 41-year-old boss at her part-time job would have her work alone and attempt to fondle and kiss her. As we talked about these incidents, I shared with her that one of the things we have learned is that when someone is sexually used as a child especially when he or she has not received help with it, the person is susceptible to later attacks. People who prey on women and children are very good at reading others' vulnerabilities. I wondered if she had been hurt or used sexually by anyone when she was younger. Cheryl began to cry.

CHERYL: Something happened but I don't want to remember it. It would be too awful.

THERAPIST: It would be horrible, wouldn't it?

CHERYL: Horrible. I can't imagine living with the thought of it. It can't be true. I don't want it to be.

THERAPIST: If it were someone you loved, could you still love him? (*Cheryl begins to cry harder.*) If we could figure how you could still love him but hate the part of him that hurt you would that be all right? (*Cheryl shakes her head "yes."*) It must be so confusing, so hard, to be hurt by some you love.

CHERYL: Yeah. (*She cries harder.*)

THERAPIST: This is real hard. Would you like me to stop or can we talk a little more.

CHERYL: Maybe stop. (*When Cheryl tells me she wants to stop, we will stop. Stopping will not be abrupt, but we will move slowly out of the intensity. So the following questions which I ask serve as a transition as she leaves the painful memories.*)

THERAPIST: What would happen if we speak more of it?

CHERYL: I would feel more horrible.

THERAPIST: Would it be all right just to share what you are feeling now with me?

CHERYL: It hurts. I am so sad.

THERAPIST: I know. I know. Is it embarrassing to talk about this?

CHERYL: Yes.

THERAPIST: Of course.

In the ensuing weeks the therapy was structured to allow full disclosure of the incest which was perpetrated against Cheryl by her father, who passed away when she was eight. Prior to mother's hearing of the incest, I worked to prepare Joyce so she could help her daughter and stop the cycle of violence.

THERAPIST: What would it be like if someone Cheryl loved molested her?

MOM: That would just be awful. I don't know if I could take any more of this.

THERAPIST: This whole thing has been awful. It's time to finally end it. Do you think you and Cheryl could become free of all this abuse if we know about all of it?

MOM: I guess it would only end if we find out everything.

I continued to work with Joyce to help her deal with the onslaught of feelings that came as she accepted that her husband (Henry) sexually abused her daughter. He was somewhat idealized in his death, and it was extremely painful to bring back the bad memories of the relationship. Yet to be connected to idealization as opposed to the real memory is in fact a disconnection. Although reconnecting both Joyce and Cheryl to the reality was a painful, slow process, I believe it was necessary to prevent a further revictimization.

Near the end of therapy, both Joyce and Cheryl wrote letters to Henry in which they expressed their anger and sadness over what he had done. Both placed the responsibility clearly on his shoulders. And Cheryl forgave him, writing "even though what you have done to me has caused me so much pain, I want you to rest, and I want you to know I love you just the same. But I will always hate what you did to me."

"FORGOTTEN" SIBLINGS

In the examples described so far, the child who has been betrayed plays a central role in the therapy. The following case illustrates how this good intention can go awry. It will also serves to open up the subject of therapeutic bias and the impact of ideas on therapeutic practice.

I was contacted by Patty Young's therapist (Dr. J), who had attended a workshop I conducted on the topic of incest. He had been working for over a year with Patty, who was 15 years old at the time. She had a host of symptoms, including an explosive rage, guilt, and dissociative and bulimic symptoms. During the past 2 years she was hospitalized several times because of suicide attempts. I agreed to see Patty and her family with Dr. J. Patty lived with her father, her stepmother, Diane, and her older brother, Billy. I also asked to include Patty's mother, who had not played a strong role in her treatment. Patty had an older sister who was living with her boyfriend and did not participate in the therapy.

During the consultation it became clear that Patty's treatment was driven by the idea that her problems and symptoms were caused by acts of sexual abuse and other abuses committed against her and that by uncovering these abuses Patty would get better. In the first hospitalization it was discovered that she was molested by her mother's previous boyfriend. Later, she briefly revealed a sexual attack by her brother. This was immediately followed by a suicide attempt.

During the consultation sessions I learned from the family history that each of the adults was very protective of his or her own parents. For example, George spoke about his father as a good man who provided for his family. Yet when I asked his wife and ex-wife about his dad, they both had much more negative descriptions of him and his relationship with his son. From this I hypothesized that in this family it was very hard for children to speak against their parents and family members. Yet, in her therapy, Patty was told that in order to get better she had to get honest about the past, which included conversation of how she was hurt by her parents (i.e., how her mother underprotected her and how she had given her up to be raised by her father).

Another thing that struck me from our meetings was that Patty's siblings and parents had serious problems that were not being addressed. I wanted to know why Patty was doing all the work. I asked the following questions during the consultation to present my hypotheses and to see if the family could understand Patty's therapeutic predicament.

"Who in this family would be most guilty to talk against his or her parents?" "Who would it be hardest on?" "What would be like for you [George] to spend each week creating a story of how your father's drinking has caused many of the problems in your life?" "What if your father knew you were doing that?" Also, "Who in the family is working hardest on his or her problems?" "Who is doing the worst?" "Would Patty do better, if the family started worrying more about her older sister or her brother?" (Her older sister was living with a boyfriend, and there were signs that he was violent toward her.) "If it would help your sister, Billy, would you take charge in trying to remember what you did to Patty?"

As the family responded to these questions, they saw how difficult it would be to do what Patty was doing. At one point Patty smiled—her first in the session. "Hey, it's no fair I'm doing all the work in this family."

The consultation changed the direction of therapy. Since Dr. J was not a family therapist, I began working with the family, and Dr. J was invited and attended many of the sessions.

IDEAS: WHIRLING DERVISH

The therapy of Patty Young is an example of how therapeutic choices can be misguided by powerful ideas. Family therapy has a tradition of recognizing the influence of ideas on therapy, which can be traced back to Bateson's use of the concept of epistemology. More recently, using the term "discourse" (from Foucault, 1979), Michael White has shown how cultural ideas both influence therapy and our families (White & Epston, 1990).

A therapist will be influenced by the ideas generated in writings, conferences, and political action taken on behalf of incest survivors. Some of the ideas will become "truths" and will greatly influence how treatment is conducted. The helpfulness of these "truths" depend on the context of the families, for families have their own "truths." For the Young family, the truth of loyalty by not expressing one's negative feelings about one's parent clashed with the "good" idea of the hospital and therapists that secrets, especially bad and sad ones, must not remain secrets. And as the professionals continually encouraged, coaxed, and even confronted Patty to remember her "bad" memories, she became more cut off from her family. Like the incest, therapy made her different. And unlike the promise of feeling better, remembering the bad only made her feel worse.

What might be a great idea for one client may be less appropriate for another. For example, the idea of confronting the father with the abuse is one to which many therapists in the recovery movement subscribe. I have dealt with a number of women who previously were coached to confront their fathers. In two of the cases after the confrontation, the women ended the therapy convinced that they were crazy and that they had made up the memories. Indeed, families of origins powerfully shape our realities.

Another problem that has evolved from the recovery movement is the belief that in order for treatment to be successful, the survivor needs to get in touch with the pain of the incest and that the pain will be extremely intense. Moreover, some "experts" suggest this work takes a great deal of time—even a lifetime. Thus, if someone who has been sexually abused does not feel this type of pain or feels it too quickly, he or she may get the idea that the pain has not been dealt with and the work is unfinished.

Indeed, remembering and dealing with sexual abuse is painful. And for some clients it will take time to go through the process. But humans — particularly children — are resilient. Additionally, applying information from the adult survivor movement to working with children may not always be appropriate. Trauma has a way of being accumulative. Thus, particularly when trauma is not attended to or is attended to poorly, it will create a context of repeated traumatization.

We are not the only experts involved with the treatment. Having clients collaborate what us during the treatment and using their expertise contributes to the agency of our clients.

REFRAMING MOTHERS

As Ehrenreich and English (1978) demonstrate in their chapter called "Motherhood as Pathology," ideas and psychological "truths" about mothers put them at the center in causing children's pathologies. Nonperpetrating mothers of families where incest has been committed are not spared from these harsh assessments. In her review of the literature, Herman (1981) points out that these mothers have been referred to as "very unattractive," as "giving reason to the husband to look elsewhere for sex," as "frigid and hostile," and as "cold" and "rejecting" (p. 43). One author, in explaining a case of father and daughter incest, states, "In simplest terms, [the father] and his daughter . . . acted out in incest the yearning to assuage the emptiness each felt as a result of inadequate close maternal 'symbiotic' care" (Steele, 1991, p. 21).

If mothers are framed as colluding, coabusing, or nonprotecting, this only weakens them and robs them of their agency. The process of mother-blaming reinforces their personal and societal oppression. Positive interpretations and framing of problems go a long way in empowering people. In my work with these families, when mothers deal with their pain, ambivalence, and conflicts, they have been the major healing allies in working with both abused children and the abusing children.

If we place ourselves in the role of a mother who is confronted with the information that her daughter has been molested by her husband, we can see just how difficult it will be for her to respond. She is faced with a multiplicity of losses. She must deal with the potential economic loss, if she chooses to believe her child and leave her husband. How does she reconcile her daughter's loss of innocence with her view of herself? A natural emotional reaction will be to view her daughter as a sexual competitor. If she thinks this, can she ever admit it or talk about it? Her husband had sex with her own daughter. Either consciously or unconsciously, she will be prone to the same mother-blaming that is so prevalent in the literature.

Helping a mother understand the real complexities of her position and giving her an opportunity to talk about these issues have a significant place during the therapy. By showing her understanding and allowing her to explore her complex position, a mother will begin generating a potential for self-understanding and self-caring. The capacity of self-care is diminished in these women. Speaking of women in general, Jordan (1991a) explains: "Many women do not develop dependable self-empathy because the pull of empathy for others is so strong, because females are conditioned to attend the needs of others first, and because women often experience so much guilt about claiming attention for the self even from the self" (p. 30). Introducing the importance of self-care for women into family sessions will help develop a new truth for women in the family: women's needs also can come first. Questions that will introduce the discourse of self-care into the therapy include the following: "How can you take better care of yourself?" "What would it would be like in this family if women put themselves first?" "How would you feel if your mother did more for herself?"

Family tasks may also be created to practice self-care. When a parent is so starved for care that she covertly asks her child to care for her, the therapist can overtly encourage the reversal of the hierarchy (Madanes, 1984). I have found that in getting explicit credit for their support of parents, children are relieved of the anxiety that often occurs in covert situations. Moreover, the parent is often very appreciative of the child's support, and she is able to give her child more.

MEN: OFFENDERS
AND NONOFFENDERS

In accepting and using many feminist-informed ideas, the therapy presented here seeks to correct social conditions wherein women have been devalued. It does not seek to redress this state by devaluing men. Men in these families, including the offender, will make valuable contributions to creating a healing context if they learn to relate in mutual and empathetic ways toward their families. By placing their abusive and negative behavior in a discourse or "truth" of masculinity, I challenge men to recreate a new ideal of masculinity. Men who behave abusively and lack empathy are not acting strong. A strong man cares for and supports his wife and children.

In the course of the therapy with the Young family, George and Billy Young explored their role as men in their family and how their behavior impacted on the women. By using anger, which created fear, avoiding domestic tasks, controlling the finances, and escaping to work and high-risk behaviors, Billy and George were acting in tradition of "strong" men in their family. Each claimed compassion for their mother or sister or wife. Each was uncomfortable in looking at his behavior. Each was challenged to give up his notions of a strong man and to create a new concept of the masculine ideal in the family.

The following is an excerpt from a session attended by Billy and George. Billy was talking about how nervous he was when his mother was telling him someone molested his sister. Later, he found out it was his mother's boyfriend, and he was relieved.

THERAPIST: Why were you so nervous and then relieved?

BILLY: I guess I thought it was me and I was feeling guilty, and then when I heard it was Dan I felt off the hook.

THERAPIST: Why do you think you were feeling guilty.

BILLY: I don't know.

THERAPIST: If you had to make a guess.

BILLY: (*long pause*) Maybe, I am guilty of something. I know Patty thinks I did something. So I must have done something.

THERAPIST: What is the something we're talking about?

BILLY: Something sexual. Something she didn't want to happen.

THERAPIST: What would it mean if you did something sexual to Patti against her wishes?

BILLY: It would mean I'm pretty screwed up.

THERAPIST: Maybe it would mean you had some things to own up to and some problems to work out. George, how would you feel if Billy did this?

GEORGE: When I first heard about this I was mad. Now I'd want him to get it out—to get rid of it.

THERAPIST: Can you forgive him? Will you love him?

GEORGE: Yeah, I . . .

THERAPIST: Tell him.

GEORGE: Billy, look, I'm not going stop loving you. I'm going to be here for you. I want you to remember. It will help your sister and it will help you.

THERAPIST: How do you feel about Dad's support?

BILLY: I'm glad he's with me and I want to help my sister. I know something happened. I don't think I want to remember.

THERAPIST: I understand that. What is it like talking about this stuff?

BILLY: It's hard.

THERAPIST: George, how do you feel about the way Billy is trying to face this?

GEORGE: I'm proud of him. I know he will remember.

Billy's remembering his molestation of his sister was viewed as a move toward a positive and mature manhood. It was a stronger Billy who was reflexively looking at what he did when he was acting as entitled "weaker" male. Billy's memory of the events returned in stages. First he remembered some details, but he had his age wrong. If he were 8, it was tolerable. He said, "It would mean I wasn't so sick." Finally, he remembered he was 13 and he was drunk. His memories matched his sister's story.

Discussion of his drinking and fast driving were contexualized in his need to appear stronger. His parents encouraged him to see how concentrating on school, helping his sister, and getting a part-time job were all signposts that he was becoming a "new" and "better" man.

The road for George was no easier. He protested having to change, claiming "I didn't molest anyone." Moreover, his father wouldn't participate in therapy. With Billy changing it became embarrassing for George not to. In a way, his son pushed him to be a better man. George worked on his temper, and he has begun to do more around the house. Although he has not been able as of yet to share financial control equally with his wife, she demanded and received credit cards in her name and received a greater amount of money as a monthly allotment.

In working with men like George and Billy, their development of empathy for those they have hurt is crucial in helping them change. Since male expression of emotion is often instrumental, the empathy is viewed as genuine if they change their behavior.

In accepting responsibility for the incest, an offending father or brother can make a significant contribution in helping his daughter or sister work out her loyalty issues (Gelinas, 1988). Thus, as Billy accepted his incestuous attack, his guilt and shame increased, and Patty was freer to talk about her feelings about the abuse. In therapy, the family helped Patty develop her voice, and as they helped Billy carry his shame, his shame lessened. Billy was becoming a more responsible young man.

CONCLUSION

Creating a healing context for families that are dealing with the problems of incest is a challenging and rewarding experience. By fostering mutuality and empathy, a family will feel safe to face the complex issues of incest. The context for healing is one of connection. Initially, building a connection between mother and daughter begins the process of overcoming the problems caused by the abuse. They begin differentiating the past from the present as a way of letting go of the past.

The therapist pays attention to how the problems' symptoms influence the system and how the system influences the problems. The therapist is aware of how biases influence the therapy, and the therapist is vigilant of family "truths" or ideas.

Helping men in the family relate in mutual and empathetic ways is an important part of their healing. Men are asked to develop new ideas about what it is to be a good man. The offender, in owning the responsibility for the abuse, not only helps himself but also helps the family member he has hurt.

REFERENCES

Beck, A. T., Rush, A. J., Shaw, B. F., & Emery, G. (1979). *Cognitive therapy of depression.* New York: Guilford Press.

Ehrenreich, B., & English, D. (1978). *For her own good: 150 years of the experts' advice to women.* New York: Doubleday.

Everstine, D. S., & Everstine, L. (1989). *Sexual trauma in children and adolescents: Dynamics and treatment.* New York: Brunner/Mazel.

Everstine, D. S., & Everstine, L. (1993). *The trauma response: Treatment for emotional injury.* New York: W. W. Norton.

Finkelhorn, D., & Browne, A. (1988). Assessing the long-term impact of child sexual abuse: A review and conceptualization. In L. E. A. Walker (Ed.), *Handbook of sexual abuse of children* (pp. 65–71). New York: Springer.

Foucault, M. (1979). *Discipline and punish: The birth of the prison.* New York: Random House.

Gelinas, D. J. (1988). Family therapy: Characteristic family constellation and basic therapeutic stance. In S. M. Sgroi (Ed.), *Vulnerable populations: Evaluation and treatment of sexually abused children and adult survivors* (pp. 25–49). Lexington, MA: Lexington Books.

Gilligan, C. (1982). *In a different voice: Psychological theory and women's development.* Cambridge, MA: Harvard University Press.

Haley, J. (1987). *Problem-solving therapy* (2nd ed.). San Francisco: Jossey-Bass.

Herman, J. C. L. (1981). *Father–daughter incest.* Cambridge, MA: Harvard University Press.

Hoffman, L. (1981). *Foundations of family therapy: A conceptual framework for systems change.* New York: Basic Books.

Imber-Black, E. (1988). *Families and larger systems: A family therapist's guide through the labyrinth.* New York: Guilford Press.

James, K., & MacKinnon, L. (1990). The "incestuous family" revisited: A critical analysis of family therapy myths. *Journal of Marital and Family Therapy, 16*(1), 71–88.

Jordan, J. V. (1991a). Empathy and the mother–daughter relationship. In J. V. Jordan, A. G. Kaplan, J. B. Miller, I. P. Stiver, & J. L. Surrey, *Women's growth in connection: Writings from the Stone Center* (pp. 28–24). New York: Guilford Press.

Jordan, J. V. (1991b). The meaning of mutuality. In J. V. Jordan, A. G. Kaplan, J. B. Miller, I. P. Stiver, & J. L. Surrey, *Women's growth in connection: Writings from the Stone Center* (pp. 81–96). New York: Guilford Press.

Jordan, J. V. (1991c). *The movement of mutuality and power.* Work in progress, No. 53. Wellesley, MA: Stone Center Working Paper Series.

Jordan, J. V., Kaplan, A. G., Miller, J. B., Stiver, I. P., & Surrey, J. L. (1991). *Women's growth in connection: Writings from the Stone Center.* New York: Guilford Press.

Luepnitz, D. A. (1988). *The family interpreted: Feminist theory in clinical practice.* New York: Basic Books.

Madanes, C. (1984). *Behind the one-way mirror: Advances in the practice of strategic therapy.* Washington, DC: Jossey-Bass.

Mollica, R. F. (1988). The trauma story: The psychiatric care of refugee survivors of violence and torture. In F. Ochberg (Ed.), *Post-traumatic therapy and victims of violence* (pp. 295–314). New York: Brunner/Mazel.

Morrison, T. (1970). *The bluest eyes.* New York: Washington Square Press.

Sheinberg, M. (1992). Navigating treatment impasses at the disclosure of incest: Combining ideas from feminism and social constructionism. *Family Process, 31,* 201–216.

Steele, B. F. (1991). The psychopathology of incest participants. In S. Kramer & S. Akhtar (Eds.), *The trauma of transgression: Psychotherapy of incest victims* (pp. 15–37). Northvale, NJ: Jason Aronson.

Trepper, T. S., & Barrett, M. J. (1989). *Systemic treatment of incest: A therapeutic handbook.* New York: Brunner/Mazel.

Wheeler, D. (1990). Father–daughter incest: Considerations for family therapists. In M. P. Mirkin (Ed.), *The social and political contexts of family therapy* (pp. 139–157). Boston: Allyn & Bacon.

White, M., & Epston, D. (1990). *Narrative means to therapeutic ends.* New York: W. W. Norton.

Winnicott, D. W. (1965). *The maturational process and the facilitating environment.* Madison, CT: International Universities Press.

Winnicott, D. W. (1986). *Home is where we start from: Essays by a psychoanalyst.* New York: W. W. Norton.

III

FAMILIES OF CHILDREN PLACED IN INSTITUTIONS

There are many reasons why children continue to be placed in institutions. The most compelling reasons are that children are endangered, either by their own behavior or by the behavior of adults who should be protecting them, and there are no safe alternatives. When safe alternatives are not available, it is usually because professionals in the helping system have not cast their nets widely enough to find them, or because the systems of safe alternatives to institutional settings have not yet been developed (as they have in the exceptional system described by Stephen Christian-Michaels in Chapter 3).

But admitting a child in an institutional setting may be the treatment of choice, as described by John Sargent. This step can be taken when it appears that a period of intense work with child and family in a focused treatment setting can mobilize a stuck system. The inpatient program at the Philadelphia Child Guidance Center has been family-focused since it opened in 1974. Programs for families in its apartments have been vividly presented in Brendler, Silver, Haber, and Sargent's book, *Madness, Chaos, and Violence,* but in this chapter Sargent describes how families can be central in the treatment of a child who is hospitalized without them.

Michael Fox takes a strict systemic approach to working with families of children in placement as a means of empowering them to take charge of their children. In doing so, he addresses layers of systems that maintain powerlessness in parents and keep families dismembered. His rendering of his efforts to make such a system work in one residential placement system underscores how difficult it is to rearrange multilevel systems.

The Mentor Hospital Diversion Program described by Julie McKenzie and Edwin J. Mikkelsen places children temporarily with therapeutic families in lieu of hospitals during a crisis. The advantage of this approach is that the child still remains in the community and in a family-like setting while efforts are being made to calm the child and work out things with the child's own family. This program previews a number of therapeutic foster care options described in the next section.

Francine Feinberg's program of including children in the residential treatment of their substance-abusing mothers is one of a few programs that recognize how mothering is often a strong incentive to get off drugs and onto other aspects of life. Feinberg presents a feminist approach to the treatment of substance abuse in women, explaining why standard approaches for men do not address critical issues for women. Women's experiences of being exploited and demeaned as children play an important role in their substance abuse, and their recovery may be strongly motivated by offering their children a different experience.

7

Children and Adolescents in Psychiatric Hospitals

John Sargent

In the past 20 years, there has been a significant increase in the use of psychiatric hospitalization for children and adolescents. During the first half of the 1980s there was a dramatic increase in the number of inpatient beds for children and adolescents. This increase in the use of hospitalization to manage disturbing behaviors in young people quickly generated a concern about the implications of hospitalization for young people. Although seriously mentally ill young people have been hospitalized in state institutions or long-term treatment facilities for the greater part of the last 50 years, the use of hospitalization only recently has been identified as a specific treatment for children and teenagers with aggressive, withdrawn, self-destructive, or otherwise disturbed and disturbing behavior. Various justifications for hospitalization of children and adolescents have been offered, including provision of safety, stabilization of behavior, development of enhanced diagnostic perspectives on the child's difficulties, and the opportunity for respite for family members (Pfeifer & Strzelecki, 1990). But many have worried about the deleterious effects of hospitalization—effectively removing the child from the family, even for a short but critical period. Several aspects of the hospitalization procedure have come into question, including identifying the child as the primary source of the disturbance, socializing the child to an inpatient treatment facility, and possibly, through excessive reliance upon hospitalization, failing to develop or utilize other potentially less restrictive and more useful treatments.

Removing a child from his or her home, often in a moment of crisis, danger, and demoralization has significant problematic implications. These include reinforcing the experience of failure on the part of parents or parent figures, labeling the child, and reinforcing the parents' sense that the child's care requires expert intervention that will replace and supersede parental care. Because the focus in the hospital is on the child and his or her difficulties, problems in the family and confusion about the child's care at home may not receive sufficient attention (Combrinck-Graham, 1985). Differences between parents may not be noticed or addressed. Excessive emphasis may be placed upon the child's adaptation to the inpatient unit milieu and management of the child's behavior solely within the hospital environment. Hospitalization can proceed without any predictable involvement of the family or the child's community-based treatment system. If the child's home context is left unchanged while the child is socialized to the inpatient unit with its specific rules, expectations, and opportunities for consistent care, then discharge of the child can be extremely problematic, reinforcing further reliance upon the hospital and its staff.

Family therapists have viewed hospitalization of the child as an outcome to be avoided, often regarding hospitalization as a failure of therapy. In this atmosphere, parents, child, and therapist are further demoralized by the need to hospitalize the child, and hospital staff will have to generate energy, alternatives, and hope for all participants. A hospital staff that responds to the family's sense of emergency and danger either prior to or during hospitalization by imposing control and replacing parental authority reinforces the expectation that the child cannot be safe and that the parents cannot be trusted to keep the child safe.

More recently, however, changes in child and adolescent mental health care have occurred that may limit excessive and inappropriate reliance upon hospitalization. Family therapy is now an expected part of inpatient treatment. The average length of stay in private or public institutions has decreased to less than 30 days. Enhanced diagnostic evaluations have improved specificity in identifying the young person's difficulties. A variety of community-based settings offer intensive treatment that allows the child to remain in the community and often in the family. Such programs include home-based treatment, partial hospitalization or day treatment programs located both in treatment centers and in schools, and community-based respite or group homes. Increased sophistication in the use of psychopharmacologic agents has shortened the duration of hospitalization, and the enhanced focus within the hospital on behavioral stabilization and disposition planning for the hospitalized young person has further defined and limited treatment. While these changes have had a significant impact on hospital admissions and lengths of stay, and while there is a general practice of acknowledging families in all psychiatric hospitalization of children and adolescents, very few centers have an approach to hospitalization that puts the family at the center of treatment, specifically addressing family difficulties with their children and enhancing the ability of family and community to maintain children outside the hospital.

This chapter will describe an approach to psychiatric hospitalization for children and adolescents that emphasizes inclusion of the child's family and community supports in the planning and implementation of inpatient treatment and will highlight specific opportunities to effect change in how the family and community respond to the child, how the child responds to his natural environment, and how family and child together view themselves as they continue through the process of development. This approach has been developed and utilized by family-oriented mental health practitioners at the Philadelphia Child Guidance Center over the past 20 years (Brendler, 1987; Brendler & Combrinck-Graham, 1986; Brendler, Silver, Haber, & Sargent, 1991; Combrinck-Graham, Gursky, & Brendler, 1982). This treatment model has been used both in the more traditional inpatient unit where the child is hospitalized individually and in two family apartments where entire families live in the hospital with the child who is the identified patient.

FAMILY-ORIENTED INPATIENT TREATMENT

Shawna, a 15-year-old, was seen for evaluation with her mother following a serious suicide attempt by ingestion of medication. She had been hospitalized for 48 hours in a medical unit and had recovered from the physical effects of her intentional overdose. She was now ready for discharge from the medical unit, and a psychiatric consultation was requested. The girl was the oldest of three sisters living with their mother and maternal grandmother. When asked why she took the overdose, she replied that she does not know and that she does not know how she could have done anything differently. Two nights previously, her mother had come home from work late and found the house a mess; she woke Shawna up to ask her to clean the house. Shawna became angry with her mother, went into the bathroom, locked the door and took the entire contents of the bottle of medication for her asthma. Following her overdose, she told her mother about it. She was observed for several hours, during which time she became lethargic, nauseated, uncoordinated, and finally lost consciousness. She was taken to the emergency room, where she was hospitalized in the intensive care unit. Her mother stayed with her during her hospitalization, and she recovered uneventfully. A psychiatric evaluation found that the mother was frightened, angry, and overwhelmed with the responsibility of maintaining her job, dealing with a conflictual relationship with her own mother, and looking after her three daughters. She was clearly angry at Shawna for taking the overdose and for being irresponsible but could recognize ways in which her daughter was unhappy and stressed. She did not have any ideas about how she might prevent her daughter from making further suicide attempts or how she might be able to help her daughter with her depression. She told the consultant, "I think she needs to be kept in the hospital until she learns how to become stronger and deal more effectively with stresses in her life." Throughout the interview Shawna's mother was worried about her job and her other children. She hoped to leave Shawna in the psychiatric hospital so that she would become happier, less withdrawn, and more cooperative.

Fred was an 8-year-old boy who was referred for psychiatric hospitalization following a several year history of disruptive behavior in preschool, elementary school, and at home. He had been diagnosed with attention-deficit/hyperactivity disorder (ADHD) in preschool and started on Ritalin, with some improvement in his behavior and his ability to pay attention in school. But he had frequently refused to take his medicine at home or to go to the nurse to receive his medicine while at school. He had marked difficulties doing his homework after school and had been identified as having significant learning problems in first grade. He had been placed in a special class in second grade but had been frequently disruptive and aggressive while in school. Psychiatric hospitalization was requested following an episode that occurred at home, when Fred had taken a knife from the kitchen and threatened both his younger sister and his mother. Since his parents had been divorced when Fred was 2½ years old, he had lived with his mother with little contact with his natural father. Fred's mother worked during the daytime and had arranged for a baby-sitter to care for Fred and younger sister in the afternoons after school. The baby-sitter had become exasperated, the outpatient therapist and outpatient psychiatrist had felt that treatment was not effective, and school personnel were wondering about private school placement or residential placement for Fred.

These situations are familiar to anyone who has worked with child and adolescent mental health problems. They are the kind of difficulties that lead children and teenagers to be referred for psychiatric hospitalization and lead professionals to believe that hospitalization is needed and could be helpful. Each situation presents immediate danger to the child or adolescent, to family members, and to other adults involved with the child. In each case there are also chronic difficulties that have not been ameliorated through community attention, outpatient mental health treatment, or the involvement of other social systems, including the Department of Human Services (DHS), the school, and health care providers. There is significant stress in the family, loss through death or removal of a family member, and the influence of poverty or severe financial demands. The family believes that they are doing all that they possibly can to resolve their problems. In each of these situations it is also obvious that the child has significant individual difficulties. The experience of depression, a lack of competency, and difficulty in meeting developmental needs as well as dealing with the stress of physical illness or academic or social demands render the child in serious trouble and in obvious need of assistance. Any attempt at treatment must take into account the child's difficulties and strengths, and his or her behavioral style and ways of coping with severe stress. The dilemma presented to the inpatient psychiatric treatment team is to respond to the child's needs while embedding that response within an approach to the family and involved community resources that facilitates the family's ability to help the child and the community's ability to support the family. We will follow these two cases through the course of hospitalization throughout this chapter, identifying ways of responding to each child's problems and his or her family's needs simultaneously.

THEORETICAL FRAMEWORK

Family-oriented inpatient psychiatric treatment requires a distinct theoretical framework. While hospitalization is required in order to assist the child and prevent further violence or danger, the hospital treatment itself is for the entire family. The family also brings their relationships with neighbors, extended family, schools, health care professionals, and other community and social agencies to the experience. All participants in the family's life should be seen as participants in the psychiatric hospitalization. The problems to be addressed during hospitalization include not only the difficulties the child has but the difficulties presented to the child and family members by the disruption in family relationships and in the relationship between the family and community agencies.

For Shawna, the hospital staff has to address her suicidality, depression, and emotional withdrawal and her inability to enlist her mother's support when she is stressed as well as her mother's difficulty responding to Shawna's stress when she herself is stressed and overwhelmed. This raises the additional issue of Shawna's mother's inability to receive support and assistance from her mother. For Fred, the hospital staff as to help his mother to understand his limitations; in managing his difficulties, she may have to work with his father, her ex-husband.

The family therefore must be involved in all decisions and all aspects of the treatment program, and an intervention is chosen based upon how it assists the family as a whole and how it assists the family to communicate effectively with community agencies and support systems. The hospital staff, including all professionals—psychiatrists, psychologists, primary therapist, special educator, nursing staff, and mental health associates—must direct their interventions to the family as well as the child. As conflicts between child and family are identified, the staff's job is to help the child and family members address those conflicts and begin a process of working together to resolve difficulties. Diagnostic and therapeutic considerations, whether they be to answer a question of medication for Shawna or psychological and educational evaluations to provide additional information about Fred's difficulties in school must be oriented to answer the questions raised by the family. The family also participates in discharge planning in an active way, recognizing that after the hospitalization the child will return home and continue living with them. This provides them with additional motivation for active participation during the hospitalization.

When hospitalization is oriented to relationships, the staff becomes a consultant to the family rather than assuming a role as surrogate caretaker for the child while the child is hospitalized. The staff might be concerned about how the child is resolving difficulties with other family members and how the family is addressing their social isolation and disconnection from their community. As one might expect, this approach can lead to an overwhelming list of family difficulties for hospital staff to address. As the staff clarifies these problems and works toward enhanced competence, setting priorities and addressing difficulties becomes possible.

There are several crucial points in family-oriented inpatient treatment. These include admission, programming decisions, decisions about evaluations and discussion of the results of these evaluations, the degree of autonomy and self-direction that the child is permitted, visits of family members, and passes and trips outside the hospital. Day-to-day programming decisions, including activities, plans for afternoon and evening, the degree of focus upon schoolwork, athletic and artistic pursuits, and other events that can enhance the child's awareness of his or her own competence, abilities, and needs are decided upon by family and staff together. Family and staff decisions about follow-up treatment, school placement, and future community relationships are actively considered throughout the hospitalization. The test of all of these decisions is how this particular aspect of the plan assists the family as well as how can it be useful to the hospitalized child. This collaboration between hospital staff and family members requires the participation of all and assists the family in understanding that the hospitalization will proceed according to directions that they wish and only with their active agreement. Small moments in treatment, such as decisions about the child's bedtime, giving the child money to buy snacks, or decisions about the child's participation in unitwide activities can be equally important in creating mutual accountability, shared appreciation of family strengths, and a sense of connection and mutual support between family members and between family members and community supports. The family must experience the hospitalization as both a powerful and important event in the family's life and as an opportunity for all family members to participate, identify, and utilize internal resources and receive support and assistance.

STRUCTURE OF THE INPATIENT UNIT

For an inpatient psychiatric unit to be structured to address problems in relationships between people, as well as those of individual children, the orientation of its leadership and the expectations and training of unit staff must reflect this approach. Documentation of the child's symptoms and need to be hospitalized must be recorded in the patient's chart, the rules and organization of the inpatient unit must meet standards of accreditation required by funding agencies and the Joint Commission on Accreditation of Health Care Organizations, and utilization review must be performed to support continued hospitalization based on appreciation of the child's need to be an inpatient. The standard guidelines for accreditation and utilization review are usually child-focused, so the family-oriented inpatient staff must simultaneously meet those standards and accomplish the relationship goals inherent in their treatment and approach.

The unit staff needs special training to work with families and assist in improving relationships between people as the primary focus of treatment. The staff of this unit will possess discipline-related skills that provide a unique perspective and when added together create a coherent picture of the situation, appreciating both the child's individual contribution to the problem and family members' strengths and difficulties simultaneously. The usual staffing for an inpatient unit includes child psychiatrists, family therapists, psychologists capable of performing psychological and neuropsychological evaluations, psychiatric nurses, consultant pediatricians, special educators with the capacity to identify each child's preferred learning style and assist with planning for academic remediation and special instructional needs, and mental health associate staff who are able to work with children, adolescents, and family members.

The special staff capacities for a family-oriented unit are best developed through training within the unit since standard training in most child-serving disciplines is primarily child-focused. There is strong emphasis on team cohesion, the integration of perspectives to create a comprehensive view of the child and family, and a willingness to collaborate throughout treatment as each situation requires. Further, staff members are offered ongoing supervision to stay focused upon the goal of helping each child or adolescent to respond more adaptively to family members, while at the same time as assisting family members in learning about and finding effective ways to parent their child. A willingness to take risks, to collaborate, and to see one's own perspective as part of a whole rather than the entire picture requires that the staff members value one another and maintain mutual support throughout their work. Difficulties such as those of the children described in the case studies, and others that result in children and adolescents requiring psychiatric hospitalization present significant risk of danger from violence, abuse or neglect, and mistrust and hopelessness among family members and community agencies are common. Staff cohesion and support is essential to ensure that the response to these difficulties embodies optimism, hopefulness, and a willingness to get to know the child and family members and the commitment to firmly insist upon the involvement of family members and all involved professionals.

The physical structure of the unit also organizes staff and family behavior. There must be, in this type of unit, enough room for family members to participate in all of the activities in which their children are involved, such as classrooms, group discussions, children's interactions with peers, and unit activities such as meals, trips, games, academic lessons, and athletic or artistic enterprises. Meeting rooms for sessions must be large enough so that the entire family can be present and so that involved staff members can participate in discussions as appropriate. These discussions may focus upon the child's participation in the unit, responses to problematic behaviors, setting goals, and periodic progress reviews during the hospitalization. The unit should also be accessible to outside referral sources so that these professionals may be able to participate in treatment sessions, team meetings, and other activities. When an existing unit is altered to include a family-oriented approach it must be done with an awareness of the way office size, sleeping areas, unit spaces, and activities rooms and classrooms encourage participation of family members. The staff should to be conscious of the need to include family members in day-to-day activities as well as sessions so that the family actually views themselves as not only hospitalizing their child but as planning and participating in an active and accountable way in the child's treatment.

Rules of participation and behavior within the unit must be designed to encourage family involvement while also regulating intrusiveness. The staff should consistently expect responsible and respectful behavior. They must also anticipate the danger of impulsivity, dangerousness, and provocativeness between family members. The staff should encourage family members to recognize situations that are stressful and to respond to them without any individuals losing control. Children and family members identified as prone to violence or impulsive responses must be actively monitored and encouraged to proceed slowly and respectfully in tense or stressful situations.

Each family is assigned a primary therapist who assists the family throughout the treatment and works with the family to ensure their active participation in treatment. The therapist should be able to understand and support individuals in the family as well as encourage effective family function and effective collaboration between staff, family, and community professionals. The primary therapist's work depends upon strong individual and family psychotherapy skills, and his or her connection to the treatment team. The therapist can intervene in small everyday events that the family engages in through their previous method of relating. He also must possess the ability to develop and articulate a comprehensive picture of the child and family, integrating the impressions of the child psychiatrist, psychologist, educator, and nursing and mental health associate staff.

Led by the primary therapist, the staff sets priorities and develops an approach to each family that encourages a steady and positive response to treatment. Often families come to the inpatient unit with many problems often outside the scope of standard mental health treatment, such as economic difficulties, job-related stresses, school problems, difficulties with extended family or noncustodial parents, and marked disconnection from community agencies and other social supports. This list of problems can be daunting to hospital professionals and can cause treatment to be scattered and diffuse. Priorities must be set to focus on the family's difficulties with their child, and additional problems are formulated as a part of the context of the family and child's difficulties.

Family-oriented hospitalizations follow a consistent time pattern. Hospital staff can use this pattern to plan the course of treatment and gauge their developing relationship with the family. The first 3 to 5 days is a time for the family to become familiar with their new situation. Symptomatic behavior often decreases as family members experience the novelty of the hospital environment and become familiar with the hospital staff and other patients and their families. Family members' anxiety and affect decrease initially due to the relief provided by hospitalization. This time is most successfully used to better understand the child and his family by asking each individual to explain his sense of himself or herself, of the family and of how they got into trouble. As the family members tell their stories, unique aspects of their situation begin to emerge and family members feel more included and more readily understood by staff. Generally, after this initial period the children and family members resume symptomatic behavior. Children may become more demanding; depression and hopelessness may reappear; and family members behave impulsively and display a sense of desperation and failure. It is during this time from the end of the first week through the second week of hospitalization that the problems inherent in the family situation become apparent and the opportunity for addressing them differently occurs. If these symptoms are properly handled, family members may become optimistic. Often at the end of the second week of hospitalization family members begin to believe that things can actually be different and can recognize positive characteristics of each other that they had neglected or overlooked in their concern about their difficulties. As family members feel more comfortable and hopeful they may bring up other concerns, including the child's relationship to a noncustodial parent or a parent's conflictual, unresolved relationship with extended family members. These concerns generally reflect longstanding problems and are often presented as impediments to improvement. The staff and the family can also begin to discuss the child's return to school and the family's return to outpatient treatment. As these concerns are brought up the family's previous sense of helplessness and their expectation of failure also re-emerges.

An essential aspect of family-oriented hospitalization is the development of a clearly defined discharge plan, outlined at the time of admission. By adhering to the plan for discharge the hospital staff can help the family maintain focus and progress with consistent participation. The final phase of treatment that can be expected by staff includes the disruption and testing of limits that occurs prior to discharge. Family members' worry about how things will go after the family leaves the environment of intense support of the hospital, provides the staff with the opportunity to assist the family in planning how they will deal with difficulties, symptomatic behavior, and stresses that are likely to resume following discharge. Everyone must recognize that during the first month following discharge the family must work hard to avoid resuming their previous patterns of interacting. Ultimately the staff must recognize that the value of their interventions is not only how the child and the family do in the hospital but also how they do among themselves without staff support. The staff can then decrease their involvement and gradually increase expectations of independent functioning by the family, leading to a smooth transition at discharge.

THE PROCESS OF FAMILY-ORIENTED INPATIENT TREATMENT

Admission Phase

The admission process sets the tone for any hospitalization. In a traditional psychiatric inpatient unit admission occurs directly following the determination of the need for inpatient treatment, with no specific inclusion of the family. Admission to a family-oriented unit provides the opportunity to determine what family goals are to be addressed and how family members will participate in treatment. Indications for hospitalization are similar to those in other child and adolescent units: (1) outpatient treatment has not been helpful in reducing serious or dangerous symptoms, (2) the child's functioning is seriously compromised, or (3) there may be risk of harm to the child, family members, or others in the community due to emotional disturbance or mental illness. Suicidality, episodes of violence, runaway behavior, an inability to manage serious medical illness, severe psychosomatic symptoms, psychosis and associated erratic behavior, or depression with severe withdrawal and functional impairment are all potential indications for psychiatric hospitalization. The hallmark of all these situations, however, is the family's inability to manage symptomatic behavior and participate in a process of problem resolution safely.

In the family-oriented unit, a referral is accepted by the admissions staff, information is collected, and an admission meeting is set up between the hospital staff and the family and referring therapist or agency professional. The child, his or her family, and involved professionals meet with the assigned inpatient therapist to discuss both the need for hospitalization and the nature of treatment. This facilitates the development of the relationship between the therapist and family members at the same time that information is obtained and a plan for hospitalization is formulated. If the hospital has an interview room with a one-way mirror, other members of the inpatient unit staff can observe the meeting, offer input, and participate if necessary in the admission meeting. If the referring therapist is included in the admission meeting, his or her impressions of the problem and goals for treatment can be heard directly by the family while the expectation of follow-up outpatient treatment is ratified. The admission session also provides an opportunity for the family members to discuss what they have tried previously to improve their situation and to identify their strengths All involved family members should be present at the admission session. Both divorced parents should be present for the admission meeting as well as grandparents, other family members, and school personnel or church personnel who have been involved in the family's difficulties. If the DHS has been involved with the family, the assigned case worker is also expected to participate. An admission meeting may last 2 hours and should be scheduled so that enough time is available.

At this meeting the family and involved professionals are expecting the relief associated with the child's admission to the hospital. Family members often feel frustrated, helpless, demoralized, and guilty about the need for inpatient treatment. Since the difficulties that lead to hospitalization are serious, it is essential that the inpatient therapist be prepared for high levels of affect, personal isolation, and an undertone of unresolved conflict and blaming among family members and professionals. Admission is often precipitated by violence or the threat of violence and occurs after a period of declining function, deteriorating relationships, and fruitless efforts at improving the situation. Supportive relationships among inpatient team members and the availability of trusted colleagues or a supervisor are extremely helpful during admissions meetings. The supervisor can help the therapist listen, be welcoming and respectful, and avoid prematurely engaging the family in discussions of conflictual issues. The primary goal of an admission session is to agree upon the need for hospitalization, to welcome the family to the unit, to provide a sense of safety, understanding, and hopefulness about inpatient treatment, and to engage the family in the process of addressing its difficulties with the support and guidance of hospital staff. Tolerance and acceptance on the part of the inpatient therapist and team, as well as respect for the resilience of the family, are essential elements of successful admissions sessions.

The strengths, difficulties, and behavioral style of the child must also be identified during the admission interview to help the staff to recognize and define the child's attributes that will be worked with during the hospitalization. The primary therapist and hospital staff help the family explain to the child the reasons for the hospitalization and what the child can expect from inpatient treatment.

The process of asking family members to discuss their problems, what they have attempted to do about these difficulties, and why their efforts have not been successful provides the therapist and team with an appreciation of how the family addresses significant difficulties, what differences of opinion there are within the family, and how effectively the family can negotiate with professionals. Directing this session requires the skill to actively enlist all participants, avoid premature conflicts and blowups, and achieve consensus about the goals and nature of the treatment. Signing the child into the hospital and agreeing upon an initial contract for treatment solidifies the sense of partnership and shared participation. The admission session should close with agreement about goals to be achieved during hospitalization, what skills are to be learned during the course of treatment, and how each participant in the admissions session will further participate during inpatient treatment. A follow-up meeting to review progress and revise the treatment plan should be scheduled during the admission meeting.

Case Illustrations

Shawna was referred for admission following hospital treatment for her suicide attempt. The inpatient therapist's goal for the admission session was to prepare Shawna and her mother for hospital treatment, which would involve both of them. Therefore, she needed to link a therapeutic response to Shawna's suicidality with an appreciation of problems in the family. It was also essential that the therapist develop a relationship with Shawna's mother that would support the mother so that she would be available to and supportive of Shawna. At first the mother did not see anything that she could do to help Shawna with her feelings of sadness and desperation or to prevent further episodes of suicidal behavior. She was angry with Shawna for harming herself and very frightened about the possibility of seeing her daughter die. As the therapist experienced the mother's anger, helplessness, and fear, she was able to direct the mother to begin to question Shawna gently about what had happened that had to led her overdose. The therapist further raised the intensity in the session so that the mother was able to say directly to Shawna that self-destructive behavior was wrong and that she expected Shawna to speak to her more openly and directly when she was upset or felt like harming herself. When pressed to tell her mother what problems had led to the suicide attempt, Shawna said that there was a great deal of tension in the house, that her younger siblings bothered her, and that she was worried about her mother working so hard and appearing so stressed. Shawna's mother became increasingly upset and angry, declaring that those kinds of difficulties ought not to lead to suicidal behavior. The therapist observed that the mother's anger and irritability when problems were being discussed seemed to reflect her feeling that the existence of difficulties might indicate that she had failed as a mother and that her efforts in raising her daughters, trying to live successfully with her mother, and working 8 to 10 hours a day to support the family in a low-paying job were not enough.

As the therapist discussed these issues with the mother, the latter sadly spoke about how difficult her life was and how frequently she felt desperate, helpless, and hopeless herself. Shawna appeared to want to protect her mother from stresses in the house by keeping quiet, and her mother felt that her job was to do as much as she could for her daughters also without asking for their support. Thus, when problems became apparent there was no escape valve in the family—the mother became angry and punitive, and Shawna became self-destructive. The therapist suggested that the hospitalization could be an opportunity for Shawna to learn other ways of dealing with sadness and stress while she and her mother together learned ways to talk about difficulties in the house and resolve them more productively. As the therapist addressed Shawna's mother she became quieter and readier to assist in her daughter's treatment. The hospitalization was defined as an opportunity for Shawna to learn how to express herself in words rather than through self-destructive behavior and for the mother to learn to hold Shawna accountable for controling violent impulses while the mother worked to resolve difficulties between herself and her own mother as well as her three daughters. The therapist developed a plan to gradually involve Shawna's younger sisters and maternal grandmother in the process of hospitalization and therapy sessions. She also agreed to work with Shawna and the mother to discuss Shawna's difficulties with her father, who lived nearby but whom Shawna had not spoken to for the past several months. Shawna was then admitted to the inpatient unit, and her mother was assisted in helping Shawna settle in, put her things away, and meet the staff and the other children and adolescents. Because Shawna's mother would have to miss some work while Shawna was in the hospital, the inpatient staff assisted her in speaking with her boss about her need to rearrange her schedule for the next 3 weeks so that she could participate with Shawna in the inpatient treatment.

Following Fred's referral for hospitalization, the inpatient therapist had asked that his mother, younger sister, outpatient therapist, and natural father attend the admission session. With everyone in attendance, the therapist noted that Fred was active, anxious, and easily excitable and that the mother and father experienced a great deal of tension between them. The father began the session by being critical of Fred's mother and defensive about his own lack of involvement. He attempted to exonerate Fred from any blame concerning his behavior. Fred's mother quickly became critical both of Fred and his dad and reiterated her fear concerning her son's potential for violence as well as her helplessness about what to do when Fred became upset or impulsive. Fred's mother and father disagreed about how to discipline him as well as about how best to help him if he became upset or angry.

The outpatient therapist presented her experience of Fred, including some of the difficulties that Fred had with frustration, learning, discipline, and direction. She discussed her diagnosis of ADHD, the trial of Ritalin, and the psychological evaluation showing serious learning difficulties that especially affected his ability to read. As the outpatient therapist brought up these issues the inpatient therapist assisted both parents in responding to these concerns and in stating their degree of agreement with Fred's intrinsic problems. Fred's father stated that he, too, often had difficulty concentrating and that his easy frustration made work difficult for him and influenced his decision not be involved with Fred on a regular basis rather than move in and out of his son's life. When asked how he had learned to deal with his easy frustration, Fred's father reported that he tried to stay calm and to slow himself down when he felt stressed or upset. Fred's mother then related how these difficulties had been part of the reason that she and the father had divorced.

Gradually, the admission session became an opportunity for everyone to begin to appreciate that Fred was experiencing specific difficulties both at school and at home, and the parents were encouraged to agree that they needed to find ways to help Fred with frustration and hyperactivity as well as to limit his tendency to become violent when angry. The inpatient hospitalization was thus structured to help the parents develop a shared appreciation of Fred's unique problems and strengths and how to manage them and to begin to work together as parents sharing responsibility, not leaving all the care to one or the other. Both parents seemed relieved with this prospect, and at the close of the admission session Fred said that he hoped that he could have more time with his father and apologized to his mother for threatening her. Both parents then helped Fred settle in on the inpatient unit. Fred's father was encouraged to stay with him in the afternoon, while his mother was asked to return for the evening. Future sessions for both parents as well as a plan for both parents to assist Fred in unit activities and learn the staff's impressions of Fred were scheduled for the upcoming days.

Middle Phase

Following admission, the development of goals for hospitalization, and articulation of a plan for participation of the family, the primary function of hospital staff is to understand more about the child and to develop, with the family, methods of implementing new patterns of interaction that effectively respond to the child's moods, abilities, and difficulties as well as define the intrinsic capacities of the family. Rapidly, the hospital staff assesses the child's responsiveness to directions, ability to interact effectively with both peers and adults, and his or her ability to learn and to direct his or her own behavior. The inpatient unit has a set schedule with times for patients to get up in the morning, eat meals, and participate in group activities. This schedule assists staff and family in planning and gives everyone the opportunity to observe the child's ability to participate in a structured program. During this time the child's intellectual and academic abilities and difficulties are also identified. Different staff members viewing the child in different circumstances usually develop different impressions of the child, and staff members with different professional backgrounds and different levels of experience may disagree on how the child is seen. These differences are forged into a shared framework for understanding the child's behavior, ways of thinking and learning, and emotional response to routine and troubling situations. The staff pays particular attention to the antecedents of difficult behaviors and assists the child and family members in appreciating these events, also. This understanding can lead to developing ways to prevent impulsive and aggressive behaviors. The staff works with the family so that they agree on what they are seeing and how they understand what they are experiencing.

Regular team meetings can facilitate staff coming to consistent impressions of each child, and family members can be invited to participate in staff meetings when their child is discussed. The parents and other family members are encouraged to speak up whenever they have something to contribute or have questions about how things are proceeding, particularly if their sense of their child is different from the staff's. During the middle phase of inpatient treatment there are also numerous opportunities to involve parents in establishing a schedule for their child and in responding to behavioral difficulties and emotional difficulties as they occur for their child. The staff may call the parent(s) when a child is disrespectful or disregarding of the schedule or limits; the parent(s) may collaborate on decisions about appropriate consequences for a child's behavior. The staff may also encourage the child to call the parents when he/she is emotionally upset or needs comfort.

Family meetings with the primary therapist and other staff members occur several times a week. These meetings offer family members the opportunity to further discuss concerns about their child, to continue the process of planning hospitalization, and to review their impressions of their child's strengths, difficulties, and treatment needs. Often parents discuss their needs for further assistance as well as more general issues within their life as a family and their individual lives that contribute to the difficulties they are experiencing with their child. The therapist and inpatient treatment team must continue to focus on the child and use articulated reasons for the child's hospitalization as a vehicle to encourage the parents to begin to resolve difficulties between themselves and within themselves that may have caused some of their current problems. Often at about 10 days to 2 weeks into hospitalization parents begin to discuss concerns in their own lives that make parenting extraordinarily difficult. These concerns may have involved previous trauma or serious hurts that have been inflicted upon them or may be issues related to their relationship with their child, their neighborhood, or their extended family that have been unresolved.

When these issues come up, the family may feel an impasse that threatens the progress of the hospital treatment. If the therapist, treatment team, and supervisor are prepared for this occurrence, however, such issues can be seen as further concerns requiring resolution over time. At times the parents may demonstrate an inability to work together, whether they live together or not. At times the difficulty of arranging alternative child care or insuring economic stability may be viewed by parents as barriers to resuming effective care for their child. It is important that the inpatient staff maintain their expectation that the family can be successful while continuing to participate in therapy and working toward the planned discharge of the child back to his or her home. The creativity of inpatient staff as well as their connection with the family's outpatient treatment team and community resources are often helpful in this regard. The inpatient team and primary therapist also can use an experience of impasse to enhance their connection with the family as well as to assist the parents in grieving what cannot be changed about their life circumstances and reorienting themselves toward living successfully with the difficulties and stresses they experience.

The staff should avoid impulsive discussion of alternative placement or living situation as well as avoid participating with the child in devaluing or disconnecting from the parents. By the middle phase of hospitalization the child may, in fact, entrust inpatient staff with his or her negative impressions of the parents, and the inpatient staff may find themselves hard-pressed to maintain their belief in the parents as they hear the child's version of previous difficulties. The child may, for example, reveal episodes of physical, emotional, or even sexual abuse at the hands of the parents or other adults in the child's home. Such revelations require that the family be reported to the DHS for additional supervision and assistance, especially in the immediate time after discharge. Once again, the more the staff can encourage the child to confront these concerns directly with the parents in family meetings with staff members present, the more readily these issues can be addressed. If everyone expects a period of demoralization and disruption in the middle of hospitalization and is prepared to persist through these difficulties, the therapist can assist the family to continue to participate actively in the hospitalization.

Especially during the middle phase of treatment, when the novelty of being in a new place has worn off, the staff should guard against allowing the child to become attached to the inpatient unit and its staff, in lieu of his or her own family members. Referring the child to parents for discussion of privileges and activities, encouraging the child to understand his or her difficulties in relationship to family, school, and neighborhood, and assisting the child to speak directly about problems with parents in meetings and during visits all facilitate the ongoing connection between child and parents. Passes can be arranged during the middle phase of the hospitalization, but these need to be planned so that demoralizing problems do not occur without everyone being prepared. Passes should also have a specific focus and goals so that everyone participates in carrying out the the objectives of the pass. The family is encouraged to stay in touch with outpatient treatment resources and the child's school so that everyone is prepared for the child's return home, to the community, to previous treatment, and to school. For children and families who entered the hospital without previous treatment the family should be helped to connect to outpatient treatment resources and school personnel so that the child's return to school is planned and as uneventful as possible.

Case Illustrations

The morning after admission Shawna was expected to join the young adolescent group in their daily activities. She was initially buoyant and friendly and an eager but somewhat immature participant in group activities. When asked by other teenagers why she was in the hospital, Shawna said in a smiling and offhanded manner that her mother had put her in the hospital. When asked why, she said in an equally offhanded way that she had attempted suicide. The staff noted that Shawna was acting as though nothing out of the ordinary had happened. They encouraged the other teenagers in the unit to question Shawna further about why she attempted suicide and why she was acting as if there was no reason for her to be in the hospital. When thus challenged by other teenagers, Shawna became abruptly withdrawn and refused to answer their questions. Shawna clearly had little ability to explain what had happened, accept responsibility for having made the suicide attempt, or identify problems that might have led to this serious behavior.

When the mother visited later that evening, the staff advised her that Shawna had difficulty speaking up for herself, staying with conversations, and clearly identifying her reasons for being in the hospital. Shawna's mother was asked to help Shawna review answers to those questions and to speak directly about what had led to her suicide attempt. The mother initially became angry with Shawna and was critical of her; Shawna became even more withdrawn and even less able to speak for herself. The staff reminded the mother that Shawna's tendency to withdraw had been a part of her difficulties in the first place. As the staff spoke calmly with Shawna's mother, she became less critical and more reflective, and even though that evening Shawna still was not able to develop answers and speak openly with her mother, the continuation of the theme of Shawna speaking for herself and not quitting or becoming self-destructive when challenged was maintained. This theme was continued by one staff person who was identified as someone who would work with Shawna on a daily basis to help her identify her thoughts and feelings. Shawna's mother was encouraged to visit daily, a reminder to Shawna of her mother's commitment, and to assist her daughter to make herself understood. The entire staff made it clear to Shawna that they would only believe her and respond directly to what she said when they felt that she was being "real." Shawna had to learn to speak when angry and pursue conversations about interests and activities as well as about concerns at home and her feelings of worthlessness and failure.

Shawna appeared to be embarrassed about the suicide attempt and worried that she was further distressing her mother and her family. In a session with the primary therapist in the first week of hospitalization,

Shawna was encouraged to discuss her worries, and the mother was encouraged to reiterate that hospitalization was essential and likely to be important for the entire family as well as for Shawna. The mother was encouraged to talk with the primary therapist about other stresses at home and about how difficult it was for her to get to the hospital on a consistent basis, maintain her work schedule, and care for her younger children.

Evaluations of Shawna's intellectual ability, academic abilities, and learning style demonstrated that she had a slightly above-average IQ, grade-level academic abilities, and no specific learning difficulties. However, everyone noticed that when Shawna did not know an answer immediately and was not able to respond in a complete fashion to a question that she would rather not offer an answer than be wrong. This tendency to withdraw rather than risk being wrong and to be less confident than other teenagers seemed to be a general behavior style of Shawna's and to represent a significant fear of being criticized or of being the focus of other people's concerns. Staff members also noticed that Shawna tended to act in a immature fashion when with other teenagers, even though her interests were similar, and did not volunteer her ideas or opinions in group discussions. Shawna's mother was invited on her day off from work to spend the afternoon in the group meeting with Shawna and the other teenagers to help Shawna speak up for herself and have an enjoyable time with the other teenagers. The children were playing some games, and the mother was able to gradually assist Shawna to participate in a more active and assertive fashion. It became very important for staff to help the other teenagers not speak for Shawna and not leave her out of discussions or activities, even though she might not speak or volunteer directly on her own. In a meeting with Shawna and her mother, the primary therapist noted that conversation was likely to be impulsive, and both Shawna and her mother had real difficulty listening to each other. The pacing of meetings with Shawna and her mother was slowed down so that they could work specifically on how to have conversations.

At the beginning of the second week of hospitalization the mother was invited to include her own mother in the treatment. The mother stated that her mother was critical of her activities and that she didn't want to bring her into treatment. The therapist stressed that this was an essential part of treatment and that the grandmother should come to the next session. The mother was so reluctant that she canceled the next family session, claiming work pressures. The therapist persuaded the mother by letting her know that she was less interested in the grandmother's impressions of the mother than she was in the mother being effective with Shawna and being able to help the grandmother know how best to be helpful to the mother. The mother did bring the grandmother to the next meeting, and the grandmother's tendency to be critical, controlling, and harsh with her daughter was apparent. The therapist encouraged the grand-mother to participate by listening to the mother to learn about what the family needed and how she could be most helpful. While recognizing the grandmother's interest in being helpful to her daughter and supportive of her daughter's efforts in raising her three granddaughters, the therapist confronted her to request her cooperation with treatment. The existence of long-standing tensions and conflicts the between mother and grand-mother was obvious, and the therapist suggested that they needed time and space to resolve these difficulties and work together more successful-ly. The grandmother was encouraged to talk about her wishes and dreams for her daughter, her sense of upset at seeing her daughter hurt by other people, pushed around by bosses in low-paying jobs, and not respected by the grandchildren. These discussions took place over three separate meetings and ultimately led to some beginning re-establishment of a mutu-ally supportive relationship between mother and grandmother.

During the second and third weeks of hospitalization, Shawna was able to speak more directly to peers, answer questions, and participate more confidently in conversations and group activities and ask directly for things that she wanted or activities that she wanted to pursue. Shaw-na's interest in music was utilized in having her participate with other teenagers in learning to dance and in discussing different types of music. Meanwhile, the mother was encouraged to get Shawna's schoolwork with instructions from teachers and to talk with school professionals about iden-tifying a primary support person for Shawna at school. The mother lo-cated an outpatient therapist in a convenient location and facilitated collaboration with the inpatient treatment team prior to Shawna's dis-charge. When the therapist that the mother had identified called the hospi-tal, she was encouraged to attend some inpatient sessions prior to Shawna's discharge. Shawna's mother was asked to bring her younger daughters to the hospital for visits and some therapy sessions, and Shawna was en-couraged by the staff to request a pass home. The pass was planned around what she would like to do with her mother and sisters while at home. The grandmother was applauded for looking after the younger children and maintaining things at home so that the mother could participate in Shawna's inpatient treatment.

Shawna was also encouraged by her mother to telephone her father, tell him what had happened and where she was, and invite him to visit and to participate in a session if he could. Her father did come for two visits to the hospital and stated to the staff that he would be happy to have Shawna visit him at his home on weekends after her discharge. He did not participate in sessions but did ask the staff for information about Shawna and her treatment. After 20 days of hospitalization, as Shawna approached discharge, the staff noted her continuing difficulty in expressing herself when she was frustrated or angry. They continued to encourage her but also noted to the mother and outpatient therapist that those skills would require continued emphasis in outpatient treatment.

After admission Fred's mother and father helped him settle into the unit, and it was noted by the staff that Fred was extremely active and had tremendous difficulty accepting limits and following directions. Fred's father stayed with him for the afternoon. He and Fred were interviewed by the unit psychiatrist, who noted Fred's tendency to become active, distractible, and impulsive and to interrupt. On that basis and the previous history of Fred having been placed on Ritalin, the psychiatrist recommended to the team, Fred, his father, and his mother that the Ritalin be restarted. The psychiatrist, however, also appreciated the need to involve the primary therapist and other staff members in the decision to restart Fred's medication as well as to involve everyone in defining specific target symptoms and goals of utilizing the medication. These considerations took place over the next 24 hours, and a list of specific behaviors for which the Ritalin was expected to be helpful was created. These included distractibility, fidgetiness, inability to wait his turn, impulsivity, and difficulty modulating his emotional response when frustrated or upset. It was also apparent that Fred was frightened and highly anxious and that he was worried about staying in the hospital. The primary therapist encouraged Fred's mother and father to plan for one of them to be with him as much of the time as possible. Fred was interested in sports and enjoyed physical activity, so he was encouraged to play games and pursue physical activities in the unit and only gradually become involved with the other children in the unit classroom or attend classroom activities. As Fred's need for calm and patient human attention was met and Ritalin began to be helpful, his tendency to be overactive, aggressive, and impulsive decreased and his fearfulness and anxiety also abated. During the second week of hospitalization, evaluation of Fred's ability to relate effectively with other children his age as well as of his intellectual and learning abilities was undertaken, and he was noted to have marked difficulty dealing with other children his age and to have a significant reading disability. The unit educational counselor spent time with Fred, further defining his severe reading disability. She requested that the primary therapist get further information from Fred's school as well as determine the resources within his school to assist him in learning to read. It was also noted that Fred went from one child to another, could not easily stay in conversation, was highly reactive to teasing or perceived slights, and tended to be a child that other children did not want to play with.

In meetings with the primary therapist, the mother and father sat together and talked about their marriage and divorce, their difficulties in working together, and the experience that each of them had of being abandoned and let down by the other. It also became apparent that the father owed a significant amount of child support and that the mother harbored resentment of the father for his refusal to pay. The father had had difficulty holding a job or maintaining his own financial and emotional stability. He cited his difficulties in organizing his behavior and reluctantly decided to seek treatment himself. As the father received his own treatment, his apprehension about being involved Fred's life decreased, and the mother was assisted by the primary therapist to make space for the father's involvement with Fred and his younger sister and to collaborate with the father if he were acting in a responsible and supportive fashion.

Meanwhile, over the second and third weeks of hospitalization Fred's difficulties in accepting limits continued, and even though his degree of distractibility and impulsivity decreased, it was apparent that he did not expect adults to be consistent and did not know how to differentiate limits from threats. Over time it was noted that the parents fluctuated between excessive permissiveness and excessive harshness in dealing with him, especially when encouraging that he go from one place to another or that he accept a limit about a snack, drink, or activity. The staff developed a more intense partnership with both parents by assisting each of them to set limits and learn the process of physically holding Fred when he became upset and then helping him stay in a time-out situation as he calmed down, prior to returning to activities. Both parents were excessively critical of or instructive with Fred and had trouble being patient when setting a limit or imposing a time out.

By the middle of the third week of hospitalization, both parents had become more competent in playing with Fred, in helping him deal with other children on the unit, in helping him attend to instructions, and in helping him accept "no." Each parent was encouraged to talk about his or her own fear of losing control with Fred and degree of exasperation with him, as well as the true difficulty that he had in accepting limits and dealing with frustration. Each parent also talked about other demands in his or her life, in particular those associated with work and attending to the younger sister, and both related how difficult they expected dealing with Fred would be after discharge. At the close of the third week of hospitalization it became apparent to both parents that Fred would continue to require special care and would continue to be a challenging child to raise. At this point the therapist from the inpatient unit contacted the referring therapist and psychiatrist to begin the transition to outpatient treatment, as well as to make plans for Fred to have passes to both the mother's and father's house as well as to return to school prior to discharge.

The Discharge Process

Discharge from a family-oriented acute care inpatient hospital is an important and often challenging process for the hospitalized child, his or her family, and the inpatient treating staff. The entire family has been involved in an active process of getting to know, trust, and collaborate with the inpatient staff as a whole and the primary treating therapist in particular. But the family has also been disrupted by the hospital treatment. The hospital staff expects that there is likely to be regression, symptomatic escalation, confusion, and sadness prior to discharge. The anxieties of the leaving as well as the difficulty in moving from relying on many people to relying on an outpatient therapist and other community supports can be anxiety-provoking for everyone. The child looks forward to leaving the hospital. Family members may not appreciate the degree to which they have become involved with inpatient staff and come to rely on them for advice, guidance, and company.

The family should recognize that things may become difficult upon returning home and that the first 2 months following hospitalization is an extremely important time for the entire family. We have found that the better the family is prepared to expect difficulties upon returning home, the easier discharge is. Often everyone expects to relax and resume "normal life" after discharge and, given the commitments of energy, time, emotion, and effort that people have put into a family-oriented inpatient stay, everyone may very much want the opportunity for a break from the need to monitor their behavior and maintain a focus upon implementing and pursuing what they have learned to be successful in the hospital. Often this is signaled by a recurrence of symptoms in the few days prior to discharge or a period of disruption and difficulty during a pass home on the last weekend prior to discharge. Often, at this point, family members and even inpatient staff can become apprehensive and wonder about the wisdom of following through with discharge plans. There is also a tendency to try to resolve problems in the hospital so that everything is stable prior to the child returning home, when in fact most problems that have led to hospitalization require a significant amount of support through outpatient treatment and monitoring in an effort to maintain changes following discharge. It is often better if problems are left obviously unresolved and requiring further work on an outpatient basis.

Often the family has been reluctant to inform neighbors, family members, or school personnel that their child was in psychiatric hospital and may wish to maintain secrecy and risk isolation of the family upon returning home from the hospital. We advise families to let important people, especially school personnel, know that their child has been in a psychiatric hospital because their child will need consistent, patient support upon returning to school. Children who have been hospitalized, especially for disruptive behavior, become anxious either prior to or at the time of discharge, leading to worsening challenges of authority and discipline-related difficulties. The adolescent who has been hospitalized will often try to deny the reality of the hospitalization and attempt to return to school and to the peer group as if nothing were wrong and he or she has no special needs for help or assistance after discharge. As stated previously, it is essential that a discharge plan and date be set as soon as possible in the course of a family's treatment in a psychiatric hospital. That allows for continued focus upon returning home and sets a schedule for saying good-bye.

The inpatient staff must also be prepared to support the child and family's decision making and to expect the family to deal with symptomatic disruption with straightforward support rather than intensive staff intervention. The more openly difficulties associated with discharge are spoken about in therapy meetings and in informal gatherings among the staff, the more straightforward family members are in identifying their sadness at leaving and their concern about their ability to continue to make progress at home. Although it is important that each child's discharge be identified and celebrated by the staff, other patients, and families, it is also necessary that the staff treat discharge as just one event among many that occurs every day. We ask the outpatient therapist to meet with the family and the inpatient therapist prior to the child's discharge from the hospital. This allows for an orderly transfer of responsibility as well as clarity among family members about the issues that the inpatient therapist is describing to the outpatient therapist and for which the outpatient therapist will take responsibility and direct his or her attention. By meeting the family in the hospital, the therapist gains personal experience with the degree of calm, order, and connection that the family has established within the hospital. Other methods of maintaining connection between the family and the hospital can prove useful in bridging the transition from inpatient to outpatient care, particularly that of encouraging the child to write about the progress at school and at home at some point after discharge, and perhaps even planning a joint meeting 1 or 2 months after hospitalization, at which point family members can demonstrate to the inpatient therapist their success at maintaining and improving their situation through the transition period to home. The outpatient therapist may also be invited to continue to call and check with the inpatient therapist when difficulties arise so that there can be continuity of approach to both the family and the child. In addition, inpatient staff can agree to make follow-up phone calls in a planned way at specific intervals after discharge.

The most problematic situations occur when there is a new outpatient therapist who has not had the opportunity to meet with the family during hospitalization. This should not happen, but some agencies do not allow therapists to meet with families prior to their discharge, and it is often challenging for that therapist to engage the family after they have returned home. In those situations, communication with the inpatient treatment team and expectations for orienting the new outpatient therapist to the structure, content, and progress of treatment can be very helpful. The reluctance of treatment programs to continue with treatment after hospitalization, especially when hospitalization has been seen, perhaps, as a way of decreasing the level of involvement is an additional problem. Treatment following hospitalization should be maintained at prehospital levels or greater. An interim period of home-based treatment or intensive outpatient treatment is often useful. The child usually needs a more intensive educational support system, such as day treatment or special education classes after the diagnostic work. Such placements can be stigmatizing for the child, so additional support is needed for this. Every child discharged from family-oriented psychiatric hospitalization should be identified as the responsibility of a designated school professional who will meet with that child regularly and work on improving social relationships within the school environment. When additional systems such as pediatricians or the legal system have been involved prior to or during hospitalization, clear plans for the involvement of those professionals with the family and the outpatient mental health therapist will need to be made. It is also useful to identify what difficulties can occur when the child goes home, what everyone might do if things became significantly disruptive, how emergencies might be handled, and what if any would be reasons for rehospitalization. These ideas often further decrease the family's anxiety as well as orient the outpatient therapist toward helping the family maintain gains made in the hospital and continue to develop. If the hospitalization has been at all successful, that success has been accrued through extraordinary effort on the part of child, family members, primary treating therapist, and hospital staff. It is also important that everyone take a minute and congratulate each other for their work.

Case Illustrations

As Shawna prepared for discharge with her mother and grandmother, there were several important aspects of the transition that the inpatient staff needed to attend to. The staff, the mother, and Shawna all spoke with school professionals. While on pass, Shawna had an opportunity to meet the counselor who would be assigned as her primary contact person in the school setting. School professionals were encouraged to enlist Shawna in pursuing academic success upon her return to school, as she was clearly able to do well in school. In the concluding several sessions held in the hospital with the mother, grandmother, sisters, and Shawna, the inpatient therapist and one staff person who had been working with Shawna focused on the ability of each individual to remain open to each other, to listen before reacting, to decrease impulsivity, and to maintain engagement and not quit on conversations or relationships when people seemed critical, stressed, or frustrated. The inpatient therapist reiterated that the family was a team that included the grandmother, Shawna, and her sisters, with the mother in charge. During the last pass home, Shawna became angry with her mother because of a restriction, and the mother, as instructed, called the inpatient staff prior to engaging Shawna in disagreement. The staff supported the mother to maintain calm, hold firm to her expectation that Shawna stay at home, and have lunch with the family prior to returning to the hospital. Upon the family's return to the hospital, the primary therapist spoke with the family about the way in which Shawna's challenge and her anger were a way for Shawna to learn whether her mother would hear her voice and experience her upset without becoming critical or giving up on her limits.

An appointment was made with the outpatient therapist identified by Shawna's mother. The inpatient therapist also spoke with the outpatient therapist, reiterating several important points: (1) continuing to talk could be painful; (2) family members should try not to burden each other while neglecting to request help and support when stressed; (3) they might feel that their need for emotional support was a sign of weakness rather than strength; and (4) the ensuing 2 months would offer everyone in the family a chance to get to know each other in a new way in which people would be more open and there would be more patient attention to a process of solving difficulties gradually, rather than attempting to fix things impulsively at the minute that they occurred. The mother was able to ask Shawna to be patient with her, especially when she was stressed by work, and at the same time to not give up on her when she was overwhelmed or tired. Everyone on the staff encouraged Shawna about returning to school, reminded her to appreciate her strengths and interests, and congratulated Shawna's mother and grandmother for their successful work in the hospital. The outpatient therapist was not able to attend the meeting in the hospital prior to discharge, but a conversation was held by phone with the mother, grandmother, outpatient therapist, and inpatient therapist reviewing these issues and outlining the availability of the inpatient therapist for consultation. Further, Shawna was invited to return to the hospital, as it was not far from home, in 2 weeks to visit and to let everyone know how she was doing. Follow-up in this case indicated that an 8-month course of weekly therapy, often involving the mother alone or the mother and grandmother alone, led to Shawna's successful resumption of normal school activities, and a 2-year follow-up after the conclusion of therapy indicated that Shawna had been doing well at age 16, with no further suicide attempts and no further episodes of significant depression or disruption at home.

As Fred approached discharge from the inpatient unit, there was increasing clarity about his degree of distractibility, overactivity, and impulsivity, his response to firm but straightforward limits and consequences, the usefulness of Ritalin for his ADHD, his ability to gradually trust adults, and his need for consistent effort in assisting with social relationships with other children his age. His difficulty in learning to read and his tendency to become frustrated when he wasn't able to perform as well as he and others hoped also was appreciated by his inpatient treatment team and his mother and father.

The primary concern of the treatment team was whether the consistency that had been developed during the hospitalization with the parents sharing parenting and involvement with Fred and the mother being patient and available to play with and enjoy her son could be maintained past discharge. The inpatient therapist challenged the father directly about his willingness to continue involvement with his son and his ability to maintain availability and to be responsible to provide child support. The therapist was careful to encourage each parent to parent Fred independently, rather than rely upon each other to help or make up for their own difficulties or areas of apprehension and concern. Fred's father was encouraged to maintain the mental health treatment that he had initiated shortly after Fred's admission, and the inpatient therapist spoke with the father's therapist about the need to encourage the father to be consistent in his treatment and consistent in his relationship with Fred. The father's tendency to become expansive, promise too much, fail, and quit was made apparent to him, and he was directly challenged that that pattern would be destructive to Fred, perhaps even more than his not being available at all. The rewards for the father in having a relationship with both Fred and his younger sister were stressed, and the father was able to talk about how much he had missed seeing his children during the period of time when he had not kept up with regular visits. Fred's outpatient therapist was encouraged to schedule separate meetings with Fred and each of his parents on a regular basis so that the therapist would be the one who was working to help Fred's father to stay involved with him rather than the mother.

Fred's mother was also encouraged to think more clearly about whether she wanted compensation for previous abandonment by her ex-husband or whether she would settle for consistent involvement in the present and in the future. During the last few nights of hospitalization, Fred's mother came to the hospital to play with her son in the evening and help him calm himself and get to bed successfully at bedtime. She was also helped to identify points at which she became frustrated and over-whelmed so that she could discuss this with the outpatient therapist when those difficulties arose. She was further encouraged to plan to involve the baby-sitter, neighbors, and her extended family in the care of her house and her daughter so that she would continue to have time to play with and read to Fred. A final review was held of the effects of Ritalin, and the mother's need to administer the medicine on a regular basis and Fred's need to be responsive to the mother's directions concerning the use of medi-cine were reiterated. Both outpatient therapist and parents were encouraged to talk with the school to arrange the development of a special placement for Fred that would support his learning to read and be able to accommo-date to his specific learning disabilities.

Both parents also were encouraged to be sure that they knew how to establish and maintain consistent time outs for Fred if he were to be-come resistant or aggressive and to maintain patience with themselves as they went through that process. Ultimately, both parents were encouraged to appreciate the sadness associated with a true recognition of Fred's differ-ences and difficulties as well as a sense of optimism that he would be able to learn and develop with their support. The parents were encouraged to attend a parents' support group for parents of children with ADHD, and they were able to attend a meeting during hospitalization as well as to plan continued attendance after discharge. There was cautious opti-mism at the time of Fred's discharge. The outpatient therapist seemed most thankful for the inpatient treatment, especially for the clarity that had been established about Fred's condition and the opportunity to involve Fred's father in a consistent way. She also appreciated the support and reassur-ance that the mother had received in the hospital. Two-year follow-up indicated that Fred continued to be overactive and impulsive but much better regulated on Ritalin. He was attending school regularly in special education class for his reading disability, but had made some improve-ment in his self-confidence and slight improvement in peer relationships. Fred had developed an interest in soccer and basketball and was playing these sports regularly. The mother continued to have primary responsi-bility for Fred and his sister, while the father had maintained monthly visits with the children and monthly attendance in outpatient therapy ses-sions. He had continued with his outpatient treatment and had been able to obtain and manage a regular job.

CONCLUSION

In all situations of inpatient psychiatric hospitalization for acute problems, the family can be involved in a spirit of respect, acceptance, and explora-tion, and the family members can be oriented to an understanding of who their child is and of what some of their child's needs may be. The parents' ability to take advantage of the support offered by inpatient staff may vary; however, the experience will remain a rich and ultimately reaffirming one for family members as long as the staff involve them, believe in them, and care about them. In no circumstance will this obviate the need for continued attention to the needs of the child and support for the family, but in many situations it may help family members be able to utilize that support effectively as they and their children grow into the future.

REFERENCES

Brendler, J. (1987). A perspective on the brief hospitalization of whole families. *Journal of Family Therapy, 9,* 113–130.

Brendler, J., & Combrinck-Graham, L. (1986). The treatment of hospitalized families of young children. In L. Combrinck-Graham (Ed.), *Treating young children in family therapy* (pp. 85–95). Rockville, MD: Aspen.

Brendler, J., Silver, M., Haber, M., & Sargent, J. (1991). *Madness, chaos and violence: Therapy with families at the brink.* New York: Basic Books.

Combrinck-Graham, L. (1985). Hospitalization as a therapeutic intervention. In R. Ziffer (Ed.), *The use of adjunctive techniques in family therapy* (pp. 99–124). New York: Grune & Stratton.

Combrinck-Graham, L., Gursky, R., & Brendler, J. (1982). Hospitalization of single-parent families of disturbed children. *Family Process, 21,* 131–152.

Pfeifer, S. J., & Strzelecki, S. C. (1990). Inpatient psychiatric treatment of children and adolescents. *Journal of the American Academy of Child and Adolescent Psychiatry, 29*(6), 847–853.

8

Organizing the Hierarchy around Children in Placement

Michael R. Fox

In the last 20 years, many improvements have been introduced in treating abused children in foster placement, yet treatment failures keep occurring at an alarming rate. Why? To some extent, there is continued confusion over role responsibilities and the meanings of the terms *treatment* and *change*. But failures continue primarily because the *process* of treatment decision making and implementations has not changed.

Haley (1977, 1980) supports this emphasis with his well-known definition of a therapist's job as not changing *people,* but changing the *context* in which their problems occur. According to Haley (1963, 1977, 1980) and Madanes (1981, 1984), change is effected through hierarchical reorganization of the systems in which the problem exists. In the context of treating abused children in foster care, this means that decision-making processes are crucial in this hierarchical reordering, and the preferred treatment goal is systemic change in the total context for decision making (Fox, 1990). When this happens, families can then take responsibility for solving their own problems.

The therapist's dilemma is a strategic one: How to direct therapy without undermining the family's sense of strength and autonomy? This chapter presents a method that *directly* empowers birth families with *complete* authority to make *all* treatment decisions while their child is in residential treatment, but only after the hierarchy of responsibility for change at various systemic levels has been clarified. This method thereby setting up a different division of labor between therapist, treatment team, birth family, social services, and the judicial system.

This chapter focuses on children in residential placement to illustrate both the necessity and the obstacles to implementing a pervasive ecological reorganization that will enable extremely disorganized families with histories of abuse and neglect to re-form and care for themselves. The implementation of this model requires that the reorganization be consistent throughout the hierarchy, from the child to the department of child welfare. I tried to implement this approach in one residential treatment center, only to find out after 14 months that it was not possible to alter the collusion in the larger system that helps the family remain out of control. However, the approach is more broadly applicable, as I will illustrate. For example, foster parents or in-home staff can substitute for "treatment system." And since parenting arrangements often differ from traditional two-parent models, when I refer to "birth parents" or "family," the reader can substitute the appropriate configuration.

FIRST- AND SECOND-ORDER CHANGE

Watzlawick, Weakland, and Fisch (1974) hypothesize that a system can change in two ways. First-order change occurs when specific individual parameters within the system shift in a continuous step-by-step manner, while the structure being impacted remains unaltered. Traditional (nonsystemic) intervention approaches usually introduce first-order changes. They reconfigure common variables: more or different medications, different foster placements, different caseworkers or therapists, changes in birth family contract. Often these changes are followed by relapse and further escalation, not resolution.

Second-order change operates discontinuously, by leaps and bounds. Watzlawick et al. (1974) defined it as a change in the rules governing the system's structure or internal order. A second-order *intervention* introduces a change in the rules governing how decisions are made and implemented, thus altering the system's structure.

So how can we introduce second-order change into the structure of the therapy process in a way that will *directly empower* families and treatment? Such intervention would require therapists to reconsider their focus of treatment and change their ideas about their roles. It would mean including in the expanded focus not just the birth family system and the social service system, but the mental health care system. It would radically reconsider the rules about how decisions are made and implemented in all three systems, not just the birth family system.

Assumptions about the problem that are not in fact part of the problem prevent effective solution finding. In unsuccessful treatment we develop solutions based on such limiting assumptions, which are then tried over and over without success. For example, many therapists believe one must understand the underlying dynamics or obtain an accurate diagnosis before starting treatment, when solutions to complex problems often have little to do with assumed causes. Similarly, when a therapist focuses on parental personality rather than the incongruent system in which they must raise children, solutions tend to keep parents and children separated until the parents are "better," instead of creating contexts in which they can function more effectively given their personalities.

Therapists who assume that the problem, cause, or solution lies inside persons other than themselves, rarely evaluate their assumptions that they are not at fault in unsuccessful treatment, and thus do more of the same interventions that ultimately contribute to relapse and failure. For example, psychiatrists treating a family member with a relapsing mental illness frequently prefer searching for a better medication rather than changing the context that undermines effective treatment or using psychosocial interventions.

I propose a system resting on three basic assumptions:

1. Change is predicated not on understanding a problem's source, but on creating a total context that allows a family to discover effective solution finding (de Shazer, 1985). Creating this new context requires structural shifts by each system in how it helps the family.
2. Second-order change is only possible after representatives of all systems accept clearly defined role responsibilities. The roles of therapist and treatment system as agents of change are clearly preserved, preventing contamination by other roles such as social control agent, researcher, or advocate (Haley, 1980).
3. Simultaneously incongruent overt and covert hierarchies structure every treatment relationship, and thus determine each system's solution-finding process. In order to effect second-order change, one must be able to neutralize these incongruent hierarchies (Madanes, 1984).

Imber-Black (1988) stated that reorganizing the family's helping ecology was the proper first therapeutic step for families with multisystem problems. This means reorganizing *how* each system's professionals provide help to the family, and most importantly, how all the professionals interact with each other. Therefore, a "helping ecology" solution to treating children in placement requires changes in the structures of the child, the family, social services, the judicial system, the treatment system, and, most importantly, the relationships among all the systems.

This model requires therapists to take responsibility for reorganizing the helping ecology in a way that respects each system's role responsibility. It reorganizes

- how the family relates to their child in treatment and to the treatment team,
- how the treatment team relates to the family system,
- how social service providers relate to family members, and
- how social service providers relate to the treatment team.

PROBLEMS FOR WHICH THE MODEL IS A SOLUTION

From my experience, five problem areas must be neutralized to treat foster care cases effectively:

1. *Confusion over each system's role responsibilities.* As Haley (1980) stated, professionals in a helping ecology are often confused. Are they agents of social control or change? Social service providers who function as agents of social control frequently prove ineffective when given the task of producing change in families. Therapists are often rendered impotent when they assume or are charged with social control responsibilities.

To facilitate treatment, a context of segregated roles is needed. Social service providers must receive adequate information from treatment teams to make decisions and exercise their legal social control responsibility, but they must also cede sole treatment responsibility to the treatment team and implement limits on birth families. Treatment teams, who function as agents of change, must be protected from an overlay of social control responsibility.

2. *Disempowerment of abusive birth parents by societal agents.* Society disempowers abusive parents to protect their children and coerces parents into learning "noncoercive" child-rearing methods. This is a fundamental incongruence. Since most abusive birth parents grew up in coercive families themselves, they respond with passive resistance and act in powerful ways that disempower treatment.

Frequently, birth parents are required to change before they are permitted significant involvement with their children in placement. Often there is little therapeutic interaction between the parents and children, and few supervised visits. With the change process segregated thus on two separate lines, systemic integration of change into the family is difficult. In addition, little responsibility for change is placed on the children. Obviously, systemic reorganization is needed to safely integrate and empower the birth parents in treatment.

3. *The isomorphic patterns of inconsistency in all systems.* All too often the inconsistency at all levels of the helping ecology is isomorphic with the family's history of inconsistency. Families usually experience the social service provider as combined policeman, judge, and jury rather than as a concerned social agent willing to assist in facilitating change. With the typical frequent turnover of supervisors and caseworkers comes altered contracts, threats, and ultimatums that cannot or will not be implemented, and a general chaos that thwarts the social worker's effectiveness as well as the process of family change. It is no surprise that the family does not take societal agents seriously.

This scenario, in turn, is isomorphic with the caseworker's complaints about birth families who have no clear, consistent plan to deal with the child's behavior. Roles and expectations change capriciously. Consequences are not forthcoming consistently. Ultimata are not followed through. Threats of separating the child from parent are used to exert control, but often remain threats until unexpectedly the child is removed by social services.

After months or years of different caseworkers, nonspecific contracts and inconsistent limitsetting, birth parents are held accountable for *their* lack of attention, and the children are put into placement. Too often children lose their families because of the helping system's lack of attention and consistency. Thus, therapists must take responsibility for reorganizing not only the family, but also the social control system, so as to interrupt destructive patterns.

4. *Difficulties in setting limits on professional colleagues who break agreements.* Just like families, professionals at all levels are often unable or unwilling to comply with contracts. In order to effectively empower the treatment process and introduce second-order change into the family, all professionals must be empowered by their administrators to consistently implement contractual consequences for irresponsibility by birth parents and their professional colleagues.

When social service providers refuse or are unable to implement previously agreed-on parental consequences, the treatment team's administrator must empower them to implement limits on the workers. In such cases, treatment should be terminated, because the family recognizes that the treatment team has no power delegated to them by social services, and change ceases. Similar dynamics arise when the team's administrator refuses to support their decision to terminate treatment. In such situations, the family's pattern of irresponsibility is replicated in both professional systems. No one in any of the three systems surrounding the child is respecting the contracts.

The birth parents again experience society as not serious in its demands, and denial increases. As a result, children learn to tolerate abuse and work the system, at least until they escape being child victims and become adult victims, or themselves the next generation of abusers.

5. *Expansion of the predominant focus of protecting children to include reorganizing families and/or relationships between helping systems.* In abuse cases, most professional empathy and protection is directed toward the child, not the family as a whole. A better system would also protect (birth) parents from abuse by the treatment and social service systems with whom they must interface.

AUTHORITY AND HIERARCHY STRUCTURES IN TREATMENT

The next step is understanding that viable solutions are derived from an interactive decision-making process within and between the family, treatment system, and surrounding larger systems. Unsuccessful solutions result from habitual static decision-making processes within and between systems at any level. Thus the ultimate key, requiring serious reconsideration, is the distribution of power and authority throughout the total system.

The power to change or maintain behavior does not lie solely within institutions or individuals, including therapists. Therapists have little if any intrinsic power to change any problem. Therapists can change themselves by utilizing their own personal authority and power, but the authority and power to change others always comes from those other individuals.

The power to change a family lies in the rules governing the process of decision making: *how* everyone involved relates to each other (Fox, 1990), not *what* therapists or caseworkers do. In order to help the birth family find and develop more successful solutions, therapists must concentrate on *how* everyone, at all levels, makes and implements decisions about *what* is done to change the disturbing behavior between the child and birth family. When treatment is unsuccessful, therapists must reconsider the hierarchical relationship between the treatment system, the social services system, and the family system regarding decision making.

Individual therapy's hierarchy usually has the therapist at the top, or in the "one-up" complementary position (Haley, 1963), because of his or her "expertise" about the problem. The patient is more "powerful" than the family, by virtue of his or her private relationship with the therapist, while the family members are "one down" because of their relative lack of involvement.

In traditional family-focused treatment, family members are involved and often given special status by the therapist. The hierarchy in family therapy can be seen to reverse the roles of family and identified patient from the traditional therapy hierarchy, with the patient now in the "one-down" position.

Madanes (1984) offers an alternative sense of hierarchy, hypothesizing that when a child becomes ill or behaviorally disturbing, the situation establishes simultaneously incongruent hierarchies. Parents are usually in a one-up position with respect to their child simply because they are being parents, for they are responsible for taking care of and providing for the child. This is especially evident when the child is ill or emotionally upset. However, as the parents desperately struggle to help their child overcome problems, the child—by virtue of her or his inability or unwillingness to change in ways that parents wish—can be seen to defeat the parents' attempts to manage him or her. The parents and child are simultaneously one up and one down.

Following Madanes's theory, simultaneously incongruent hierarchies also operate in treatment situations. Traditionally, the treatment team is viewed in the one-up position, with the patient and the family being placed in the one-down position by virtue of needing the team's help. But when a treatment team appears unable to change the patient effectively, it is hierarchically configured in the same one-down position that was experienced by the family prior to seeking treatment. As the treatment team persists ineffectively, the "recalcitrant" child or family rises in apparent power in the hierarchy.

In family therapy, there are simultaneously incongruent hierarchies that place each component (treatment team, family members, and identified patient) in any of the three hierarchical positions (one up, one down, or in the middle), depending on how the actors in the system view who is more or less powerful. Often, especially with children who have been neglected or abused, the treatment team will form a coalition to protect the child, placing the family in a one-down position and almost guaranteeing the failure of any reunification efforts. When the child does not respond to the treatment process, however, the child may be viewed as one up, and the team and the family struggle to disclaim responsibility for the treatment failure.

These simultaneously incongruent hierarchies operate in all treatment situations, but are usually denied by all involved. Operating only from the position that the treatment team should be in charge, as the correct approach with children in placement, leaves the child and family members only covert ways of influencing treatment and usually leads to struggles for control and the manifestation of the other hierarchical arrangements that are unrecognized. Even when a child is severely ill or disorganized, the effect of these simultaneously incongruent hierarchies is paradoxical: It empowers the child or the family members, leaving them covertly in charge of the treatment process, and the team disempowered. As the end result, treatment is rendered ineffective.

THE UNIQUE HIERARCHICAL ASPECTS OF FOSTER CARE

Treating children in placement or under protective supervision creates additional hierarchical issues. From my perspective of the treatment team, there are two care providers — the social service system and the treatment team — and three consumers of the team's services — the child, the social services, and the birth family. But from my experience of the social services system, the caseworker usually sees only the family as the focus and consumer of treatment.

The model proposed here views social services as the primary consumer of the team's services, and the child and family as secondary consumers. Social services admits the child into treatment with the family and pays the fee. The treatment system agrees to the purchase of its services by social services, as long as both social services and the family desire admission and comply with specific contracts.

Space does not allow description of all possible simultaneously incongruent hierarchies. When the team cannot achieve the change desirable to the other systems, a common hierarchical organization emerges that seems to be run by the judicial system, followed by the social services system, the identified patient (child), family members, and, finally, the treatment team, in the ultimate one-down position.

Terry was a 6-year-old boy referred for residential placement after failing in foster care homes for the past year. His continuing problems included temper tantrums, inappropriate sexual behavior and urinating, running away, "night stalking," and setting fires. The father was a recovering alcoholic who previously abused the mother. The mother lived separate from the father, acknowledged past drug abuse and was being evaluated for Dissociative Identity Disorder. Child care was done by the mother and her mother, often with bitter arguments. At age 3, Terry was found performing sex acts with little girls on two occasions, which led to Terry disclosing he observed the father watching pornographic movies. There was little behavioral change after a psychiatric hospitalization, two years of treatment, and Ritalin.

After an initial intense struggle between the team, social services, and the family, and a threatened denial of admission, treatment went relatively smoothly. For the first time, the mother and father worked collaboratively and incorporated the staff's concerns. The grandmother had some difficulty with the father's limit setting and great difficulty getting Terry's uncle to attend sessions. Terry rapidly progressed in privilege levels, but lost his first home visit privilege the week before his annual judicial review. His parents and grandmother were devastated and found fault with the staff's strict adherence to the rules that had been established by his mother.

The therapist was unable to attend the judicial review hearing, because of illness. No substitute was available. With the foster care worker present, the mother explained the situation from her perspective and requested the weekend home visit that had been denied according to the contract. The judge ordered the visit, anyway, and the staff permitted him to go. Thus the hierarchy described above was instituted.

As this was early in the program's development, the team's disempowerment by the family, social services, and judicial systems was handled differently than a subsequent disempowerment (to be discussed later). We assumed the problem arose because of boundary testing and lack of information. In a meeting with the family and the foster care worker, the therapist reiterated the importance of everyone maintaining agreements, despite disappointment on everyone's part. The staff informed them that if any similar problems were to arise, Terry would be discharged to the custody of social services. In a meeting where the program's philosophy and procedures were explained, the judge apologized and affirmed his support for the program, agreeing to inform the other judicial staff. Treatment progressed satisfactorily.

AN ALTERNATIVE SOLUTION

The therapeutic challenge is, how does a team acknowledge the reality of its one-down position yet empower the birth family and safely effect treatment? One way follows Haley's (1977, 1988) recommendation that therapists arrange the treatment situation to approximate the dynamics that normally occur with families: That is, families occupy the hierarchical level between their child and society's supervisory systems, who remain in the background as long as the family is responsible and uses nonabusive child-rearing methods. This model strives for a hierarchy that places family members at the same level with the judicial and social service systems: That is, guiding the treatment system, with the treatment team subordinate to them, and the child in the ultimate one-down position, appropriate to his or her age and station.

When the family and larger systems are reorganized with clear roles and responsibilities for everyone involved, and the reality of the treatment team's one-down position is accepted, the family members will find their own solutions. From another perspective, when the systemic configuration for a nonabusive family is created in the abnormal situation of treatment, the abusive family will find its own solutions.

In this approach, the goal of safely reuniting abused children with their birth parents is achieved through *direct empowerment,* after specifically designed contracts between the family, treatment team, and social services are developed, to neutralize the problems described above. When contracts are completed, the treatment team gives real power to the birth family by delegating its authority to make all treatment decisions concerning their child to the involved family.

The team is hierarchically placed between the family members and child because it implements the family's decisions about the child, and the child has no authority to change the family's or team's decisions. The team is the implementing agent for the family, after the family has accepted contractual agreement that highly structures their relationship with the larger system, the team, and their child.

In summary, the four steps to arranging this hierarchy are:

1. Posit the family as the most important resource of the helping ecology.
2. Change the process of team treatment (meta-rule intervention, see below).
3. Change the process of family decision making/implementation (decision-making intervention, see below).
4. Develop specific contracts with defined consequences for noncompliance, binding on all three helping systems: treatment, social services, and family.

THE META-RULE INTERVENTION

I began utilizing the meta-rule intervention (Fox, 1985, 1988, 1990) in 1978 after realizing I was confusing the power to change patients with my medical authority to make treatment decisions. Clearly, family members have more power than I previously acknowledged. So, under safe conditions, why not give the family my authority to make the decisions, since they have the ultimate power to decide what they will do anyway? The cornerstone for therapists is the acceptance that they are powerless unless they accrue power from the family.

The intervention changes the process of therapy in a way that neutralizes the simultaneous incongruent hierarchies. It requires therapists to acknowledge overtly that while the team has power over the process of *how* therapy is conducted, everyone else but the team has power over *what* will and will not be done in treatment. It changes the process of *how* the family system and the team work together in deciding *what* will be done to treat the child and family, in a way that directly empowers the family. The meta-rule is explained to families as follows:

Our goal is to create a different treatment experience for you and your child and to increase the likelihood that change will proceed in the way you desire and will be maintained after discharge. In order to assure those goals, the treatment team is willing to change how it makes and implements decisions about your child's treatment, in exchange for your help.

If you agree, the staff will do *what*ever you, as parents, decide is the best treatment for your child, as long as the team is allowed to prescribe exactly *how* those decisions are made and implemented by you. You will make all treatment decisions about what you and the team will be doing to help your child and family. We will keep this agreement, as long as

- everyone involved, professionals and family, maintain their commitments to the contracts that will be developed between social services, the team, and the family;
- the decisions do not expose anyone to grave risk of harm or liability; and
- the family makes the decisions according to a process the team prescribes.

The team is comfortable accepting your right to decide what is in your best interest, so we support your right to refuse this treatment. However, because we believe any other approach will likely not be successful, we cannot in good faith accept your child without this agreement. If you and your caseworker disagree over the propriety of this approach, we will attempt to help you resolve the difference or, if necessary, suggest alternative placements.

The team maintains complete medical and legal responsibility for all the family's decisions, but is protected from extremes because the decisions cannot expose anyone to risk of harm or liability. Team members function as consultants in the purest sense of the word. They educate and advise the family on the alternatives available and their comparative assets and liabilities, and on the family's right not to make a decision. The team can never veto the family's decisions and is responsible for implementing the family's treatment plan without deviations.

Once agreement is reached on all the contracts, the team must be able to follow through. This is not an engagement strategy. Rather, it is an acknowledgment that the team has no direct power over *what* the family decides to do and that the team is willing to delegate the authority given them by society to the birth family as long as their decisions are within safe, normal practice and legal.

As a result, family members are engaged very differently and feel hopeful and enthusiastic. They usually fight less with the team, except to test whether the team's authority is really delegated. Once they realize the team's commitment and support for any workable decision, families tend to work collaboratively and reasonably with the team — at least until a crisis arises.

However, in order to get this opportunity, the parents must in exchange allow the team three changes it needs to empower the treatment process and change the family. The parents must accept the contracts negotiated with social services, incorporate the team into their system, and delegate to the team their authority over *how* they make and implement decisions regarding their child's behavior.

For example, during the initial visit to the program and exploratory conversations with the mother and grandmother of Terry (described above), both were very excited about the opportunity to be actively involved. They assumed it would be like other psychiatric treatments Terry had received, but only now they would have control over the decisions. There was a great disappointment and concern when they were informed that the father would also be involved, as would any others who lived in the grandmother's home, where the mother currently lived. They were informed that contracts must be agreed on between all three groups, before admission would be confirmed. A meeting between the social service worker and therapist was set. (See also Tanya and Billy, p. 202)

THE FAMILY DECISION-MAKING INTERVENTION

The decision-making intervention (Fox, 1988, 1990, 1991) changes the family's decision-making process based on an assessment of the child's developmental needs, the cyclical sequences between the parenting figures, and their habituated decision-making process regarding the child, which has proven so ineffective. The intervention should create a situation where each parent must participate differently in solution finding with both the child and other parenting figures. Thus, each parent is provided new role responsibilities based not on stereotypical gender-role ascriptions, but on what will effect different role behavior.

Conflict always arises between parents whenever their decision-making process is not clear and previously agreed on. This is especially true when each parent believes he or she has the right to make and implement rules acting on his or her personal authority. As a result, each parent undermines the other's rules and neither supports the other.

In my opinion, parents rarely make and implement decisions regarding their children by mutual consensus. Usually that responsibility is divided. At any one time, one parent is delegated the authority to make and implement decisions, or one is authorized to make the decisions and the other partner is given the authority to implement the decisions. When the process is agreed to in advance, role responsibilities are clear, every family member is empowered to hold the others accountable for maintaining their role responsibilities, and children experience their parents as co-equal authorities.

The decision-making intervention was devised in 1980, in part inspired by Stuart's work (1980), as well as my own frustration with traditional mutual consensus decision making and the sexist aspects of putting one partner in charge and the other on vacation. This intervention divides parental roles into "decision making" and "decision implementing." The "decision-making" parent is authorized (by the therapist or team) to make final decisions on the treatment plan. But he or she can do so only after obtaining input from the team, the child in treatment, and, last, other family members. The decision-implementing parent is authorized to monitor the child's behavior and decide when to implement the decision-making parent's plan. Thus, the child experiences each parent as having different functions, yet co-equal authority.

By the time of referral, each parent believes his or her approach is right and necessary to counteract the other's approach, which leads to a symmetrical escalation as each parent feels defeated by the other's refusal to change. All the while, the child is in effect defeating both. It is a no-win game, seemingly without end. Both parents feel powerless in relation to each other and their child, but usually one is feeling and acting more overtly powerless than the other. That parent is more emotionally escalating, actively provocative, loud, controlling, openly critical of the child and other parent, and intrusively attempting to change the child. This parent is usually the abuser. The other parent is usually more quieting, passively provocative, sympathetic to the child, views the other parent as the problem, sets few limits, tends to talk as a way of helping the child, and acts less abusively.

The therapist prescribes each parent's new role responsibilities based upon his or her pre-treatment behavior. The actively escalating and intrusive parent, who is doing too much and experienced most negatively by others, becomes the decision-making parent. As a result of being given the authority to make all treatment decisions, he or she is encouraged to do less and become more positively involved with the child. The passively escalating parent, who tends to avoid limit setting and withdraws when a conflict arises, becomes the decision-implementing parent, and is delegated authority over when to implement the decision-making parent's plan. As a result he or she becomes more actively engaged in limit setting, less sympathetic, and more supportive of the previously out-of-control parent. The decision-making parent is left free to develop a more positive relationship with the child, since he or she agrees to avoid all overt disciplining.

The team must always follow the decision-making parent's treatment plan. When a decision needs to be made or modified, the team addresses their concern to the actively-escalating decision making parent, who has the authority to accept, modify, or reject any advice given. Similarly, when the team questions whether the child should receive a consequence, they address their quandary to the decision-implementing parent and follow his or her decision.

The goal is eventually for the actively-escalating parent to be completely and overtly supported by the passively-escalating parent and the treatment team, who implement that parent's plan. Simultaneously the actively-escalating parent gives the other parent and the team what they desire: positive and caring involvement.

Once the "out-of-control" parent experiences influence, he or she usually regains control of his or her own behavior, cooperates, and becomes more nurturing toward the child. When the "quieting" parent finds his or her partner changing, becoming more available and less threatening, he or she engages more actively in limit setting. In effect, dynamically and structurally, the assumed covert pattern prior to treatment is reversed.

Terry's parents provide an example of such pattern. The father was very empathic about the difficulties with Terry and preferred to talk with him over setting any limits, as he had had similar problems in childhood. He explained Terry's problems as being due to the mother's erratic and confusing behavior that led to verbal and physical abuse. After Terry's admission, the father offered good advice on the behavioral plans and increasingly supported the mother's decisions and implemented consequences, as he saw the mother change. She became more appropriately nurturing and consistent with Terry and more firm in setting limits on the grandmother's intrusions, insults directed at the father, and noncompliance with attendance contracts.

ARRANGEMENTS AT THE FACILITY AND ROLE OF THE TEAM

The clinical team is all the professionals hired by the administration of the facility to staff the unit and provide direct care to the children and their families, regardless of their degrees or education (this includes nurses, social workers, mental health counselors, psychologists, psychiatrists, and child life specialists, recreational personnel, and psychiatric technicians and aides).

I was hired by the executive director as program developer, after we mutually agreed that I would be the sole decision maker and have final veto power on the program's policies and hiring. After consultation with the administration team, I developed the program's policy and procedures, which were authorized by the administrative team.

The unit director (an MSW) was then hired by me after consultation with the four members of the administrative team — the executive director (an MSW), the assistant to the executive director (an MSW), the admissions and programs director (an MSW) and the child life specialist supervisor. Other program staff members were hired by mutual consensus between the unit director and me. There were twice-monthly meetings between the unit director, director of admissions and programs, the child life coordinator, and me, where administrative problems were resolved by mutual consensus. Decision-making authority on clinical matters remained with me. When the unit was functional, I assumed the roles of program consultant and trainer, and psychiatric consultant. I was directly responsible only to the executive director and assistant director. Training was done via workshops, group and individual one-way mirror and verbal supervision of ongoing cases, case conferences, and staff meetings.

The clinical and administrative functions of the program were patterned after those used with the family. For example, once there was a consensual agreement between the social services agent and the clinical team, the family was admitted, and the parental subsystem was divided into decision-making and decision-implementing functions. Similarly, after there was consensual agreement between the executive director and myself that I was authorized to be the program's decision maker, the functioning of the team's leaders, the unit director and I, was divided. The unit director was given administrative responsibility for the team's functioning and implementing the clinical policy and procedures that had been previously decided by me.

Similarly, any modification of the clinical policy could be decided by only myself after consultation with the administration, the unit director, and other team members via staff meetings and informal discussions. Thus, the pattern utilized with the family was isomorphic with that used in the team's functioning. I was the decision maker and the unit director was the decision implementer, just as one parenting figure was the decision maker and the other the decision implementer.

The unit director authorized the therapist to be the treatment team implementer for each specific case. The therapist was charged with monitoring the progress of treatment and ensuring that every one involved maintained their prescribed roles — that the child's plan could be changed only by the decision-making parent and that the child life staff, decision-implementing parent, and the therapist were implementing the decision-making parent's plan. The Child Life staff were responsible for implementing the decision-making parent's plan while the child was in their care or during a visit where the decision-implementing parent figures were absent. Both the unit director and myself were responsible for monitoring the performance of the therapist and staff.

PREADMISSION AGREEMENTS BETWEEN SYSTEMS

During the initial inquiry phase, before any significant history is obtained, the therapist briefly explains the admission process, treatment format, and the meta-rule intervention to the caseworker and family members. Visits to the program are arranged.

The first negotiation phase involves the caseworker only, and focuses on gathering information concerning the following:

- the social and treatment history of the child,
- the family's past style of dealing with agencies,
- what has been successful in the past, and
- any anticipated compliance problems.

It concludes with agreements outlining expectations and consequences regarding the following:

- behavior that social services and the treatment team expect of each other,
- behavior social services expects of the family, and
- behavior the treatment team expects of the family.

The social services agreement with the treatment team must

- exclude the team from any social control responsibilities,
- exclude the caseworker from any therapeutic responsibility, and
- maintain a commitment not to place the child or deny parental rights, unless the family has demonstrated an inability or unwillingness to change as defined by the agreements.

To insure the viability of these commitments, most aspects of the agreement are nonnegotiable. Social services must incorporate at minimum the following into their agreement with the family, or admission will be denied:

- Any family member living in the child's future home or whom the team believes is important must attend family therapy.
- The family must visit the child at least once per week in addition to participating in a weekly family therapy session.
- Substance abuse is directly addressed; timelines for abstinence must be defined. Attendance at Alcoholics Anonymous and Al-Anon is required in most cases.
- Once home visits are in effect, the birth parents must manage all

behavior nonabusively in their home, instead of returning their child as a punishment or respite.

- The child will be discharged when social services is unable or unwilling to implement previously agreed-on consequences for parental noncompliance or does not keep commitments to support the family or team.
- When problems arise, the caseworker must meet with the team within 14 days; otherwise, the child will be discharged.
- The agreement must outline to the family what information social services and the court require the therapist to divulge, leaving all else confidential. There can be no secret passing of information. If the therapist is ordered by the court to violate confidentiality, which is an intrusion of the court into the treatment, treatment is usually terminated because the family construes it as forcing the therapist into the role of a social control agent.
- Confidentiality must be protected, unless overruled by a viable mutually agreed-upon contract or a law that takes precedence.
- The family must know the caseworker requires the therapist to report any undisclosed abuse and violations of the agreement.
- Violence or intimidation toward *any* family member is violence against children as well as a crime that requires family members to file criminal charges and follow through in court. The consequence for not doing so is the same as for violence toward a child.
- If the family calls a caseworker to ask for advice, the worker must (1) listen and gain information, (2) tell the family to contact the therapist for advice, (3) refuse to give treatment advice unless there is imminent danger, and (4) tell the family he or she will also immediately call the therapist.

Karen's father was a long-standing alcoholic who had been abstinent for the past 6 months following her removal from the home after two previous foster care placements. The father worked inconsistently and the mother suffered from recurrent depressions but refused medication. There had been some substantial change in the 4 months since admission, and Karen had progressed to having brief home visits.

The mother called the caseworker, seeking assistance with the rent payment, and disclosed that the father had started drinking again and was spending most of the rent money. Questions to gain clarity about the situation raised concern that there may have been another episode of spousal abuse. After determining that there was not an immediate safety issue, the caseworker provided the mother with the necessary information, told the mother to call the therapist, called the therapist herself, and recorded the information for future reference, as the drinking and suspected spousal abuse were violations of the contract.

The mother did not call the therapist, so the therapist called the mother. At an emergency session, the mother's safety was confirmed and the details recorded. The resulting crisis over losing home visits and the possible permanent loss of custody of Karen because of the contract violations caused a second-order reorganization in the marital relationship. The father continued to drink, and the mother became more active in Al-Anon and left the home and the father. She later obtained her GED and started a supported employment program.

After the caseworker accepts these conditions, he or she is asked to outline parameters of family behavior, such as the following: How is a missed session/visit defined? How many are allowed within what time frame? What are consequences of substance abuse and positive urine tests? Who is allowed to be with the child? What constitutes adequate housing? What are allowable punishments? and so forth.

Admission is accepted tentatively only when the team is satisfied that the agreements sufficiently hold everyone accountable for irresponsible behavior and, as a result, empower the team and protect them from social control responsibilities.

The next phase is negotiation between the caseworker, family members, child, therapist, and the team member who will be the family's liaison with the team. First, the meta-rule intervention is restated. Then, the caseworker outlines to the family the expectations that the team and social services have of each other, the consequences for noncompliance, the expectations social services has of the family in treatment, and the consequences for noncompliance.

Regardless of pressures from social services, admission is finalized only when the family accepts the meta-rule intervention and the preceding agreements. It is openly discussed, with no hidden agendas. There can be *no* renegotiation about what the optimum treatment plan is. Once the family and the caseworker accept the agreements, the social worker is excused and family therapy begins.

When a caseworker backtracks on the expectations of the family, the therapist must interrupt the meeting and excuse the family until the breach is repaired in a way that protects and empowers the treatment. If agreement cannot be renegotiated, the admission is canceled as per the meta-rule intervention. If the family refuses the agreements, it is rejecting a once-in-a-lifetime opportunity to have nearly complete control over treatment. A therapist should never commit a family or their team to a disempowered treatment process. Therefore, if either the family or social services is unwilling to accept what the therapist believes are optimal treatment conditions, admission is denied until they accept the conditions.

The following case illustrates how mishaps occur even when the protocol is followed, especially when there is role confusion, isomorphic inconsistencies, and professional inability to set firm limits. The importance of using the meta-rule intervention and program policy to manage a crisis and promote systemic change is demonstrated.

After initial program visits and negotiations, Terry's admission session was arranged. There were many surprises. First, two caseworkers arrived, as the case was being transferred. So, the family was excused and expectations of social services and the family were reviewed again. Tension markedly increased as the guidelines for "missed sessions" and "family visits" were negotiated. There was obvious disagreement between the two caseworkers around setting firm limits, especially referral to the Foster Care Review Board, to "show cause for denial of parental rights." Eventually, three missed sessions was set as the limit. Next, reticence over requiring the mother's therapy to be done in the program was resolved by our agreeing to her completing the evaluation.

The session erupted as we restated all family members living in the home must attend treatment sessions. First, grandmother's attendance was an issue. Then we discovered uncle Sam had moved back into the home when Terry entered foster care, despite his chronic PCP and marijuana abuse, erratic work pattern, and violent tempers. The team restated their position. Either Sam must attend or move out permanently. The initial caseworker vehemently protested that he had asked Sam to be involved and enter drug treatment, "but we can't force him," to which the therapist responded, "but Mother can put force on him. Without this agreement, we cannot admit Terry." The caseworkers refused to take that position, and said Terry's mother would have to make that decision.

When the family joined in the session an intense emotional barrage followed, as the mother and caseworkers attempted to change the team's position. The mother initially denied any influence in the grandmother's home, claiming that her mother would have a nervous breakdown if Sam had to leave. The team stated they were powerless to make an exception to the policy. The caseworkers attacked the model as excessively demanding. The mother refused and angrily left the session twice, while the staff patiently waited with the caseworkers. She soon returned with her mother to plead their inability to control Sam. After 45 minutes, the therapist definitively announced that the admission was not possible, but the program would reopen negotiations whenever the family and social services were willing to accept the program policy. As the team got up and left the room, the mother called the team back and agreed to the conditions. Admission was arranged 3 days later. The staff later commented that it was the most intense session they had ever experienced.

IMPORTANCE OF CRISIS POINTS IN THERAPY

Understanding how to utilize crisis in treatment is crucial. When treating seriously disturbing behavior, especially that which is involuntary or coerced by authorities outside the family, little change occurs until a crisis develops. Intermittent small changes may occur, similar to those in previous treatments, but entrenched family structure and solution-finding methods dominate. Whether the crisis is spontaneous or introduced by the team, second-order change occurs only when the crisis is resolved differently, either because of or as a result of a significant change in the structure of the family (i.e., in the assignment of authority and power in decision making).

Usually after the contracts are signed and the behavior plan developed, there is a honeymoon period during which everything goes well. This illusion of a harmonious transformation in the family is only one segment of a multifaceted circular sequence, which prior to treatment normally lasted a few moments or hours and was followed by relapse, that is, by the resurgence of other segments in the systemic circle.

The family's agreement to change their structure with the decision-making intervention in exchange for control over decisions eventually provokes a crisis, when the long-term effects of the intervention become apparent. What actually makes a difference and precipitates second-order change is that family members have agreed to be incorporated into the treatment team in exchange for complete control over decisions. But their inclusion is contingent on maintaining new role responsibilities during this crisis. As a result, the conflict is not between family members and the team, but between family members only where it should be, since they are the ones who will reap the benefits and suffer the havoc of resolving the crisis differently.

The crisis usually occurs when the decision-implementing parent blatantly does not implement the decision-making parent's plan; the old behavior cycle reinstates itself. During the crisis, the team maintains its role responsibility and commitment to the decision-making prescription, and follows only the decision maker's plan. The team provides both parent support and strategies to help them maintain or recapture their role behavior throughout the crisis until the basic family structure has changed. To effect such change, the decision-making parent is supported to detach emotionally and maintain a positive caring involvement with the child and the other parent and to avoid returning to old reactive patterns. The structural change at this point takes one of three forms. Either (1) the family violates their social services contract, which leads to denial of parental rights, permanent placement, or adoption, or (2) the decision-implementing parent returns to consistently implementing the plan, or (3) one parent makes an unequivocal move to change the marital relationship. Whatever occurs, there is a structural change in the family.

The crisis can occur, however, when another member of the larger social system also acts in disregard of the agreements. Often this is an individual who has not directly participated in the agreement, as is true of the judge, in Terry's case. In this instance, the administrative and clinical teams effectively collaborated to neutralize the judge's potential undermining of the treatment process.

INSTITUTIONAL STRUCTURAL AGREEMENTS

During 1988 and 1989, this model was utilized in a foster care residential facility that had previously functioned virtually as an orphanage. Little was done to encourage family reunification. After years of discussions, the director asked me to develop a program. Over the next 3 months, discussions centered on changes the institution would undergo in order to effectively respond to reactions in the foster care system that the program would evoke. After 4 months of staff workshops, writing the treatment and research protocols to deal with those reactions, and hiring staff, the program as outlined in this chapter was approved. The following vignette illustrates how crucial these institutional structural agreements both empower and disempower the processes of change.

Tanya and Billy, ages 10 and 7, respectively had already been residents in the facility for over 18 months with little involvement of their mother, a severe alcoholic and addict who had abused them since birth. Their father was not known. They were only moderately disruptive on the unit, but lost control whenever foster home placement was discussed. The administration hoped the program could entice the mother's involvement, since she was attempting detoxification and treatment. Otherwise, the children were doomed to long-term residential placement. The mother quickly responded and the children were admitted.

Within 8 weeks, the situation deteriorated. The mother nearly violated the missed session provisions, was verbally abusive on the unit, and was asked to leave once because of suspected intoxication. At the mother's urging and with strong support from the caseworker, a brief home visit was arranged, because the children had met their home visit criteria. The mother returned the children severely beaten. There was subsequent difficulty contacting the caseworker, who reluctantly agreed to bring the case before the Foster Care Review Board after the staff threatened to call her supervisor. The staff continued attempts to contact the mother, who made no further visits. Home visits were denied.

While the team mobilized their administration to deal with the caseworker's noncompliance, the mother went for her annual judicial review and requested a weekend visit with relatives in another state. With the caseworker present, and not protesting, the judge ordered the staff to release the children for the visit in the custody of an uncle whom no one knew, or had met. Since the social service's violation of the contract was so egregious, the team informed the administration of their reasons for discharging the children in 14 days, with another placement or not. Immediately, the administration informed the team that it would not authorize the discharges.

The program's power to produce change was first challenged by the mother's violation of her contract with the team and social services. Next, the social service system's contractual noncompliance and overt support of a weekend visit in the face of recent abuse made treatment impossible. When the team's own administration withdrew its authorization by abrogating on policy, the program and its change process were disempowered. What was thought to be second-order change in the treatment system was in fact only first-order change. Under pressure from other elements in the larger system, the administration withdrew decision-making authority from the program and forced its return to the previous structure—an orphanage for abused children.

There were three possible responses: (1) accept the reversion back to an orphanage, (2) engage the administration in dialogue to re-establish the policy, or (3) abandon the program. Six weeks of attempted renegotiation failed. The administration was unwilling to set limits on social services, allegedly because it would endanger the placement of children and cause further upheaval in the foster care system. Despite having forecast these problems and addressed them in the initial phases of the program, they now viewed it as an unworkable concept. I resigned as program consultant, according to a protocol we mutually agreed on. The program apparently continued, but with only a shadow of its previous family involvement.

Trainers must always work at the interface between themselves and the agency system that hires and authorizes them. Even with that interface in view, even with contingencies mutually agreed upon early in the endeavor, trainers fail. Their impact is undermined by the dominant organizational structure and its response to the vicissitudes of change that underlie the treatment problems of children in placement. As a result, second-order change in the child's family system is difficult, if not impossible. In my opinion, continuing treatment within a flawed organizational system does not allow a team to empower families in any direct way, and should therefore be avoided.

WHEN THE MODEL WORKS: AN ILLUSTRATION

The experience in the residential placement system illustrated and confirmed the hypotheses about organization and hierarchy being the underlying essentials of perpetual dysfunction in the families whose children inhabit this system. While, for a time, I was able to influence these structures within the institution and at its immediate interfaces with families and caseworkers, in the long run I did not have the power to influence the larger administration of the child welfare system. Yet the model is an effective organizing tool for difficult families, as the following vignette, from an outpatient context, illustrates:

Mr. K and his family were referred by Child Protective Services (CPS) to the Johns Hopkins Hospital Family Therapy Clinic (JHH) for treatment. Teachers had noted extensive bruises on the 9-year-old son, Charlie. The abuse was reported anonymously, because, when confronted, Mrs. K refused to file a complaint against her husband, out of fear of more severe violence.

Mr. and Mrs. K had been married 15 years. He was employed and supported the family of five children living in the home. Five adult children from Mrs. K's first marriage lived out of the home. Mr. K had a long-standing history of alcoholism and physical abuse of his wife and the children. He was a strict, but ineffective disciplinarian who claimed to abuse only when drinking. Mrs. K's history of abuse preceded both of her abusive marriages.

In the first session with the CPS worker, alone, the following treatment agreements were developed:

- Any replacement worker was bound to implement the plan.
- Mr. K had chosen JHH for treatment, so was mandated to attend regularly and follow all directives.
- If Mr.K decided not to participate with any part of the plan, once developed, CPS would obtain an order of protective supervision to remove him from the home.
- If Mr. K abused the children or his wife, Mrs. K was to seek safety, inform CPS and the team, file charges against her husband, and follow through with a court trial. If she failed to take these steps, she should be described as colluding with the abuse and endangering her children.
- The team would expect alcohol abstinence and mandatory reporting of AA and Al-Anon attendance. Mrs. K was to report any violations.
- The team was required to report any new or newly disclosed abuse and violations to the CPS worker.
- Any individual treatment for Mrs. K would be done by the team.

As the CPS worker informed the family of the conditions of treatment, Mr. K appeared visibly defiant, and Mrs. K looked frightened, while the children were noisy and demeaning toward the father. After clarifying questions were answered, the worker left the session. When the therapist asked each family member what changes were needed to reestablish the family's integrity and end the abuse, the father responded that he didn't think he wanted to start and would appreciate it if we go on to the others and come back to him, later. After being told several times to take his time because we were interested in his perspective, he denied abusing his children, stating that a father just has to smack kids on the backside to teach them right. Initially the therapist challenged his denial, but later accepted Mr. K's definition of the problem as the children needing discipline that was not being adequately provided by his wife. Mrs. K quickly noted that the problem was Mr. K's drinking, but she confirmed that the children misbehaved, but it was not a problem for her. The children all concurred that their father needed to stop hitting them.

Mr. K was noncommittal about returning, though he understood that he was constrained to return or leave home. In closing, the team acknowledged that there was validity to each family member's perspective on the problems and that our responsibility was to create a situation where people could find effective solutions to problems in an atmosphere free from violence, fear, and intimidation. We underscored that future violence or intimidation must be reported and that Mr. K must address his abuse by attending AA meetings, and his wife, by attending Al-Anon.

In the next meeting, two weeks later, Mr. and Mrs. K were seen separately. Mrs. K unleashed a barrage of complaints about her husband's alcohol and physical abuse, beginning with their first dates. She married him because he promised to stop drinking when they had children. She reported that things were much better now that the worker was coming around. She reported that he was doing more with the kids and not calling them names. Occasionally he would slip, but apologized, something he had never done before. Incidentally, she noted that he was still drinking. When pressed, she added that two nights ago, when drinking, he had picked up Charlie and banged his head against the basement ceiling, but "it wasn't that hard." When pressed further, she guessed he was drunk, but it's hard to tell sometimes, but when he's drinking, the kids irritate him. When asked how this episode was different from the past ones, and why it was less serious, she said that Mr. K didn't really hurt him and, besides, the kids were using the worker's involvement to take advantage of him.

When asked whether she could tolerate things as they were, she indicated that it was OK. The therapist reflected that it seemed to be "OK if Mr. K drank a little and bashed the kids softly," and she said it was OK as long as he didn't cause any trouble. She was unable to say how there would be any predictable lasting improvement after the workers left. The therapist suggested that perhaps the worker would need to stay in the house for the next 10 to 15 years.

Mrs. K didn't think her husband would like the worker being involved for so long. The therapist continued to push the issues reminding Mrs. K of her own responsibility, finally informing her that it was time to stop saying she loves her kids without protecting them, and show that she loves them by protecting them.

Mr. K was asked what needed to change in the family so that he wouldn't be tense and drink or hit, he answered that when his children are doing something wrong or dangerous, like climbing on fences, he knows what happens when kids get hurt. He added that he didn't hurt Charlie.

The therapist reflected that Mr. K was seeing that the kids needed to learn discipline, and Mr. K eventually agreed that the disrespectful way the kids treated him was a problem. He observed that whenever he cautioned or scolded them, they talked back. The therapist wondered whether, if the kids were more respectful, he would feel better and feel more in control and less likely to drink and get violent. Mr. K thought this would work, particularly if he had his wife's help, so when he corrected the kids, they would stay corrected. The therapist impressed on him the need for patience and forbearance, reinforcing the fact that he risks losing his children—that if CPS thinks he has a problem, he has a problem.

With the parents together, they were informed that treatment would proceed in stages. In the first stage there must be a cessation of drinking and violence. Attendance at AA and Al-Anon were mandatory, otherwise treatment would stop. Neither parent would get any support for violence or for tolerating or excusing violence.

It was also observed that the children were taking advantage of Mr. K and probably of Mrs. K, as well, and the children would very likely develop their own problems of substance abuse, violence towards spouses and their own children or be beaten by someone they loved. Thus the therapy would offer a different way of dealing with the kids. They were then given the decision-making intervention, with Mr. K making the rules and Mrs. K being the one to implement the discipline. Mr. K seemed more comfortable with this role, while Mrs. K uncomfortably reported that the kids didn't mind her, either, and then asked, "What if they act just like their father?" The therapist stated that she should do the same as when you deal with their father, stick to your agreements and give them the consequence you committed to from the start. They were given instructions to talk for 15 minutes each day about the proposed rules for discussion in the next session.

In two days the worker reported that Mrs. K had filed an abuse report, and they were in the process of obtaining an order of protective supervision, but allowing Mr. K to remain in the home unless there was another episode. Over the next two sessions a reasonable and safe behavior plan was developed, and over further sessions problems with implementing the plan were resolved. AA and Al-Anon meetings were attended, and the father achieved abstinence. Treatment focused on strategies to deal with containing and defusing conflict, expression of caring and support, resolving ineffective communication, and reviewing and renegotiating decision making in all areas of their marriage.

At the end of 9 months, the team and family met with the worker who was hesitant to change her involvement, since she doubted the degree of change over such a short time. The worker was asked what she needed to see change, and for what time, to end the order of protective supervision. The family had to acknowledge and accept their powerlessness over changing the worker, and use what resources they had to meet her requirement of continuing the present level of functioning for an additional 6 months with reduced observation visits. At the end of this period, the case was recessed, Mr. K not having been drunk or violent, and both parents actively involved in their self-help groups.

For the next seven years we had no further contact with CPS or the family. Recently, we heard from a colleague who evaluated Charlie for school problems and substance abuse that Mrs. K did act on a promise she had made early in treatment—that she would leave Mr. K when the kids grew into adolescence and young adulthood.

CONCLUSION

Three components distinguish this method from earlier models:

- Explicit contracts between the three systems are negotiated prior to treatment and are rigidly maintained by the treatment team, often at painful cost to all. Their purpose is to clarify each system's role responsibility.
- The meta-rule intervention is a rigidly imposed rule about how decisions in treatment will be made, implemented, and changed. Its purpose is to empower the family and treatment through second-order structural alteration of the treatment system.
- The decision-making intervention serves to interrupt the family's previous decision-making process and ineffective solution-finding patterns. Its purpose is to provide new and clearly differentiated role responsibilities that alter the structure of the family.

The approach has rigid and flexible components. It protects children rigidly, yet empowers abusive birth families and maintains the team's legal responsibility. Within rigid role responsibilities, expectations, and consequences (e.g., limits on the team's ability to intervene), there is tremendous therapeutic flexibility. While motivating families who experience themselves largely as victims, this approach separates out those families unable or unwilling to change, without disempowering the team with inappropriate social control responsibilities. Paradoxically, staff who often feel powerless in the face of passively noncompliant families are empowered as agents of change.

Even in abusive families, change is not only possible but inevitable. This is especially true when empowerment is activated through partnership of people helping other people to help themselves in a way that respects the authority of the family. Long ago I learned that first step: relinquishing my illusion that I possessed personal power that could change people. Doing this clears the path for people under treatment to empower themselves. Being in charge means knowing when not to be in control, and holding others accountable.

REFERENCES

de Shazer, S. (1985). *Keys to solution in brief therapy.*New York: W. W. Norton.

Fox, M. R. (1985). *Placing families in charge of hospitalization.* Unpublished manuscript.

Fox, M. R. (1988). Treating families with a member diagnosed as mentally ill. In E. W. Nunnally, C. S. Chilman, & F. M. Fox (Eds.), *Families in trouble* (Vol. 4, pp. 39–55). Newbury Park, CA: Sage.

Fox, M. R. (1990). Strategic inpatient family therapy with adolescent substance abusers: The Fox system. In T. Todd & M. Selekman (Eds.), *Family therapy approaches with adolescent substance abusers.* Boston: Allyn & Bacon.

Fox, M. R. (1991, December). Helping parents take charge. *The Family Therapy Networker,* pp. 75–78.

Haley, J. (1963). *Strategies of psychotherapy.*New York: Grune & Stratton.

Haley, J. (1977). *Problem solving therapy.* San Francisco: Jossey-Bass.

Haley, J. (1980). *Leaving home.* New York: McGraw-Hill.

Imber-Black, E. (1988). *Families and larger systems.* New York: Guilford Press.

Madanes, C. (1981). *Strategic family therapy.* San Francisco: Jossey-Bass.

Madanes, C. (1984). *Behind the one-way mirror.* San Francisco: Jossey-Bass.

Stuart, R. B. (1980). *Helping couples change: A social learning approach to marital therapy.* New York: Guilford Press.

Watzlawick, P., Weakland, J. H., & Fisch, R. (1974). *Change.* New York: W. W. Norton.

9

The Role of a Home-Based Mentor Program in the Psychiatric Continuum of Care for Children and Adolescents

Julie McKenzie
Edwin J. Mikkelsen
Wayne Stelk
Gerald Bereika
Donald Monack

Mentor Clinical Care is a 12-year-old national corporation providing specialized health and rehabilitation services to diverse patient/client populations who are in need of residential, day, or outpatient services. In general, services are designed to be an alternative to hospital or institutional care and are provided in natural or normalized community-based settings.

Over the past few years, a specialized program has been developed to meet the needs of third-party payers (health maintenance organizations [HMOs], insurance companies, and others). These funding sources are particularly concerned about inpatient psychiatric admissions for children and adolescents. Recent statistics show that an extraordinary percentage of the health care dollar is being spent for inpatient psychiatric admissions for children and adolescents. Additionally, there is evidence that many of these admissions are unnecessary or result in unwarranted lengths of stay. Other problematic aspects of psychiatric hospitalization include the following (Scahil & Riddle, 1990):

- inhibition of the learning of new skills and behaviors due to the artificial environment of a hospital or large group facility, and generalization to other settings;
- contagion effects;
- negative modeling;
- limits on program's ability to individualize care and treatment; and
- difficulties in trying to design services that can simultaneously meet the widely diverse needs of patients/clients and their families.

The Mentor Hospital Diversion Program utilizes specially trained lay individuals who work in conjunction with a multidisciplinary treatment team. In this chapter we will describe the program, elaborating on the following:

- the theoretical framework from which the model is derived and the key operational components of the program;
- empirical data that compares the efficacy of the program to the results obtained with psychiatric hospitalization;
- our experience in involving stakeholders, professionals, funders, and clients in the program; and
- case vignettes that illustrate the clinical impact of the program's theoretical framework.

The Mentor program model is based on the principle that emotionally disturbed children should be treated in as normal an environment as possible, and in a manner that does not alienate them from their families, is nonstigmatizing, is cost effective, and maximizes the potential for the child to return to his or her parental home.

This program may at first appear to be a variation of foster care. While there are similarities to specialized foster care, we believe that functionally the program is more similar to psychiatric hospitalization. As with psychiatric hospitalization, the goals of the program include short-term stabilization, thorough diagnostic assessment, pharmacologic intervention when necessary, active case management, and intensive psychotherapeutic treatment involving both the family and the child (Jemerin & Philips, 1988). All of the children and adolescents admitted to the program are either diverted from psychiatric hospitalization or admitted from a psychiatric hospital. An important theoretical underpinning of the program derives from the observation that while psychiatric hospitalization represents an important treatment modality on the spectrum of care, it is overutilized given the existence of effective, less restrictive alternatives. This program aims to achieve results that are the same as or better than those of psychiatric hospitalization without the restrictiveness, stigmatization, or cost of hospitalization. Naturally, selection becomes a key factor in utilizing this treatment modality rather than hospitalization. Key factors that would necessitate psychiatric hospitalization rather than this model include the need for a locked door to contain the child or adolescent, the need for continual 24-hour-per-day awake supervision, either due to lethal suicidality or erratic unpredictable dangerous behavior, and/or a high degree of impulsive aggressiveness that would require restraint by several staff members or mechanical restraint. For example, a highly aggressive, 18-year-old, 200-pound male in the midst of a steroid or other drug-induced psychosis would not be a likely candidate for this program. However, we do find that, in general, children with aggressive histories do better than expected because they do not have to compete for the mentor's attention (there is only one child placed in a home at a time), and they are not exposed to other aggressive children who might incite them.

PROGRAM MODEL OVERVIEW

Admissions to the program can be arranged 24 hours a day upon referral from a hospital emergency room, crisis intervention team, utilization review clinician, or other source. A clinician completes an intake assessment and arranges placement into a treatment home within a few hours of referral. Each patient is under the care of a team of mental health professionals, including a psychiatrist, while residing in the home of a mental health technician, known as a "mentor." Only one patient is placed in a treatment home at any one time, thereby allowing truly individualized and intensive care.

The mentor treatment home is a structured but natural environment in which to provide comprehensive assessment, crisis stabilization, and treatment services. As an integral member of the treatment team, the mentor is responsible for observation and documentation of patient status, behavioral management, life skills training, therapeutic activities, and support and supervision of the patient. The child typically does not attend school while in the program. The mentor is responsible for working in conjunction with the child's family to obtain his or her school work and keep the child as current as possible with the class. The team of professionals is responsible for assessment and diagnosis, treatment planning, comprehensive case management, individual and family therapy, crisis intervention, and psychopharmacologic services. Twenty-four-hour-per-day backup to each home is also provided.

The program, which has an average length of stay of under 30 days, combines the following critical elements of effective psychiatric treatment.

- *Orientation and training:* Comprehensive orientation and education regarding all aspects of the program is provided for referral organizations, including utilization review and case management staff.
- *Crisis intervention:* Skilled clinicians provide timely intervention into the crisis situation.
- *Assessment:* A multidisciplinary team under the medical direction of a child psychiatrist provides comprehensive evaluation and diagnostic services.
- *Stabilization:* Acute situations are effectively stabilized through active support, supervision, and structure within a mentor treatment home.
- *Brief treatment:* Short-term, goal-oriented treatment for the individual and family focuses on resolution of the specific problems that precipitated the crisis.
- *Active case management:* Clinicians call upon the full therapeutic impact of community resources and the patient's natural support systems.
- *Utilization review:* Each case is frequently reviewed by a multidisciplinary team under the direction of a psychiatrist.
- *Discharge planning:* Successful long-term outcome is maximized through careful discharge planning.
- *Reintegration:* The integrity of the family unit is preserved by facilitating a successful transition back home at the earliest appropriate time. As indicated, Mentor Clinical Care can provide in-home follow-up services to minimize the possibility of recidivism.

REFERRAL AND ADMISSION PROCESS

Most patients are referred to Mentor Clinical Care by a psychiatrist, a mental health case manager at an HMO or an insurance company, or other mental health professionals in the community. At times, patients or family members may contact Mentor directly. Referral procedures are as follows:

1. The referral agent evaluates the patient and determines that the patient can benefit from a mentor treatment program.
2. The referral agent reviews the program with the patient and, if needed, the patient's family, then obtains approval to make a referral.

3. The referral agent contacts the admission coordinator for the Mentor Hospital Diversion Program.
4. An immediate telephone screening interview takes place to determine the presenting problem, preliminary diagnosis, psychiatric or substance abuse history, and other critical information.
5. A clinical coordinator reviews the information, consults as necessary with the medical director, evaluates the patient regarding appropriateness of admission, and begins the process of matching the patient to the most appropriate mentor home.
6. The clinical coordinator arranges an on-site intake evaluation interview typically within 24 hours of the initial telephone referral. The clinical coordinator, the mentor, the referral agent, the patient, and the patient's family may be participants in this interview.
7. The admission can be completed at the conclusion of this meeting. All releases and other necessary chart documents are completed and signed. The patient and, if necessary, the patient's family proceed to the mentor home and begin the treatment program.

Admission and ongoing treatment in the Mentor Clinical Care Program is on a fully voluntary basis. Normally, admissions occur during the hours when Mentor's admission coordinator is available—between 8:30 A.M. and 5:30 P.M., Monday through Friday. After hours there is a clinical staff person on call to evaluate a potential admission, and after-hours admissions can be arranged.

ADMISSION CRITERIA

Mentor's Hospital Diversion Program is geared for child and adolescent patients who

- are between 3½ to 21 years of age;
- have serious to severe symptoms of a psychiatric disorder, based upon DSM-IV criteria;
- have serious to severe impairments in attending to age-appropriate responsibilities in one or more major life skills functional areas, as a result of the psychiatric disorder;
- manifest significantly impaired judgment and/or thought processes;
- require frequent professional intervention and high and consistent levels of structure, supervision, and behavior management on a 24-hour-per-day basis;
- are not in need of emergency inpatient psychiatric treatment due to acute danger to self or others; and

- are medically stable, and not in need of intensive nursing services and/or detoxification from alcohol or other chemical substances.

The program model has demonstrated success with treating patients with dual diagnoses, including those who in addition to their emotional problem, have a diagnosis of substance abuse, developmental disability, traumatic brain injury, and the like.

COSTS

The Mentor Clinical Care's Hospital Diversion Program is capable of producing substantial cost savings as a clinically effective alternative to inpatient treatment for children and adolescents. Mentor's per diem cost is inclusive of all charges and can save 40% to 60% of the typical charges for inpatient psychiatric treatment.

PROFESSIONAL STAFF

The patient's team may include psychiatrists, psychologists, psychiatric social workers, case managers, nurse clinicians, and other allied health professionals in addition to the patient's own mentor, depending upon the patient's special needs. The important distinction here is that the services of these professionals are brought to the patient in the mentor home or elsewhere in the neighborhood setting, incorporating treatment into a normal pattern of life and living.

Mentors (Mental Health Technicians)

Mentors are at the heart of the treatment team, providing the day-to-day patient contact and ensuring that the treatment plan is followed. They are typically, but not always, women who are second-wage earners in the family and prefer to work at home. Many mentors have worked in the caring professions at some time in their lives and have a devotion to community service. In all cases, mentors are very carefully trained to handle a wide range of behaviors, and they are in constant contact with the other professionals on the patient's treatment team. Every effort is made to match the mentor's ethnic and socioeconomic background with that of the patient's, so that the child begins to feel at home right away.

Like paraprofessionals in psychiatric or substance abuse hospitals, mentors are mental health technicians. They are identified through professional recruiters, through print advertising, radio, and word-of-mouth.

(Existing and past mentors are the most consistent and cost-effective method of attracting qualified mentors.) A detailed review of each candidate's background is then performed and a comprehensive analysis is undertaken regarding the suitability of the individual's current home environment, including all individuals living there.

Once accepted into our program, the mentor recruit is trained over a 30-day period to deliver treatment in a home environment. The beauty of this training is that the new and positive behaviors children learn occur in a setting most like their own home. Real-life situations, such as eating meals together, cleaning up, and grooming, are not simulated, as in an institutional setting, but are the actual activities of everyday life.

Child Psychiatrist

It is often important for a child to see a physician or psychiatrist to rule out underlying disorders that may be causing behavioral problems. For example, a child exhibiting angry outbursts may require a neurological workup to rule out a seizure disorder that is best treated by medication. In addition, children and adolescents sometimes require psychological or sensory testing that can only be done by a specialist. Each patient in the Mentor program has a clinical coordinator who is responsible for his or her care and who accesses the appropriate specialist for the child's treatment. Mentor's medical director, a board-certified child and adolescent psychiatrist, orders and oversees these specialty referrals. All attending psychiatrists are board-certified as child and adolescent psychiatrists

Clinical Coordinators

Clinical Coordinators are licensed social workers or psychologists who, in combination with mentors, form the core of the treatment team. In addition to supervising, the clinical coordinator develops the child's treatment plan, establishes the clinical team and schedule, and works with key people in the child's world, including teachers, outside therapists, and family physicians to ensure smooth transition back to school and family life. When the program was first established, each coordinator would supervise up to four mentors with acute cases. Experience indicated that this was too heavy a caseload given the clinical and logistical demands of the program, and each clinical coordinator now supervises no more than two acute cases.

Psychologist

Psychologists are licensed mental health professionals who provide direct clinical care, clinical supervision, and, when appropriate, psychological testing. There are several types of testing available, depending on the kind of information needed. These include tests of intelligence, academic achievement, vocational skill, emotional functioning, and/or neurological functioning.

DAILY OPERATION

It is difficult to convey the fast-paced day-to-day operation of this program. The time constraints placed on the Program are similar to those for psychiatric hospitalization, and yet the operational logistics of this program are much more complex. Typically, clinical coordinators will visit each mentor home twice a week for individual sessions with the client and for supervision of the mentor. In addition, an effort is made to have twice weekly family therapy sessions. During the later stages of treatment the client's parents are frequently invited to the mentor home to observe the interactions and behavioral techniques developed by the mentor. Depending on the geographical location of the mentors and families, a clinical coordinator will often spend a few hours per day in the car. Car phones are utilized to make this time as productive as possible. A weekly meeting brings all of the members of the interdisciplinary team together to track the progress of the patient and modify the treatment plan. The child psychiatrist is available to evaluate new admissions and to follow up with those clients requiring pharmacologic intervention.

Although the logistics of the program model are taxing, they do produce a beneficial attitudinal shift on the part of the professional staff, *vis-à-vis* those who work on inpatient psychiatric units. In our experience, the nature of the configuration of inpatient services can lead to a certain egocentrism, as everyone "comes to" the hospital unit, which is the source of all treatment. In this home-based program, the professionals are continually "going out" to the mentor home, to the family's home, to meet with outside agencies, and so forth. This outward looking to the community leads to a greater degree of hands-on case management than is often done by inpatient-based professionals. It also generates a more "real-life" assessment of the child's family home and his or her functioning in another home. It is not uncommon to see a child's negative target behaviors completely disappear in the mentor home, thus providing important information on the locus of psychopathology.

FAMILY INVOLVEMENT IN TREATMENT

Unique to the mentor program is our ability to involve the family in a direct and positive way, including active involvement in the treatment planning process. While the family may need a period of "respite" from disruptive behaviors, the child or adolescent will ultimately need to be reintegrated into the family. To this end, Mentor seeks to establish a bridge between the mentor home and the family from the very beginning. Mentors provide valuable training, when necessary, to family members in a setting that directly models their own home. Additionally, family members are expected to participate in regular, intensive family therapy facilitated by their clinical coordinator.

CASE EXAMPLES

Chris H. was a 5-year-old boy who presented the following behaviors:

- acts of violence against mother (throwing objects, hitting and biting her) and yelling at mother, "I hate you," or "I'll kill you,"
- excessive preoccupation with genitalia,
- exposing himself to other children,
- inappropriate displays of affection toward strangers, and
- discharge from a special education school because of violence toward other children.

Chris had been separated from nurturing grandparents at age 2, and went to live with his parents. He frequently witnessed his father's physical abuse of his mother. After his mother left the father, Chris's behavior changed dramatically. He began having nightmares about "Uncle Fred" hurting him, and his mother alleged that Chris's paternal uncle had sexually abused Chris from the age of 14 months to 2½ years. Chris's mother was unable to control his increasingly impulsive and violent behavior, and she surrendered him to voluntary custody with the public child welfare agency.

Chris was referred to Mentor by the case manager at the HMO for a full diagnostic evaluation, emergency stabilization, and an assessment of his mother's capacity to care for him. Within 2 hours of the referral, Chris was admitted to the home of a 31-year-old mentor, who lived with her husband, two children, and several pets. Within 48 hours of the referral, Chris's treatment team met to develop his Individual Treatment Plan.

The treatment team consisted of a primary therapist with a master's degree, the program director, an LICSW, the medical director, a psychiatrist certified in general as well as child and adolescent psychiatry, the mentor, who had 7 years experience as a mentor and several additional years in other human services, Chris's mother, her personal therapist, and a case manager from the Department of Social Services.

The team focused on the following issues:

- Chris's frequent acts of violence against his mother and peers,
- his inappropriate sexual behavior (exposing himself, touching other children's genitals),
- his impulsivity and inability to concentrate on routine tasks,
- his mother's inability to provide basic parental care, and
- filing charges of sexual abuse against Chris's paternal uncle.

The treatment plan for Chris included a medication evaluation by the medical director and twice weekly individual therapy sessions with his primary therapist. He had a highly structured daily schedule to assist him in settling into a stable home routine and received frequent praise and other rewards from the mentor for any positive behavior. He was given clear expectations and labeling regarding age-appropriate expressions of affection and sexuality.

His mother was involved in weekly individual sessions with the mentor primary therapist and weekly conjoint sessions with Chris, the primary therapist, and the mentor. The mother had regular visits to the mentor home, during which she was engaged by the mentor in parenting activities, especially in relation to setting limits and handling Chris's resistance to limits. She was also assisted to file the necessary papers requesting an investigation of the paternal uncle relative to the allegation of sexual abuse.

During the first 2 weeks of placement in the mentor home, Chris had frequent episodes of biting and hitting. He responded to administration of methylphenidate by being less hyperactive, but he continued to test the limits. Within 25 days of treatment, Chris was much more tolerant of limit setting, but he continued to require close one-to-one supervision. Meetings between the Mentor primary therapist and Chris's special education school resulted in an agreement that Chris could resume school activities, and he was referred for the evaluation of a hearing problem detected by the mentor.

Chris's mother made several visits to the mentor home and attempted to imitate the mentor's efforts to set limits on Chris, but she proved unable to do this on her own, even with close supervision. In her individual therapy sessions, she showed only a limited understanding of her son's behavior. Papers charging abuse were filed and the investigation of sexual abuse by the uncle begun, and the mother was given support by the Mentor primary therapist regarding the investigation of abuse by the uncle.

In light of these developments, the treatment team recommended continued out-of-home placement for Chris. The state child welfare agency assumed payment of Chris's placement in a less intensive, specialized foster care setting.

David P is a 12-year-old boy who presented with the following behaviors:

- threatening his mother with a kitchen knife,
- frequent threats of physical harm to mother,
- physical fights with younger brother, and
- refusing to attend school.

David was given up for adoption at birth and was adopted by Mr. and Mrs. P at the age of 5 months. One year later, Mrs. P gave birth to a son and 8 years later to a daughter. After his daughter's birth, David's father had an affair and left the family. Mrs. P was hospitalized several times for depression. David, who was very close to his father, quickly became withdrawn and combative, and though he had previously been a good student, he began to fail in school and refused to attend classes. David was further estranged from his father when Mr. P remarried. He became explosive at home—punching out windows, breaking dishes, fighting with his brother, and threatening his mother.

David's examining psychiatrist recommended acute psychiatric hospitalization, and the HMO managed-care provider determined that David could more appropriately and cost effectively be treated in the Mentor program. The Mentor primary therapist assessed David in the HMO emergency room, and within 2 hours David was admitted to the treatment home of a mentor with 8 years of experience in counseling adolescents.

The treatment team included the primary therapist, an LICSW, the program director, the medical director, and the patient's mother. The team focused on the following problems in developing the treatment plan:

- David's anger and depression, as manifested by sarcasm, fighting, low self-esteem, poor personal hygiene;
- the impact of divorce and remarriage and the loss of a close relationship with the father;
- pervasive role confusion in the recently reconfigured family, with the mother inappropriately empowering the patient with father-like expectations;
- the mother's inability to set limits and the patient's constant harassing her to do so; and
- the sudden drop in academic performance, and an avoidance of school, as manifested by skipping classes.

The treatment plan consisted of a medication evaluation by the medical director, three individual therapy sessions per week with the primary therapist, a highly structured day, and immediate feedback from the mentor about verbal and physical aggression. David was given alternative physical outlets for aggression (e.g., a punching bag), and the Activities of Daily

Living (ADL)/personal hygiene schedule was rigorously supervised by his mentor.

A schedule of weekly contact was established between the school guidance counselor, mother, and patient, and the mother was involved in reviewing David's Individual Education Plan with the guidance counselor.

Family therapy sessions were held three times per week with the primary therapist, mentor, and all members of the family, including the father. The goals were to teach the mother how to set limits on David's negative behaviors and reinforce positive behaviors, to sensitize the parents about David's sense of loss (adoption, geographic relocation, divorce), and to refer the parents for longer term family mediation therapy.

David established a positive relationship with the mentor and responded positively to firm limits by behaving with improved self-control. He expressed his grief over the breakup of family and the loss of his relationship with his father. He also confronted his mother about her inattention to his feelings and fears. He expressed fears of abandonment related to his adoption and his parent's divorce, and role-played with the mentor a more constructive relationship with his father's new wife.

The school guidance counselor agreed to facilitate a review of David's Individual Education Plan, working with David's mother. Both David and his mother expressed feelings of encouragement about the increased level of support at school.

Attending the Mentor program was the first time the entire family had ever met together in therapy. The sessions were difficult but positive. The father identified feelings of guilt about not keeping promises to his family and a lack of awareness of the effects of the broken promises on the family. The mother admitted her inability to manage David's behavior and her need to improve her parenting skills, and David admitted that he was hurting himself to get back at his father. The parents agreed to meet with a family mediator in an effort to resolve their mutual anger around issues of divorce and family management.

In 21 days, David returned home to live with his mother. The treatment team recommended continued outpatient counseling for the family.

FOLLOW-UP DATA

In order to assess the effectiveness of the program, extensive data are collected at discharge and at 3-month intervals post discharge. In comparing this program to psychiatric hospitalization, we reviewed the literature concerning diagnostic categories of children and adolescents admitted to psychiatric inpatient units. The diagnostic groupings for the Mentor program are compared to that data in Table 9.1.

TABLE 9.1. Comparison of Diagnosis Categories

Disorders	Turner et al. 1989 N=100 A[a]	Pyne et al. 1985 N=69 C & A	Mentor N=112 C & A	Blinder et al. 1978 N=106 C	Shafii et al. 1979 N=145 C	King & Pittman 1969 N=60 A	Mansheim 1990 N=34 P
Disruptive behavior	22%[b]	49%	48%	20%	36%	—	62%
Mood	18		30		—	35	—
Anxiety			16		—	2	6
Personality	7		4	19		15	—
Sexual	—		1	8	10	10	
Psychotic	18	19	1	8	10	10	
Adjustment	13			26	5		
Neurotic	7		—	9	16	7	
Developmental	4		—	20			
Psychophysiological	10			5	17	5	
Neurological with behavioral effects	2	7		10		20	
Mental retardation				2	6	—	—
Other	1	—				6	5

[a]A = Adolescents, C = Children, P = Preschooler.
[b]Not all percentages = 100, due to rounding off to nearest percentage.

In this report we will describe the results of a follow-up study assessing treatment outcome at discharge and at 3 months and 6 months post discharge. The study cohort includes at 6 months 89 children who were either admitted from a psychiatric hospital (28.7%) or were diverted from an emergency psychiatric hospitalization (71.3%). The average length of stay was 17.9 days. The average age was 12.8 years; 8% were under 6, 33.3% were ages 6 to 12, and 57.5% were ages 13 to 18. Only one child, 1.1%, was over age 18; 60.9% of the cohort were male and 39.1% were female.

The discharge data for the study group indicates that 96.4% of discharges were planned, while 3.6% were unplanned; 72.3% returned home to a biological family or relative; 15.7% were discharged to a less restrictive setting, such as foster care or a group home; and 4.8% were discharged to a comparably intensive setting, such as a residential treatment center. The remaining 7.2% were discharged to a more restrictive setting, such as an inpatient psychiatric unit. There were no discharges due to unauthorized absences or runaways despite the unlocked home-based nature of the program.

Both the 3-month and 6-month follow-up data were obtained by a structured telephone interview implemented by a master's-level clinician who was blind to the actual cases. At 6-month follow-up, 48.4% were living with their parents, a relative, a family friend, or an adoptive home. Only 6.7% were residing in inpatient psychiatric units, 13.5% were in residential treatment, and 31.4% were in other, less restrictive settings such as foster care and group homes. Within the 6 months, 14.6% had been psychiatrically hospitalized (average number of episodes 1.5 and average length of stay 34.9 days), 59.6% had received outpatient treatment during the 6-month follow-up period, 4.5% had received day treatment, 19.1% had received foster care or specialized foster care, 15.7% had received residential treatment, 10.8% of the follow-up group were attending public schools, and 13.5% were attending a residential or inpatient-based school program.

In order to assess the correlates of different outcomes, the data were analyzed with regard to the patient characteristics of age, sex, admission source, documented history of sexual abuse, utilization of postdischarge outpatient services, and diagnostic category. Of these, only the following factors had a significant impact on outcome: history of abuse, post-discharge outpatient treatment, and psychiatric diagnosis. The data from the 3-month follow-up study are presented in Table 9.2, and the 6-month data are presented in Table 9.3. In order to assess the relative effectiveness of this program as compared to psychiatric inpatient care, we reviewed the published outcome and follow-up data concerning psychiatric hospitalization of children and adolescents. The 3-month Mentor follow-up data are compared to the psychiatric hospitalization data in Table 9.4.

STAKEHOLDERS, HMOs, THIRD-PARTY PAYERS, AND OTHER PROFESSIONALS

The public sector has funded Mentor Clinical Care Programs for 12 years. Historically, they have believed in and advocated for a continuum of care for their clients that includes alternatives to the more traditional outpatient or inpatient care utilized by private payers.

The recent crisis in the health care industry has forced private payers to look at ways to reduce or maintain levels of spending. They are aggressively attempting to put together a continuum of care that includes cost-effective alternatives to inpatient care.

As a result of these factors, the usual resistance one would expect to a new program model was diminished considerably, and we found many private payers willing to consider purchasing these services. We were impressed with their emphasis on securing competitively priced services with a high standard of quality. They were particularly concerned about safe-

TABLE 9.2. 3-Month Follow-Up Data $(N = 61)$

Respondent's relation to patient	# Clients	Percentage
Self	7	11.5
Birth parent	46	75.4
Adoptive parent	1	1.6
Public agency case manager	5	8.2
Other	2	3.3
Living at time of follow-up interview	# Clients	Percentage
Not specified	1	1.6
Birth family home	39	63.9
Home of relative	2	3.3
Psychiatric hospital	3	4.9
Substance abuse treatment facility	1	1.6
Residential treatment facility	3	4.9
Foster care	7	11.5
Specialized foster care	3	4.9
Other	2	3.4
Participation in mainstream school/job	# Clients	Percentage
Not specified	3	4.9
Attending regularly	45	73.8
Attending perdiodically	1	1.6
Capable, but unwilling to attend	7	11.5
Not yet school age	2	3.3
Attending hospital/residential school	3	4.9
Postdischarge community services	# Clients	Percentage
Outpatient services	40	65.6
Day treatment services	1	1.6
Foster care	11	18.0
Specialized foster care	1	1.6
Residential treatment	9	14.8
Postdischarge inpatient psychiatric services	# Clients	Percentage
Number of patients hospitalized	5	8.2
Avg. bed days per hospitalized patient	[21.8]	

ty issues, not only because of liability concerns but also as a quality-of-care issue. One of the major mechanisms utilized in overcoming the understandable reluctance about using a new program is the rigorous quality assurance and clinical follow-up work that is conducted on an ongoing

TABLE 9.3. Six-Month Follow-up Data (N = 89)

	Residence at time of follow-up			% Psychiatrically hospitalized	Regular attendance at school	
	Home	Less[a] restricted	More[b] restricted	Hospitalized within follow-up period	Public	Residential
Age:						
12 & under (41.3%)	47.3%	31.6%	21.1%	15.8%	84.2%	5.3%
13 & over (58.7%)	49.1	31.3	19.6	13.7		60.8
Female (39.1%)	60.1	22.8	17.1	17.1	65.7	14.3
Male (60.9%)	40.8	37.0	22.2	13.0	74.1	13.0
Admission source:						
Diversion (71.3%)	49.1	33.3	17.6	14.0	75.4	10.5
Step down (28.7%)	52.0	19.2	28.0	16.0	60.0	20.0
Substantiated physical or sexual abuse:						
Abused (12.4%)	9.1	45.4	45.4	36.4	63.6	27.3
Nonabused (87.6%)	56.6	28.4	15.0	15.1	67.9	11.3
Outpatient treatment postdischarge:						
Yes (59.6%)	56.6	37.7	5.7	9.4	83.0	1.9
No (40.4%)	36.2	22.1	41.7	22.2	52.8	30.6
Major diagnostic categories:						
Behavior disorder (44.9%)	32.5	41.0	27.5	17.5	72.5	17.5
Mood disorder (24.7%)	40.9	31.8	27.3	13.6	59.1	22.7
Anxiety disorder (12.4%)	72.7	27.3	0.0	18.2	81.8	0.0

[a]Less restricted refers to a nonparental home living arrangement (e.g., living with a relative or friend) that would be considered less restrictive than the mentor placement.
[b]More restricted refers to a nonparental home living arrangement (e.g., living in a residential school) that would be considered more restricted than the mentor home.

TABLE 9.4. Comparison of Discharge and Follow-up Data

	N	Age range	Discharge disposition	Recidivism	Follow-up (3 month)
Mentor short-term residential	61	3–21 yr	72% family or relative 17% less intensive (foster care) 5% comparative 6% more restrictive	5 admitted to psychiatric hospital during follow-up period	67.2% family or relative 4.9% specialized foster care 11.5% foster care 16.4% other
Blinder et al.	130	3–13 yr	72% Home 5% Foster home 6% Group home 7% Residential 1% Death	7 readmitted during 2-year course of study	Discharge & readmit data only
Turner et al.	100	Adolescents	69 Home 10 Part home 21 Not home	Not stated	6 mo. follow-up 47 Home 13 Part home 19 Not home 21 unknown
Davis et al.	74	14–19	Not stated	Not stated	1-yr. follow-up 84% Home 40% At school 37% Employed 29% Psych. residence 62% Psych. residence since discharge
Shafil et al.	145	2–16 yr	82% Home or previous residence 16.5% Place out of home 1.5% Long-term state facility	7.5% (11) readmitted during course of study	Discharge & readmit data only
Pyne et al.	70	Adolescents	42 Planned discharges 17 Unplanned child–parent 11 Expelled	Not stated	65% living w/parents 13% independent living Information not available on remainder. Length of follow-up not stated.

basis. In attempting to find comparable data for psychiatric hospitalization of children and adolescents, we were surprised at the relative paucity of studies in this area, despite the billion dollar size of the industry.

The follow-up studies have been useful in neutralizing concerns about a new program not only because of the results, but also due to the commitment to clinical excellence that is inherent in this demanding quality assurance program.

Mentor Clinical Care considers families major stakeholders. Whatever their level of functioning, they are pivotal in the treatment of their children. Families clearly are not as invested in cost issues. Quality of care, clinical excellence, and safety weigh heavily for them. They need assurance that Mentor Clinical Care is the optimum level of treatment for their child. Because most families are in crisis prior to their child's admission, the family physician or a professional must play the role of advisor to help the family make the appropriate decision regarding treatment for the child.

Physicians or professionals, then, have considerable influence regarding utilization of the Mentor Clinical Care Hospital Diversion Program. We have found that this group shares the private payers' concerns, particularly regarding quality of care, safety, and liability. The sophisticated quality assurance and clinical follow-up systems alleviated many of these concerns. It has been Mentor Clinical Care's experience that once a physician or professional makes his or her first referral, they will become ongoing advocates of the program.

We have not found clients themselves necessarily difficult to persuade (except for the normal adolescent opposition). Many of our children/adolescents have been institutionalized prior to referral to us and prefer the less stigmatized mentor model. Although many of our clients have little real choice and are dependent on their family and the professional community to choose the right level of care for them, an attempt is made to fully involve them in the decision making and admission process.

In summary, the crisis in the health care industry has provided Mentor Clinical Care an opportunity to demonstrate the efficacy of this level of care. The adherence to delivering high quality, clinically effective services to children and adolescents and their families has allowed the program to be considered as a credible, fundable standard of psychiatric care.

REFERENCES

Blinder, B. J., Young, W. M., Fineman, K. R., & Miller, S. J. (1978). The children's psychiatric hospital unit in the community: I. Concept and development. *American Journal of Psychiatry, 135*(7), 848–851.

Jemerin, J. M., & Philips, I. (1988). Changes in inpatient child psychiatry: Consequences and recommendations. *Journal of American Academy of Child and Adolescent Psychiatry, 27*(4), 397–403.

Mansheim, P. (1990). Short-term psychiatric inpatient treatment of preschool children. *Hospital and Community Psychiatry, 41*(6), 670–671.

Pyne, N., Morrison, R., & Ainsworth, P. (1985). A follow-up study of the first 70 admissions to a general purpose adolescent unit. *Journal of Adolescence, 8,* 333–345.

Scahil, L., & Riddle, M.A. (1990). Psychiatrically hospitalized children: A critical review. *The Yale Journal of Biology and Medicine, 63,* 301–312.

Shafi, M., McCue, A., Ice, J. F., & Schwab, J. J. (1979). The development of an acute short-term inpatient child psychiatric setting: A pediatricpsychiatric model. *American Journal of Psychiatry, 136*(4A), 427–429.

Turner, T. H., Dossetor, D. R., & Bates, R. E. (1986). The early outcome of admission to an adolescent unit: A report on 100 cases. *Journal of Adolescence, 9,* 367–382.

10

Substance-Abusing Mothers and Their Children: Treatment for the Family

Francine Feinberg

Utilizing a residential treatment model called Meta House, Our Home Foundation, Inc., has been treating substance-abusing women in Milwaukee, Wisconsin, since 1963. The Meta House programs went through an evolutionary process that significantly departed from traditional treatment and eventually culminated in the opening of specialized residential treatment facilities for substance-abusing mothers. Two programs currently exist for mothers and their children. One residential facility houses substance-abusing pregnant women, mothers, and their young children. Another program houses substance-abusing pregnant women and mothers who have lost custody of their children. Both programs focus on the family as a unit.

Traditional modes of treatment for alcoholism and drug abuse are rooted in a philosophy that emerged to meet the needs of men. Unfortunately, this traditional treatment modality often runs contrary to the needs of substance-abusing women, especially as it relates to the attachment process between the mother and child.

Bowlby (1958) first conceptualized the phenomenon of attachment as essential for the survival of the human infant. The concept was defined with regard to the infant's behavior toward the mother. Klaus and Kennell (1976) introduced "maternal–infant bonding" as the concept of "attachment and attachment behaviors in the context of human mothers' relationships to infants" (p. 84). We have come to understand this early relationship between the mother and child as the paradigm for all ensuing relationships for the child. But this intricate, life-long dance performed by the mother and child defines more than the sense of self in the personality of the child. Although not often considered, the woman's sense of self is also being formed as she develops into the role of motherhood. As a society we place an extraordinarily high value on a woman's ability to mother; therefore, a woman's perceived success or failure in this endeavor formulates an important aspect of her self-concept which invariably impacts upon her child. For the pregnant substance-abusing mother and her children, this is paramount. After all, she believes, as does most of society, that she is an "unfit mother."

It is interesting that a difference has been noticed at the Meta House programs in the level of self-esteem demonstrated by the mothers who have not lost custody of their children compared to the mothers who have lost custody or whose children have died as a result of their drug abuse. There is also a noticeable difference in the cognitive, affective, behavioral, and social functioning of the children who have been separated from their mothers. Both mothers and children appear to suffer more when they are separated from each other.

Pregnant and postpartum women who abuse drugs are currently the focus of much controversy. In the last few years some people have come to view these women as criminals who victimize their children rather than as victims themselves. There has been an astonishing increase in the number of pregnant women charged with a crime because their drug use potentially or actually injured their babies. It appears that despite the trend to keep families together, when faced with substance-abusing, pregnant women and mothers, punitive action prevails and families are torn apart.

One solution to this problem is to provide substance abuse treatment services to pregnant women and mothers while keeping the family intact. Despite the growing problem of substance abuse, there is a dearth of services for substance-abusing women, especially pregnant or postpartum women and mothers. Programs attempting to treat this population report that these women do not readily access treatment and, when they do, they have a high failure rate. The reasons for this lack of progress are rooted deeply in societal values, including the view that these women are criminals. After all, the image of the addicted woman conjures up a negative stereotype that is a major barrier to recovery for most women. This is the reason why women are not offered services that are delivered in a context that is compatible with their psychological functioning and fully addresses their needs. It is also the reason why children are taken away from substance-abusing mothers before attempts are made to maintain the family. Substance-abusing mothers and pregnant women are viewed as self-centered reprobates and are often punished by having their children removed in the name of protecting them. It is not likely that much time or effort will go into developing empathic treatment services for a population of people who are viewed with such repulsion. In effect, substance-abusing women, and especially pregnant women and mothers, do not access treatment because treatment is not accessible. They do not "fail" treatment, treatment fails them.

Women have different treatment needs than men precisely because they have grown up female in this society. The childhood of substance-abusing women has typically been more disruptive and traumatic than those described by the same population of men. These women are more likely to have lost a parent, grown up in a substance-abusing family, and have been sexually and/or physically abused (Gomberg, 1976). The role of caretaker is often passed on to female family members at an early age. Along with this responsibility comes the young woman's belief that it is her fault that she cannot create harmony in the family. It is also very likely that she believes she has, somehow, brought the sexual and physical abuse upon herself. Before the substance abuse even begins, this female child is likely to grow up feeling guilty and worthless.

In addition to the perplexities inherent in being born female, women of color, and especially those brought up without adequate financial means, carry the emotional and physical scars of racism and poverty. As a result, the woman who abuses drugs and alcohol is often attempting to obliterate painful emotions. Because of the stigma attached to the addicted woman, she may hide her abuse and deny its existence even more than her male counterpart. Often, her inappropriate behavior is attributed solely to depression and anxiety. Indeed, it is not unusual for the substance-abusing woman to be hospitalized repeatedly for depression and multiple suicide attempts. Of course, this rarely helps. The abuse problem gets worse, the sense of self-disgust increases, and the woman is pushed deeper into the cycle of substance abuse.

When substance abuse is finally recognized, the treatment barriers for women become quite apparent. The therapeutic communication styles needed to engage and motivate substance-abusing women usually do not recognize the histories and resulting characteristics of the population. The life experience of many of these women is such that they do not believe that anything they do will make a difference. Their goal is to merely survive, not to maintain or regain control over their lives, since they never had control over their lives in the first place. These women must be approached in an empathic, noncombative manner to allow them to reveal their pain, especially the pain that has resulted from the shame and guilt that comes with the continued use of illicit substances despite the knowledge of the destructive consequences for them, their children, and their unborn children. Defensive stances by this population do drop away quickly when these women are valued despite their histories.

In addition, treatment programs for women need access to a broad scope of services. Substance-abusing mothers tend to have a multitude of very practical problems. They often have housing difficulties, lack of education, vocational needs, financial needs, medical needs, social needs, legal needs, and all the other issues that define their lives as women and mothers.

Perhaps most importantly, effective treatment must address the significance of the mother–child relationship. The idea that substance-abusing women do not care about their children must be abolished. There has been much speculation about the effects of drug abuse on what is commonly called the "maternal instinct." Cocaine, in particular, has gained the reputation of being a substance that appears to literally wipe out the innate attachment a mother is expected to have for her fetus. The experience of the staff at the Meta House programs does not support the notion that cocaine, or any other drug, debilitates the "maternal instinct." Appropriate feelings and nurturance are often expressed by these women in clinical interviews. They appear to have similar thoughts for and feelings about their fetuses as non-substance-abusing pregnant women. A research study by this author confirmed that on overall scores of maternal–fetal attachment there was no significant difference between the substance-abusing and non-substance-abusing groups of pregnant women (Feinberg, 1991).

Likewise, substance-abusing mothers also express appropriate concern and love for their children. The mother and her children do, however, carry the emotional and behavioral scars of a very dysfunctional relationship, along with the mother's devastating knowledge that her behavior may have harmed her child.

Research indicates that infants born to cocaine-using mothers often exhibit a decreased rate of *in utero* growth, prematurity, microencephaly, perinatal morbidity, and low birth weight (Chasnoff, 1989; Cherukuri, Minkoff, Feldman, Parekh, & Glass, 1988; Petitti & Coleman, 1990). Crack-cocaine-exposed infants are characteristically fragile, hyperexcitable, fussy, and unable to be consoled. Drug-exposed toddlers are more impulsive, less goal directed, deficient in play skills, and less securely attached than non-drug-exposed toddlers (McRobbie, Mata, & Kronstadt, 1989).

When considering the effects of drug exposure in the home, the information is even more startling than the information concerning prenatal drug exposure. A recent study concluded that children who were exposed to cocaine use in the home had more serious behavior problems than those exposed in the womb (Youngstrom, 1991). Interestingly, Cole

(1989) concluded that the difficulties exhibited in a sample of preschool, *in utero* drug-exposed children were neither atypical nor dissimilar from other children who are vulnerable because of disruptive and chaotic lives.

If we are truly seeing a major negative environmental influence contributing to the dysfunction of children of substance-abusing mothers, then it is possible to intervene on behalf of the family even after children have been exposed to drugs prenatally.

A common behavioral problem for children with substance-abusing mothers comes as a result of the mother's intense guilt for perceiving herself as an "unfit" mother. The child is exposed to the extremes of sudden, harsh punishment, often recognizable as child abuse, along with guilt-ridden overindulgence and gentle kindness. The defense mechanism usually observed in children exposed to this inconsistency is called "splitting." The child splits the mother into two people, the sober, "good" mother and the inebriated, "bad" mother. Out of fear of abandonment, the child may deny the rage he or she feels toward the "bad" mother. In society, these negative feelings may be expressed in the form of anger at others, school problems, antisocial behavior, and chemical dependency. As a direct result of these problems, the children of substance-abusing mothers often appear pseudomature or "parentified." Such children will parent the mother and become overly responsible. Since these children are constantly lied to and denial is a persistent defense mechanism in their relationship circles, they do not trust their innate sense of reality. They tend to be isolated, and the inebriated mother is their only link to reality.

The Meta House programs recognize the benefits for substance-abusing women and their children in keeping the family as intact as possible, while providing coordinated treatment services. This program allows the residents the time and opportunity to work together in an appropriate mother–child relationship. The development of this relationship takes place in the very real context of day-to-day life. Women are treated for their substance abuse within the context of their family situation and everyday stressors. The children reap the benefits of a mother who will no longer be attempting to cope through abuse and neglect, while receiving prevention and intervention services for themselves. This program provides the greatest opportunity for recovery, growth, and change for both the mother and the child who have fallen victim to substance abuse.

The Meta House programs are based on three primary assumptions:

1. Successful treatment for substance-abusing mothers and pregnant women must include the undeniable fact that these women are intimately involved in relationships with their children (and vice versa).

2. Treatment must be presented in a context that is compatible with female psychological functioning.
3. A healthy mother will impact positively on her children.

With these three assumptions in mind, the program has been developed to offer a myriad of services to mothers, children, and families, delivered in a manner that places the mother and child in the highest respect, regardless of their past.

Most of the programming at Meta House is based on the principles of group dynamics. Instilled in each woman from the time she enters the program is a sense of belonging. This helps motivate mothers to stay, despite their feelings that they may not have the power to make changes. Acceptance and respect, despite past and current behaviors, provide mothers the opportunity to take the risks of self-disclosure. Powerful feelings are experienced and accepted by staff and peers. The women quickly find out that feelings will not overwhelm them, that they are not alone, and that they are not responsible for every injustice that has been bestowed upon them and their family. New perceptions, feelings, and behaviors are explored as a group, and attitudes and behaviors start to change.

The parameters of treatment for the family are defined by very structured days. The day begins early, when mothers get their children ready for day care or school. It is expected that all children will be clean, fed, and properly dressed when they leave the building. Mothers will then spend the day in scheduled activities that are defined by individualized treatment plans. The day will always include individual counseling, group therapy, education, exercise, and chores. When the children come home at approximately 3:30 P.M., families spend supervised time together. Some children may be seen individually by a child specialist for evaluation or therapy at this time. Dinner, which is cooked and served by the assigned residents, is served. After dinner, mothers assist their children with homework, if appropriate, or spend time with their younger children. After the children are put to bed, the mothers meet again informally and spend free time in close proximity to their sleeping children.

The potential ability of a family to replicate their new patterns of interactions and daily life schedule is paramount. For example, staff never takes on the responsibility of child care, unless there is clearly no other alternative. It is perfectly acceptable for a mother to ask a peer or a relative to care for her child at Meta House, since this is probably what she will do when she is no longer at the program. Dependence upon and support from the other mothers is highly encouraged, since most of the mothers are single and do not have another person upon whom they can rely.

The children are sent to day care at 6 weeks of age. This is done for a number of reasons. The women are more able to concentrate on their specific task for the day if their attention is not divided because of actual or anticipated needs of the children. Sometimes the feelings that come out in a therapeutic situation feel overwhelming. If children are in the building, the mothers are not willing to take the emotional risk of feeling like they are "falling apart," for fear they will not be available for their children. In addition, one of the goals for every mother is to be engaged in some activity that will lead to eventual employment. In keeping with the philosophy that everything learned should be replicable, it is very likely that the children will continue in day care after the family is discharged.

The other reasons for removing the children from the building and utilizing day care are based on some assumptions about the needs of the children. Depending on the age of the child, there are varying levels of attachment dysfunction. Many of these children have been extremely isolated from their peers. Day care provides these children with the opportunity to experience age-appropriate structured time with other children. They have the opportunity to be away from their mother without the fear of abandonment, since mother will always be there, on time, as planned. As their mothers become more and more consistent and predictable, the children begin to show more trust and attachment. When children are able to anticipate their day through regular routines, they begin to feel more in control and demonstrate less anxiety, depression, and other disturbances.

In addition to the communication style and the emotional work that must take place, there are very specific services that must be provided to these families. Survival services such as discharge to safe, affordable housing, financial assistance, food stamps, other welfare benefits, transportation, and vocational and educational rehabilitation is included. Health services are provided to women and children including prenatal, medical, and dental care. Human sexuality is discussed and taught, especially in light of the risk of HIV infection. Mental health treatment addresses depression, other affective disorders, phobias, and eating disorders. Issues that occur as a result of incest, sexual assault, and domestic violence are not overlooked. Support networks in the community for self-help and leisure-time are encouraged.

The children need access to the necessary safety education, learning experiences, and play equipment. They are also assessed for their physical and emotional development. When appropriate, treatment is provided for the children. Coordinated services and communication take place with the children's outside services, such as the public schools. In addition, the mother–child relationship is assessed and treated. Mothers get education about parenting, child development, and nutrition.

The actual plan of action utilized by the Meta House programs to address the treatment needs of substance-abusing mothers, pregnant women, and their young children is conceptualized into three components: the treatment needs of mothers and pregnant women, the treatment needs of the mother–child relationship, and the treatment needs of the children.

This plan is designed to address the specific risk factors that place many of the central-city drug-abusing mothers of Milwaukee in jeopardy. These risk factors are low socioeconomic status; unemployment; illiteracy; homelessness; pregnancy; single parenthood; minority status; inability to gain access to treatment; history of sexual and domestic abuse; poor or no prenatal care; limited knowledge of child development, parenting, and other child care associated skills; other psychiatric disorders; poor physical health; and legal difficulties. Of course, the children are also affected by their mothers' risk factors. As a result, the children are at high risk for future substance abuse, and suffer the physical and emotional results of *in utero* drug exposure as well as the negative affects of child abuse, neglect, and the myriad of other repercussions that result from a dysfunctional mother–child relationship. These may result in impaired cognitive, social, and behavioral functioning common to children of substance-abusing mothers. It should be understood that every interaction that takes place during treatment affects the mother, the mother–child relationship and the child. These categories have been delineated only to provide structure to the reader.

TREATMENT NEEDS OF MOTHERS

Substance Abuse

Through the experience of treating substance-abusing women for 32 years, the staff at the Meta House programs have identified a number of generic distinctions that lead to positive outcomes for most clients. Utilizing individualized treatment plans, each mother and pregnant woman is provided with a basic gender- and culturally specific program for the maintenance of sobriety. This includes participation in the Meta House programs and necessitates (1) the completion of an assessment utilizing criteria that takes into account the patterns of female (vs. male) and minority substance abuse; (2) an individualized program including resources that provide child care, transportation, and the support of other women; (3) referral to in-house and community Alcoholics Anonymous, Narcotics Anonymous, and Cocaine Anonymous meetings that are regarded as sensitive to the needs of women and minority groups; (4) all residential services including group and individual counseling; and (5) substance abuse education.

Educational/Vocational

If a substance-abusing woman is expected to maintain sobriety, she must be confident that she can financially support herself and her children. The program provides the opportunity to be gainfully employed at an appropriate time in each woman's life. To accomplish this, each woman is assessed for her interest in or need to return to school, develop skills necessary to enter an educational setting, do better if enrolled in school, get specific job training, and develop realistic vocational expectations. The agency advocates for the women with potential employers and Employee Assistance Programs, so that working mothers can be gainfully employed and earn enough money to afford child care, health care, and an adequate life style.

Housing Objective

Safe and affordable housing must be available for any family. For the substance-abusing woman to maintain sobriety, it is also imperative that she not return to the environment that can trigger the urges to use drugs. This usually means that she must find housing that is not only physically safe, but is relatively free from the chaos of the drug-using culture. For many women this means that they are attempting to find housing in neighborhoods in which the housing is not affordable.

While in treatment each woman meets with her Alcohol and Other Drug Abuse (AODA) counselor and/or her vocational counselor on a regular basis as specified in her treatment plan to analyze the family's financial capabilities; to explore resources such as energy assistance, low-income housing, and utility discounts; and to determine her need to develop money management skills as well as those related to home responsibility, including housekeeping, cooking, repairs, care of children, and personal hygiene. Assistance is provided for a housing search, acquisition of furnishings, setting goals for saving money for a security deposit, and budgeting. The agency advocates for the clients by developing a list of landlords who acknowledge the needs of these families and are willing to establish a relationship whereby the women can negotiate for housing that is safe and affordable. All graduating families leave the Meta House programs with enough money saved for a security deposit, rent, and some furnishings.

Social Objective

Substance-abusing women tend to have lived isolated lives and often have little experience with successful interpersonal relationships. They may have difficulty with authority figures.

Each woman is assessed for the following: her need to improve interpersonal relationships with friends and authority figures; her need to change inappropriate emotional responses to interpersonal interactions; her need to develop attitudes that will lead to successful integration back into the community; and her need to increase social contact. These issues are addressed *in vivo* as part of day-to-day interactions as well as through individual counseling, group sessions, and house meetings.

Psychological Objective

Substance-abusing women have extremely low self-esteem. They are often clinically depressed, display some antisocial behavior, use food for emotional purposes, and have other diagnosable psychiatric disorders. These women are provided the opportunity to address issues of self-concept, sexual identity, behavior disturbances, incest, violence, sexual assault, and co-occurring mental health disorders. While in treatment each woman is assessed for co-existing psychiatric disorders and the extent of her concerns regarding self-concept and sexual identity. Also addressed is the woman's need to change behavior disturbances such as failing to keep her word, disrespect for others, compulsivity, inability to delay gratification, excessive dependency, inappropriate aggressiveness, hostility, and antisocial and avoidance behavior. She needs to learn to work within the limits of any psychiatric disorder and to express her fears and concerns regarding incest, sexual assault, and victimization. All identified issues are addressed in individual counseling and group therapy. Special groups are held for eating disorders and issues related to incest and rape.

Medical Objective

Substance-abusing women tend to have a high a incidence of health-related problems. This results from the direct effects of the alcohol or drugs, years of health care neglect, and the risks of sexually transmitted diseases.

Each woman enters the Meta House programs with a current physical examination. The need for medication, medical attention for pre-existing conditions and potential future medical problems, and the need for ongoing prenatal care are assessed. Nutritional needs, caffeine and nicotine intake, exercise, and the monitoring of a defined psychiatric disorder, as well as her ability to identify and take care of her own health needs are evaluated. Each woman is assisted in utilizing affordable health care from her HMO or other community resources.

Legal Objective

Substance-abusing women often have many legal entanglements, including custody issues, debts, fines, and the more serious charges associated with drug abuse. This may include the legal consequences associated with child abuse, neglect, or the death of a child.

Each woman is assessed for a need to resolve outstanding legal involvements. Individual counseling sessions and consultation with volunteer lawyers are utilized to help resolve problems. Department of Health and Human Services workers are consulted when appropriate. AODA counselors advocate and make court appearances on behalf of the women and their children.

Leisure-Time Objective

Free time, if not used appropriately, can be very dangerous to recovering women. In the past, free time, and often all time, was used in the acquisition or the recovery from the ingestion of substances. Recovering women usually do not know how to structure free time.

Each woman is assessed for how she manages her free time, the need to make free time, and her ability have fun in sobriety. Organized activities are arranged for women through in-house events and other community-related activities.

Expected Outcomes

- Upon discharge each woman will have a program for the maintenance of sobriety appropriate to her needs and life style and will know exactly what she must do if she feels the urge to use alcohol or drugs.
- Each woman will become actively involved in activities that lead to eventual education or training, or will have a job by discharge.
- Families will have suitable, safe, and affordable housing and will be able to survive within their financial means.
- Each woman will show improvement in her ability to interact appropriately in a variety of social situations, and will no longer keep herself isolated.
- Each woman will have higher self-esteem. Sexual identity issues will be openly addressed and processed for resolution, and behavior disturbances curbed. Women will have been thoroughly assessed and treated for concurrent psychiatric disorders. Issues of incest, rape, and violence will have been treated and understood, especially as they pertain to substance-abusing behavior.
- Each woman will be discharged with some or all of her legal entanglements resolved, and she will have learned how to be responsible within the legal system.
- Each woman will use her leisure time in ways that are not self-destructive. She will have learned to spend comfortable leisure time with her children and that it is possible to have fun in sobriety.

TREATMENT NEEDS
OF THE MOTHER–CHILD RELATIONSHIP

Cognitive Objective

Substance-abusing women need to become aware of how their behavior affects every aspect of a child's development and identify what has gone wrong so that they can eventually work toward normalizing the relationship. Many substance-abusing mothers come from families that did not have appropriate role models for parenting, nor do they typically surround themselves with people who model appropriate parenting skills. The behavior toward their children varies between being abusive or neglectful and guilty and overindulgent. They may also have limited knowledge of good nutrition for children and the effects of drugs on their own reproductive systems and on their unborn children.

At the Meta House programs we provide each mother with information about child development, especially as it pertains to mother–child attachment issues and the resulting behavioral and emotional outcomes. We teach how to improve child management and parenting skills, and we provide information about nutrition and self-care, the physical care of children, and the effects of drug abuse on the reproductive system and the unborn child, including AIDS education.

Specific education includes classes on the emotional and physical development of children, a parenting and child management class that addresses nurturing skills, a Head Start nutrition course, an in-house program on well-baby care, and sexuality classes. The latter classes present information about the effects of drugs on the reproductive system, the effects of prenatal drug and alcohol use on unborn children, and up-to-date information about AIDS and safe sex.

Affective Objective

Substance-abusing mothers carry tremendous feelings of guilt regarding their children. If they have custody of their children, they feel guilty about making their children unhappy and perhaps causing them serious physical and emotional harm. These feelings are exacerbated if they have lost custody. Many mothers feel deeply depressed because they define themselves and are defined by others as "unfit mothers." Sobriety cannot be achieved unless these feelings are addressed and the mothers can feel a sense of competence and enhanced self-esteem. In addition, substance-abusing mothers tend to have poor boundaries with their children and tend to feel overwhelmed by them. If mothers are ever to be reunited with their children and maintain sobriety, they must have time with their children and other children in a structured environment where they can learn and practice newly acquired skills and feelings of competence as a mother.

The Meta House programs provide an atmosphere for (1) improving self-esteem through resolving guilt feelings pertaining to the children and improving the depression that results from a lack of satisfaction with self and life circumstances; (2) developing a sense of identity separate from the children; (3) improving feelings about the restrictions imposed by the parental role; (4) Preparing for the maintenance of sobriety while living with the stresses of raising children.

Tied into the psychological portion of treatment, each woman attends individual counseling and group therapy that specifically addresses her issues as a pregnant woman or mother. In addition, a new program is about to be established whereby mothers who do not have custody of their children will spend structured time with other children at our own specialized day care center. These mothers will also have supervised times with their own children so that parenting skills can be practiced and they can begin to feel a sense of competence as parents.

Behavioral Objective

Substance-abusing mothers tend to neglect the health care of their children. They may cycle between neglect and overindulgence. Mothers who have lost custody of their children have little time to spend with them in a home-like environment. They also tend to have unrealistic ideas about how, and if, they will be reunited with their children. At the Meta House programs, we provide the time, space, and supervision for mothers and children who do not live together to spend extended periods of time together.

Social Objective

Substance-abusing mothers tend not to trust other women and instead see them as rivals. They isolate themselves in fear of judgment. Consequently, they do not have a network set up for their own emotional support and the care of their children. This may add to child abuse and neglect. They also lack the self-esteem to demand quality relationships with significant others. They tend to cycle through abusive relationships with men and other women, which also victimize their children.

Each woman lives in a community-based residential facility with other women over an extended period of time in a therapeutic milieu. The women are constantly encouraged to depend on and trust other women for practical and emotional support. Strong friendships are encouraged and naturally occur as women become more open about their past and their emotional pain. Mothers learn to ask for child-related help from other women, since staff is not available for routine child care responsibilities. Therefore each mother is provided with the opportunity to eliminate her social isolation, find relationships that will help with child care responsibilities, and develop healthy relationships with significant others.

Expected Outcomes

- Each mother has been given an understanding of the emotional and physical development of children and a more empathic understanding of them. She has improved her parenting skills and has developed a knowledge of nutrition and physical care. She can better nurture and discipline her children, has learned skills and gained knowledge of proper well-baby and sick-child care, and has developed the ability to make informed choices about her own sexuality.
- Upon discharge each woman has addressed the guilt she feels regarding her children in an appropriate manner and has found activities that help her develop an identity separate from her role as a mother. She has improved her feelings about being restricted by the parental role and has prepared for the maintenance of sobriety while living with the realities of raising children.
- Each woman who does not have custody of her children has spent extended, supervised time with her children and has had the opportunity to bond and practice parenting in a sober state. She also has allowed staff to observe interactions and suggest appropriate changes in the mother–child relationship. Developmental problems have been assessed for all children.
- Each woman has begun to trust other women and to develop a network of support for herself and her children. She has also been able to choose more appropriate partners for herself.

TREATMENT NEEDS OF CHILDREN

Cognitive Objective

Research has shown that children whose mothers abuse drugs have lower intellectual and educational functioning. This contributes to lowered self-esteem, impaired school performance, and difficulty in coping with daily life and activities. These children need accurate information about alcohol and drugs, and they need guidance to know what is normal regarding basic nutrition, health care, sexuality, and physical boundaries. Because children of drug-abusing mothers have not been able to trust their innate sense of reality, they need to have their observations affirmed by other people so that they can begin to trust that what they perceive is real. This will help them toward individuation and healthy decision making.

Each child is assessed within the first 30 days of residence for age-appropriate intellectual and educational functioning. This provides a baseline and information for an individualized treatment plan. Each child is introduced to an age-appropriate stranger-awareness program, a safety-at-home program, and sex education. To improve the children's reality testing, the staff works informally with them and sensitizes the mothers and the children's other institutional personnel, such as schools and foster parents, to continue to affirm the children's perceptions.

Affective Objective

Low self-esteem has been identified as the most common psychological trait among the children of substance-abusing mothers. They often have difficulty following tasks through to completion. They may lie when it is just as easy to tell the truth. They constantly seek approval and affirmation and are impulsive and unable to understand the consequences of their actions. They feel a lack of control over their environment and often have difficulty with appropriate expression of feelings. To survive in a substance-abusing family system, the child often isolates himself or herself from the outside world and becomes overly dependent on the mother.

Each child participates in play therapy, children's groups, and daily activities that provide opportunities to be goal oriented, follow through on tasks, and anticipate consequences. The program provides an atmosphere of unconditional positive regard. In addition, the children are encouraged to participate in Head Start, public school programs, and group cultural and recreational outings with other Meta House program families.

Behavioral Objective

Children of substance-abusing mothers statistically show higher incidence of physical impairment. They may have been impaired because of the mother's prenatal drug abuse, poor prenatal care, and/or physical abuse and neglect. Because of their families' social isolation, these problems may have gone unchecked. Each child is assessed and treated as needed for possible impairment of gross motor skills, fine motor skills, or language acquisition, and for Fetal Alcohol Syndrome, drug-induced, *in utero* maladies, and neglect of preventative health care.

Social Functioning Objective

Children with drug-abusing mothers tend, as do their mothers, to develop few skills in social interaction and as a result become socially isolated. Each child is assessed throughout his or her residency. Play therapy and monitored playtime are used to observe and intercept inappropriate behavior, such as confinement to dependent, nonproductive roles, and poor communication and conflict. Staff then demonstrates alternative coping methods. The staff of outside programs attended by these children are alerted to their special skill-building needs.

Expected Outcomes

- Each child's intellectual and educational functioning has improved. He or she has an age-appropriate cognitive understanding of alcohol and drug use and its consequences and age-appropriate information about sexuality. The child has learned the importance of self-care and how to protect himself or herself and avoid dangerous situations.
- Each child has improved self-esteem, demonstrated through higher levels of self-confidence, motivation, perseverance, and commitment to personal goals. He or she is able to accurately identify, justify, and act appropriately on feelings and show behavior that indicates age-appropriate identity formation.
- Physical problems not previously diagnosed have been recognized and children are referred for treatment. Their mothers have been educated so that the children get checkups and immunizations.
- Each child is better able to communicate his or her needs, solve conflicts without the intervention of mother or staff, show empathy for others, and exhibit team-building, group maintenance, and cooperative skills.

AFTERCARE

The Meta House programs also have an aftercare component. Long-term, consistent follow-up and aftercare can help minimize future problems. When an individual or family has therapeutic support, an appropriate intervention can be made when the pressures of everyday stresses are felt. Also, aftercare can help mothers live in a society that may condemn substance use yet be unsupportive of their sobriety. Supporting these families over an extended period of time helps insure successful transition and long-term stability. Aftercare can also help mothers overcome some of the fears they may have about living alone without the supportive peers and staff of Meta House.

Each mother attends weekly family sessions at the Meta House programs. The case manager and/or other identified specialists meet with the family in their home once every 2 weeks to continue education and support. Children's interaction with the mother during structured play is observed. Staff also continues to monitor fine and gross motor development, language acquisition, self-help abilities, and social and emotional development. Mothers also attend weekly support groups with other graduates of the Meta House programs.

PERFORMANCE

The mothers and children's program at Meta House was established in 1988. About 40% of the women leave Meta House before completing treatment; some of these may return and go through a complete treatment at a later time. Of women who complete treatment in all of the components of Meta House (all gender-specific treatment for women substance abusers, but not all involving children), 90% do not have to return for treatment. About 40 women live in the five residences of Meta House with 20 of their children. Up to 70 additional children are in foster care, but included in the programming. Women remain in the program for 9 to 18 months, and about 25 women graduate from the program every year.

Eight of ten residents of Meta House are single and nine of ten are unemployed. Most residents (85%) are between ages 22 and 44—about one third are between ages 30 and 35. Alcohol is used by nearly all the residents; about two-thirds use cocaine.

Case Example

Dorothy came to Meta House when she was 6 months pregnant. She was admitted with her two children, Tiffany, age 16 months, and Curtis, age 11 years. Dorothy was 32 years old at that time. She grew up as one of eight children. Her father is a binge drinker who becomes physically and verbally abusive while intoxicated. Her mother is also alcoholic. Dorothy remembers being terrified by her father during most of her childhood.

Dorothy's parents were divorced when she was 15 years old. She was a good student in elementary school; she graduated from high school, but not before dropping out for a period of time in the tenth grade. She missed a lot of school because of needing to take care of herself and others in the family after her father's binges and abusiveness. She attended a business institute after high school and received certification. She also attended a community college for 1 year and worked for the State of Illinois for 5½ years. She married at age 22 and moved to California, where her husband was stationed in the Navy. Curtis was born in 1980. After 3 years of living in a drug-using, abusive relationship, Dorothy was divorced and moved back to Chicago.

About the time of her parents divorce, when she was 15 years old, Dorothy began drinking beer and smoking marijuana. By age 19 her drinking had increased to a six pack of beer daily, some wine, and an increased use of marijuana. While living in California, Dorothy began taking amphetamines to lose weight, and this was quickly followed by what was the beginning of her cocaine use. Dorothy lived and worked in Chicago as her drug use escalated.

After Tiffany was born, Dorothy moved her family to Milwaukee in the hope that she would get away from her abusive patterns. Her drug use continued. She no longer worked. She received benefits from the State of Wisconsin and used these resources to obtain drugs. Her drug use had completely taken over her life.

Pregnant and feeling awful about her two other children, she called Child Protective Services and told them what she was doing. This was the beginning of a new life for Dorothy.

Dorothy's children were put in foster care. She received inpatient treatment at a local hospital. She then went to a shelter for 30 days until she could enter Meta House. When she entered the program her children were returned to her. During the next 16 months Dorothy and her children faced their lives together learning to live drug free. This was a particularly difficult experience.

Much of Dorothy's immediate emotional pain centered around her children. She loved them and cared about them, but viewed them as a burden. She had a tremendous amount of guilt for actual and fantasized harm she had done to them. In addition, Dorothy's baby was born with a significant chromosome deficiency. Some of his features looked as if Fetal Alcohol Syndrome might be involved. The medical staff could not make a definite diagnosis. Dorothy has had to learn to accept the possibility that she may have contributed to her son's severe developmental delays.

Dorothy became completely involved in all aspects of the Meta House program. Stemming from her own childhood, Dorothy's biggest issues had to do with trust, negative feelings about herself, and her feelings about her children. It became clear that Dorothy felt her children were a burden primarily because she did not know how to parent them. She participated in parenting and child development classes. She learned from the staff and other mothers how to discipline her children without being physically or emotionally abusive. She took responsibility for their physical care while attending to the newborn, who needed multiple surgeries. Through all the changes and trauma, she had the support of the staff and other residents. Slowly she began to trust others and recognize her own strengths and accomplishments. She was able to take responsibility for the things that were within her control, and stop blaming herself for her childhood and other things that were not of her doing. Her older son began doing well in school, while her daughter was blossoming at the Meta Munchkins Day Care Center. Despite the fact that Dorothy used drugs during all her pregnancies, her two older children appeared to be quite bright intellectually and showed no signs of developmental problems.

Dorothy graduated from the Meta House program and was accepted at a program that trains people to become Certified Alcohol and Drug Abuse Counselors. She lives around the corner from one of the Meta House programs with her three children. Her two younger children continue to attend Meta Munchkins, and Dorothy is currently an intern in one of the other Meta House programs. She hopes that someday she will become one of the Meta House staff.

FUNDING

Meta House's 2 million-dollar annual budget is funded from a 4.7 million-dollar 5-year federal grant begun in 1991, and from Milwaukee County, the State of Wisconsin, the United Way, and a number of other sources.

In Wisconsin, the licensing and funding of programs is separated for adults and children. While the women's and children's program was being developed, an interesting dilemma occurred. On the one hand, a license was needed to treat the adult women, and, on the other hand, some kind of sanctioning was needed if children were to be housed. The Child Care Institution License demanded a high staff-to-child ratio, court-ordered placement, and responsibility for the children placed with the agency. Besides the prohibitive cost, the philosophy of treatment would have been undermined if the children were to become wards of the state and the mothers were not responsible for their children.

Since the primary mission of this agency was the treatment of alcoholism and drug abuse for adults, the adult division of the various levels of government were approached for opinions and funding. Every person approached was very supportive and cooperative in helping see this program come to fruition. Milwaukee County strongly advocated for this program in recognition of its long-term fiscal benefits. The State of Wisconsin offered a grant that covered the concept of treatment for the family. Eventually the federal level of government became involved, with a grant from the Center for Substance Abuse Treatment. The child welfare agencies are extremely supportive of the concept and the program. It was difficult, however, to find funding through the child welfare programs, since it is licensed as an adult program. It was not until the licensing of the child day care center that funding was forthcoming from the Child Welfare Agency.

Our Home Foundation, Inc., has done many things to muster the recognition and support it needs to continue programming. Nothing speaks louder than success, however. Much of the acknowledgment and resulting funding has come from the women who have been through the program and their families. As these people trickle back into the community, they have taken it upon themselves to speak out about how important the treatment experience was to them and their children. They will often accompany invited speakers and other staff who are attempting to educate the community about the program.

Of course, the financial support received does not match the demand for services. Funding for women's treatment has never been very popular. It was not until the children entered our program that recognition and support increased. This is a sad statement about how we view women. It appears that the welfare of women only becomes important when they are needed to properly care for children. As a result, this agency will be actively seeking future funding from grants that specifically target the welfare of women and children.

REFERENCES

Bowlby, J. (1958). The nature of the child's tie to his mother. *International Journal of Psycho-Analysis, 39,* 350–373.

Chasnoff, I. J. (1989). Cocaine, pregnancy, and the neonate. *Women and Health, 15*(3), 23–34.

Cherukuri, R., Minkoff, H., Feldman, J., Parekh, A., & Glass, L. (1988). A cohort study of alkaloidal cocaine ("crack") in pregnancy. *Obstetrics and Gynecology, 72,* 147–151.

Cole, C. (1989, December). *Following drug-exposed babies to school.* Paper presented at the Drug-Free Pregnancy Conference, San Mateo, CA.

Feinberg, F. C. (1991). *The maternal–fetal attachment of drug-abusing pregnant women.* Unpublished doctoral dissertation, Wisconsin School of Professional Psychology, Milwaukee.

Gomberg, E. (1976). Alcoholism and women. In H. Begleiter (Ed.), *Social aspects of alcoholism* (pp. 217–238). New York: Plenum Press.

Klaus, M. H., & Kennell, J. H. (1976). *Maternal–infant bonding.* Saint Louis, MO: C. V. Mosby.

McRobbie, J., Mata, S., & Kronstadt, D. (1989, December). *Proceedings paper from a conference on drug free pregnancy.* Presented at the Proceedings of the Far West Laboratory for Educational Research and Development, San Mateo, CA.

Petitti, D. B., & Coleman, C. (1990). Cocaine and the risk of low birth weight. *American Journal of Public Health, 80,* 25–28.

Youngstrom, N. (1991, October). Drug exposure in home elicits worst behavior. *American Psychological Association Monitor,* p. 3.

IV

FOSTER CARE OPTIONS

So-called "therapeutic" foster care has existed for some time for more seriously disturbed children who are placed away from their own families. The two approaches to foster care presented here add important systems components. Patricia Minuchin describes how a collaborative connection between foster and biological families can alleviate problems that arise in traditional foster care systems, such as separation trauma and loyalty confusions for the child and the humiliation and disempowering of the parents, and can enhance the possibility of family reunification in the future.

Marcia Eckstein's program of "foster family clusters" is a remarkable synthetic extended family, where every family in the cluster has a role in every child's life, offering extensive support and a safety net. While much of the work with these challenging children is focused within the cluster, efforts are made to keep the children's own families involved, as well.

Foster families can be a viable alternative to children's own families when children cannot live safely at home. But the expectation that placing a child in a "nice" family environment, better than the chaotic one from which they have come, will have immediate salubrious effects has long been disappointed. Addressing issues of children's loyalty and building an elaborate system of involvement make some of the more difficult placements work.

11

Foster and Natural Families: Forming a Cooperative Network

Patricia Minuchin

Maria was living in a welfare hotel with her 2-year-old son and an infant of 9 months. She and the children's father kept contact, though he lived with his mother. He was unemployed and enrolled in a job training program; she was on welfare. Maria had smoked crack, over the years, but she claims that she was not, in fact, using drugs when an unknown person called protective services to accuse her of neglecting the children. She points to the terrible conditions of life in the welfare hotel as the major problem in caring for her family.

A caseworker was sent to investigate, returning 2 days later to take the children. In a subsequent court hearing, Maria was informed that the children were in foster care, and she agreed to enter a 6-month drug program as a condition for their return. As Maria and Cary, the children's father, told the story some 3 months later, they had been trying all that time to find out where the children were. With the children gone, Maria lost her room at the hotel and moved out. In a series of events that are both unique and typical, the agency in charge of the children had been unable to locate her until now.

By the time the parents actually see the children, the baby is a year old and the older boy close to 2½. The parents meet with agency work-

ers, the foster parents, and the children. The foster parents busy themselves taking off the children's sweaters, changing the baby, setting the
older one up with toys to play with. The natural parents are passive. Maria
reaches for the baby, then withdraws with uncertainty. She talks with the
older child, who stares at her and does not respond.

The process is in motion. The foster parents are in charge, and they
function with competence. They assume that the natural parents have been
disqualified. The natural parents are disempowered, uncertain of their
rights and functions. They hide their anger and their pain. The children
are young, 3 months have gone by, and it is hard to know what they make
of the reappearance of their mother and father.

In this system, visiting times are biweekly and are on the agency
premises. The children are already uncertain. If there is no change in the
quality and quantity of contact, it is possible that the parents will become
detached and that the later reunification of the family, if it comes at all,
will not be successful.

Is this situation in the best interests of children and family? Unlikely.
The family is disqualified and disempowered, hemmed in by rules that
limit their contact with the children, even as they struggle with drug dependency and destructive living conditions. If they become alienated and
uncooperative during the placement period, it seems likely, as Kates and
her colleagues (Kates, Johnson, Rader, & Strieder, 1991) have suggested, that the behavior is basically iatrogenic (that is, caused by the system). Even if they keep contact through biweekly visits, interaction is
minimal. Parents and children will not be growing and changing together,
mutual patterns will not evolve, and it will be difficult for the parents to
cope effectively when the family is reunited.

The effects of separation and placement on children are not easily
summarized. Children who are taken into care via charges of family neglect
or abuse may or may not be sturdy to begin with, but there is little question that the process is inherently traumatic, despite the positive intent.
Children must cope with the basic uncertainty of "Whose child am I?"
(Kates et al., 1991), and some show the kind of disturbances that are
predictable: difficulties in establishing relationships, hostility and acting
out, uncertain sense of self, and confusion over identification figures.
Others are more resilient, and are judged to be functioning adequately
(Fanshel, Finch, & Grundy, 1990; Fein, 1991; Wald, Carlsmith, & Leiderman, 1988). However, the question is not whether some children can function adequately despite the trauma, but what they must cope with in this
situation, and how the negative impact can be minimized. How can policies and procedures within the system be changed so as to minimize trauma and enhance the possibilities of a constructive outcome?

The foster care system varies by states and regions, and efforts to create change have generally been local, arising in welfare and protective services, foster care agencies, private groups, and regional legislatures. However, some policies are set by federal legislation. The Child Welfare and Adoption Assistance Act (PL 96-272) of 1980 aimed at limiting the drift of children within the foster care system. It focused on permanency planning within a reasonable time frame, the review of cases to keep them moving, and preventive services. Fein (1991) notes that the law was broadly effective for a period, decreasing the number of children in care and the length of placement, although it was also evident, in some cases, that the time frame and the emphasis on permanency planning hastened decisions to terminate parental rights and place children for adoption. By 1984, the positive trends were reversed, reflecting the rising pressure of social problems and the decreasing availability of relevant funding. As the number of children in care went up and the supply of foster families went down, the emphasis shifted, in the late 1980s, highlighting family preservation and the provision of intensive preventive services for families at risk. The trend is exemplified by the growing strength of such agencies as the National Association for Family Based Services and by the federal Family Preservation and Family Support Initiative, passed and funded in 1993 as part of the administration's Omnibus Budget Reconciliation Act.

The change in emphasis is unquestionably positive. Too many children are taken into care too swiftly. Intensive services for Maria, the children, Cary, and the extended family might well have kept the children in the family and held it together through a period of difficulty. It is clear, however, that the quality of such services will determine the outcome, and it is also clear that foster care will not disappear in the foreseeable future. For a variety of reasons, ranging from a legitimate concern for child safety to the regrettable dearth of adequate preventive services, some children will continue to be placed in foster care. It is essential, therefore, to improve the process, from the first moment of decision through all the subsequent stages.

If, on careful consideration, it were deemed necessary to take the children of Maria and Cary into care, a more enlightened procedure would have reduced the shock and confusion for the children and the pain and resentment of the parents. And a different structure of contacts and services would have protected the integrity of the family during the period of placement and increased their ability to manage once they are reunited. The basic purpose of foster placement is not to rescue the child, but to offer respite for the family until life becomes manageable and the adult family members can safely care for the children themselves. That conception of purpose is, in itself, a focus of change, since it is not automatically shared by professionals and participants in the system.

In this chapter, I will describe an ecological model for foster care.

The model is based on systemic, psychologically constructive principles and includes a revision in traditional policies, procedures, and training. Kates et al. (1991) have pointed out that the issue for the foster care system is "Whose child is this?" and that in the fragmented structure of most systems, the answer is confusing and competitive. In the framework of an ecological model, the response would necessarily be "This child is ours"—denoting a coordinated network of agency and foster and biological families, mutually responsible for the child and to each other. The focus of the model is on connections, rather than the fragmentation that characterizes most systems; on empowerment of the child's family, rather than the reverse; and on the expansion of roles for both professionals and the members of foster and biological families.

THE ECOLOGICAL MODEL

If one thinks of families as complex systems, composed of people who are connected and interacting, it is a natural extension to look at larger networks in similar terms. During the 1980s, Salvador Minuchin, the director of Family Studies, a New York City training center, developed an ecological approach to foster care. Minuchin and the staff of Family Studies subsequently embarked on a consultation and training project with foster care agencies in New York City.[1] The ecological perspective guided both the conception of foster care and the efforts to change policies, procedures, and skills.

When a decision is made to remove children from a family and place them in care, an ecological framework shapes the way one understands what is happening. Assuming that all families are complex systems, even if they seem disorganized, it is clear that separation breaks up familiar patterns. The transition brings confusion and the imperative need to establish new patterns. The biological family must function without the child; the foster family must reorganize to incorporate the new member; the child must find a place in the foster family. In the foster home, the patterns of daily life, from breakfast to church attendance, may be very different from those of the child's biological family, and familiar roles, for instance, claiming the prerogatives of the oldest child, may not be appropriate or welcome in a family with a different structure and an organized sibling pattern of its own. Adaptation is difficult, but success has a paradoxical feature. If the biological family settles into a pattern that does not include the child, and if the child and foster family create a comfortable way of life together, the viability of the biological family will be increasingly threatened.

It is clear, also, that separation and placement have created a new, superordinate system. The ecological model highlights the triangle of agency, foster family, and biological family as the basic reality of foster care. As soon as the child is placed, this new system comes into being. It is not always recognized as such, in traditional child welfare systems, and its importance is seldom recognized. Removal and placement often create an adversarial atmosphere that separates the two families, and subsequent services are often fragmented, sending the biological parents, the children, and the foster family in different directions with different professional workers. But the new system is there, nonetheless. The two families coexist in the mind of the child, and members of the two families often have unexplored attitudes about people in the other family, even though they have little contact. It is a basic tenet of the model that the connection between the two families must be acknowledged and that, whenever possible, the unit must become a collaborative system. It should function as a constructive problem-solving network around the child through the period of placement. The impact on child development and the possibilities of family reunification depend, in large measure, on whether that happens.

BASIC THEMES AND SKILLS

In translating the model into a form for training and consultation, the Family Studies staff formulated a "credo" of relevant themes and skills. These describe the ideas and attitudes that foster care professionals and participants must carry, in order to implement this approach, and the skills they must develop for working with disempowered biological families. (For a fuller discussion of these concepts and skills, see P. Minuchin et al., 1990; S. Minuchin & Fishman, 1981).

The Themes

Of the five themes, three concern the perception of the biological family. They focus on resources and potential, rather than failures and difficulties.

Family Preservation

It may seem paradoxical that family preservation is a major theme, since the family unit has been broken, by definition, when children are removed and placed in foster care. "Keeping children in the family" is not a literal possibility when that happens, but it is a symbolic possibility, if family members can preserve the sense of a unit that includes children not living at home. Continuing contact is an essential medium for preserving the integrity of the unit. It provides family members with a sense of immediacy about each other, rather than memories, and with live data about growth and change in the children. If family identity can be preserved through the placement period, there is an increased likelihood that the family can be successfully reunited and that it will be able to maintain viability.

Family Empowerment

Family empowerment is, arguably, the core of this approach. It involves facilitating a family's sense of competence and control. When the children of poor, multicrisis families have been taken into care, it is important for the parents to regain the sense that they have rights and responsibilities in relation to their children: That means that they are listened to and respected as parents and concerned family members, that they are encouraged to participate in decisions affecting their children, that they are credited with the ability to learn and change, and that there is some recognition of their skills and their efforts to cope with difficult life circumstances. If the goal of foster care is to reunite the natural family, empowering that family during the placement period is not only humane and practical, it is psychologically sound. Only a family that feels some control over its members' lives can become more functional as an environment for growing children.

Outreach to the Extended Family

Protective services and courts often apply tunnel vision to a family under investigation, concerning themselves primarily with mother and children. The extended family may be difficult to reach and may not be willing to take on full responsibility for the children. However, the family may well include people who have strong ties to parents and children, who are concerned about placement, and who share the goal of bringing the children back home. They are a potential resource, and, if they are contacted, they may be able to support the household informally or in periods of difficulty. This theme is crucial for agency personnel, but it has special import in training foster parents and redefining their role. Foster parents are often particularly effective in reaching out to the extended family. They may know the community more intimately than professional workers, may find more relaxed ways of establishing contact, and may be more readily trusted by the family, once mutual stereotypes and initial wariness have been overcome.

The last two themes concern the process of foster placement and the developmental realities that shape its impact.

Periods of Transition

The foster care process is marked by periods of transition, from the first separation, when the children are removed and placed, to the final resolution, when the family is reunited, as well as any moves in between. All transitions imply upheaval for children and families, and these periods must be seen as crucial. It is necessary to recognize stress as inevitable and to tolerate disturbances in functioning as part of the transitional process. The issues are similar in all transitions, even though the first separation is especially traumatic and family reunification is essentially a happy event. In every move, the participants must relinquish former life patterns, give up or modify old attachments and establish new ones, and find a viable way to live as a family with different members and characteristics. The toll on children may be especially great. The ability of adults to function supportively is crucial, and it is essential to provide intensive supports through each transition.

Developmental Stage

The child's age and stage shapes every aspect of the foster care experience. The impact of separation, adaptation to a new family, and the possibility of maintaining a sense of the original family while accepting new people are all affected by the reality of being an infant, a 4-year-old, a school child, or an adolescent. Foster parents must know something of the characteristics and needs of children at different developmental stages, but it is important for them to understand also that children of different ages will integrate the experience of placement in different ways. The trauma of separation and the process of placement may cause them to behave differently than children of similar age in the life experience of foster parents. The concept of developmental stage applies particularly to the child, but it is useful to apply the concept, as well, to foster and natural families, which may be at similar or different stages of the family life cycle. The fit between the developmental realities of the two families will shape the nature of their contact and the form of their cooperation on behalf of the children.

The Skills

Foster care workers and foster parents are not family therapists. However, the family therapy repertoire includes some skills that are particularly relevant for the foster care situation, and these have been selected for emphasis in the training. They are the necessary skills for connecting and empowering. They enable the foster parents to make constructive contact with the biological family, and they are essential, as well, for the optimal functioning of professional staff.

Joining

Joining is a matter of conveying interest, respect, and acceptance of other people. It is carried partly by warmth and friendliness and may seem more like a natural part of social contact than a skill, but joining also involves an ability to listen well and to accommodate to the experiences and viewpoint of the other person or family. That is not automatic for many people, and it takes some practice.

Mapping

Mapping, the most specific skill, is a mechanism for thinking in terms of extended families. It is a simple technique for recording in graphic form the members of a foster child's extended family (or any family), including ages, gender, and relationships. In more complex versions, the map indicates subgroups within the family and lines of closeness and conflict. Even a simple map provides foster parents with a concrete picture of the composition and developmental stage of a biological family, and allows some inferences about the availability of extended family, the developmental issues the family must be facing, and the family's potential resources. If foster parents are able to create the map together with the foster child or members of the family, the process itself becomes an act of joining.

The Search for Strength

The search for strength operationalizes the emphasis on the positive aspects of individuals and families. When children have officially been removed from a family, foster parents may find it difficult to perceive the family in positive terms. However, it is useful for them to understand and act on the idea that court judgments of yes or no about parental adequacy are necessarily oversimplified; the family almost always has some strengths and resources. Searching for strength, as a skill, is part of the empowering process. Foster parents help to redress the uncertainty and resentment of the natural family if they can regard the parents as experts on the characteristics and history of their children, acknowledge the accomplishments that are usually ignored, "reframe" the family's self-critical preoccupation with failure, and solicit information on the parenting methods that have worked with the children.

Working with Complementarity

Complementarity is a complex idea and working with it a relatively self-conscious skill. It is based on the concept that people in interaction create a systemic equilibrium by balancing their behavior. If A makes quick decisions, B is less active; if B takes over, A does less. While the balance can be either healthy or dysfunctional in ordinary circumstances, the complementarity between foster and biological families is inherently skewed. Society assigns more weight, competence, and social approval to the foster parents, who tend, as in the opening vignette, to take charge of the child care situation. The natural parents, essentially disqualified, are often passive. If the latter are to be empowered, however, the foster parents must learn to hold back, giving space, crediting the potential of the natural family, allowing competence to emerge. The search for strength and working with complementarity build on the same underlying attitude, and, as skills, they develop together.

IMPLEMENTING THE MODEL: THE LIAISON BETWEEN FOSTER AND NATURAL FAMILIES

The liaison between foster and natural families is at the core of this approach. As noted earlier, the two families become part of a new superordinate system as soon as the child is placed in care. The thrust of the model is to make their relationship functional: to create a kind of extended kinship system, in which members of the two families are united not by blood but by their mutual involvement with the children. Since traditional procedures customarily separate the families, this is a fundamental change in philosophy and practice. It requires training at the level of staff, administrators, and foster parents, as well as a different way of involving the biological family.

The various forms and levels of training are discussed below, but it is informative to start at the end of the process, with a meeting of foster parents, social worker, and a natural mother whose three children are in foster care. The foster parents and social worker have been part of the Family Studies training project. They are oriented toward connecting and empowering the biological family, and are functioning with the perspective and skills described earlier.

Forming a Cooperative Network

Clara and Laura are the foster mothers of three children from the same family. Clara is the foster mother of Bobby, 12, and Malcolm, 5. The middle boy, James, 10, is more difficult to handle and has been placed separately with Laura. Maude, the social worker, has recently been assigned to this family.

The mother, Jana, had brought the children in for voluntary foster placement, concerned about their care and safety. She felt that her former husband was a threat, that her life was out of control, and that she was on the brink of resuming her previous drug habit. After the children were placed, she visited them every 2 weeks at the agency, in keeping with agency procedure at that time. At some point, Jana began to complain because the agency would not permit her to take the boys off the premises. They were active, and she maintained that the family could not enjoy the visit if they were cooped up in a small room. Having brought the boys in voluntarily, she was hurt and resentful about the lack of trust, becoming so angry that she stopped coming for visits, refused to deal with the agency, and could not be reached by agency workers.

The events that led to the meeting were, in themselves, part of the change in attitude and procedures among participants in the training project. On the initiative of the two foster mothers, supported by the social worker, the training group discussed a new effort to set up a liaison with Jana. Living in the same neighborhood and untainted as agency professionals, Clara and Laura were able to contact her, and she agreed to come in to meet with them and the social worker. In preliminary discussions, the team agreed that the two foster parents would carry the meeting, and that the social worker would intervene if and when she thought it necessary. The goal was to establish contact, to get past the stalemate between Jana and the agency, and to begin the formation of a cooperative network that would be productive for the children and all the families.

The following excerpts are from the first 15 minutes of the meeting. They demonstrate a variety of ways in which the foster mothers join and empower Jana (acceptance and respect, telling and asking, complementarity and eliciting strength), as well as the surprisingly swift conversion of their efforts into a genuine, mutually useful dialogue.

The meeting begins with Jana sitting between Clara and Laura. Maude is on the other side of Laura. Through the settling down pleasantries, Jana sits with arms folded tightly across her chest, stiff, conveying a deliberate distance from the proceedings. She is wary, and says nothing.

Clara starts by saying, "Jana, I just want to tell you . . . you have two beautiful sons."

(She conveys that she likes and appreciates the children, and that—like any parent—Jana has the right to be proud of them and of the part she had in making them likable children.)

Jana smiles and relaxes a little. Laura makes a joke about James being a handful, and Jana comments that everybody petted the oldest and the youngest, but James was the middle one and things were harder for him.

Clara asks, "Do you like the way I'm taking care of your boys?"

(This is a clear communication that Jana has a right to judge that by her own standards, that she is not disqualified as a parent, and that, of course, she will care about their welfare.)

Jana says, yes, and that she knows Clara is spoiling them. It's good humored. They both laugh, and Jana is visibly relaxing.

Clara begins to describe the reactions of Malcolm, the youngest boy, when the children first came to her. "He was very emotional. I really needed to give him a lot of time . . . he's stronger now. . . . "

(She's sharing information with a matter-of-fact attitude that of course Jana is interested in the details of how her children are adapting and progressing.)

Jana now begins to talk at some length about the boys: how she explained the situation to the older two; never hid anything from Bobby, the oldest, who is responsible and smart; how Malcolm didn't really understand, and so forth. It is now a dialogue.

(As she talks, Jana is revealed as an intelligent, observant parent, concerned with her children, attuned to their personalities and differences. She is sharing information, and that is useful per se to the foster parents, as well as an important step in the process of creating a network.)

Laura enters to describe the fact that James gets into fights. She says, "So, I'm having a little problem with him right now. With you, when he had tantrums, the way he does . . . I mean, how did you deal with it? What did you do?"

(She is asking for help in solving a problem of child care and management, acknowledging that Jana has experience with her son and has some ideas and skills that can be useful. It is a first step in forming a cooperative adult system that can pool resources on behalf of the child.)

Jana responds by saying that he does the same with her and that he doesn't like people to tell him what to do. Then she describes what she does to manage him. By now, these three parents are in contact, discussing the children and the situation.

It is important to note that there is no "script." The foster parents have not learned their lines. The contact flows naturally, in their own words and style, based on the fact that they have absorbed certain attitudes about the biological family, understand the importance of contact, and have developed some skills for joining and empowering. The reward is that they tap, in a very short time, the strength and knowledge of the natural mother, and begin the process of constructive communication.

It is also worth noting that the social worker has said nothing, allowing this contact to unfold. With less trained foster parents, or if Jana were not responsive, the social worker would have a more immediately active role. In this situation, she will be available to coordinate developments and to handle the many issues that will arise over time. She and the foster parents are a team, however. Ideas about complementarity and strength apply to their subsystem as well, and the social worker will give the foster parents space and support to develop their relationship with the biological mother.

Training

How do the participants reach this point? The following sections summarize training and consultation for direct service teams, agency administrators, and foster parents. The descriptions are based on the work and experience of the Family Studies staff and are offered as examples. The procedures are modifiable in different local situations, but it is important that the basic principles be implemented even if the details change.

Direct Service Teams: Caseworkers and Foster Parents

The project began in agencies that expressed interest in the approach. Training for direct service teams took place in weekly meetings over a period of approximately 2 years. The first phase was for professional staff and included theoretical discussions about family systems, illustrative material about interventions, and practical demonstrations with agency families. The structure of the second phase was more unique. Professional staff were joined by foster parents, and subsequent training was for the combined group. Caseworkers and foster parents met together with the trainers to discuss basic ideas, clarify their roles, and work, in teams, with biological families, implementing the skills they were learning.

In all this work, the concept of a network was predominant, and the relationship of foster and biological families was considered the critical feature. The meeting between Jana, the two foster mothers, and the social worker that took place in the course of the training is a good illustration of the process, though in other meetings there would usually be an effort to include the children and other members of the biological family.

It is beyond the scope of this chapter to discuss the issues that must be worked out when professional staff and foster parents function as a team in relation to the natural family. It is evident, however, that the collaboration and orientation expand both roles. The professional worker becomes the facilitator and supervisor of contact, in addition to his or her usual functions, and the foster parent moves beyond child care to outreach and continuing contact with the natural family, as well as a new form of collaboration with the social worker.

Agency Administration

Intensive training of staff and foster parents can change attitudes and skills, but traditional procedures do not change unless the innovations are supported by administrators. Behind the usual procedures are attitudes, history, assumptions about legality, and a sense of familiarity with the specific arrangements. Constructive change usually requires a shift in the organizational features of the agency and specific attention to key points in the foster care process.

In consultation with administrators and supervisors, the following areas were emphasized:

- *Intake* should begin with a meeting that includes caseworker, foster parent(s), at least two adults from the biological family, and the child or children, in order for participants to exchange information, set goals for the child, clarify the involvement of the biological family, and discuss next steps.
- *Policies and procedures for visiting* should create flexible conditions, reflecting the realities of the individual case, and provide for contact and communication between the two families, as well as private time for children and family.
- *Organization of services* should involve the coordination of services to biological family, foster family, and children under a single case manager, both to improve efficiency and to enhance the view that "this child (and situation) is ours."
- *Focus on transitional periods* should recognize the traumatic implications of separations and placements for children and families and provide for concentrated services through periods of change at the beginning and end of the process, as well as transitions in between.

In our project, the exploration of agency structures and policies took the form of scheduled and informal meetings with administrators and supervisors. The need for administrative change was inherent in the model, but alternatives were most usefully discussed in the context of plans for particular children and families. Most agencies, for instance, provided for visits between the natural family and the child every 2 weeks on the agency premises, and that policy was taken for granted. When we explored the possibility of flexibility in particular cases, however, it became evident that the policy was not written in stone. It was clearly possible to allow more leeway in setting up the frequency and location of family meetings. In the same way, some administrators were able to expedite the first contact between parents and children after placement, overcoming the usual bureaucratic delays in the interest of minimizing the trauma of separation. In these and other matters that came to discussion, administrators and supervisors were able to clarify the difference between law and habit and to modify rigid procedures.

It would be misleading to imply that policies and procedures shifted easily in response to psychological logic. It is difficult to change an organization, particularly when it is set within a powerful larger system, such as the welfare and protective services of city or state. Resistance and drift are to be expected, and a variety of approaches, beyond the scope of this chapter, are necessary (see Imber-Black, 1988). The basic point, however, is that the effort to implement a new model in a complex organization must take place at multiple levels. Procedural changes require administrative flexibility, just as the implementation of administrative changes depends on line workers capable of putting new policies into practice.

Foster Parents

Out of the experience in working with foster care agencies, the Family Studies staff has created a training manual to prepare foster parents for participating in this approach (P. Minuchin et al., 1990). The Training Manual for Foster Parents is intended for the use of trainers and assumes that the institution is basically in accord with the ecological model. The first part of the manual is theoretical, outlining the view of families, foster care, major themes, and skills. The second part describes eight training sessions, covering activities, purpose, and goals for each. The activities of the sessions are experiential, including role play, small groups, simulated cases, and discussion.

The first four sessions concentrate on understanding and attitudes: on the way families function and vary, on the involvement of the whole foster family in foster care, on attitudes toward the natural family, on the foster child's roots, expectations, and adaptation to a new family culture. Woven through these sessions are the themes described earlier, concerning preservation and empowerment of the child's extended natural family, the impact of transitions, and the reality of foster care for children at different developmental stages.

The remaining sessions focus on contact with the biological family and the collaboration of foster parents with agency case workers. These sessions invoke the skills that are relevant for joining, eliciting strength, and empowerment. For example, the fifth session deals with visiting. It includes a consideration of foster parent involvement before, during and after a visit; discussion of the child as a "traveler," carrying images and expectations back and forth between families; and role play of a first meeting between a biological mother, her young child who is in care, and the foster mother. Subsequent sessions explore the coordination of foster parents and caseworkers as they work with the extended natural family, and the complex issues and feelings that arise when the child leaves the foster family and returns home.

Working with agencies in the foster care project, we have been impressed with the strength of many inner-city foster parents. They are often wise in the ways of the community, though not highly educated, and, with training, many are able to expand their roles, accepting and implementing the idea of outreach to the child's family. In a similar vein, we have found that inner-city foster parents are responsive to the training described in the Training Manual for Foster Parents. They are able to discuss, explore attitudes, role play, challenge procedures, and learn. We have also found, logically enough, that the orientation and skills dissipate, in time, if they are not potentiated by the foster care staff. The message is unavoidable. Carefully chosen and trained foster parents can be an invaluable, essentially untapped, resource for an enlightened foster care system. However, their integration into such a system depends on a coordinated approach, involving administration, professional staff, and foster parents in interaction with each other and with the biological families of the foster children.

KINSHIP FOSTER CARE

For the most part, children are sent into foster care with families they do not know. Sometimes, however, they are placed with kin, and the effort to arrange such placements is growing. Certainly, if children must be taken from their homes, kinship foster care is the preferred solution. It minimizes the shock for family and child and maintains the structure of a familiar world with predictable boundaries, even if the children must move about within it. It also maximizes the possibility that the "foster family" will provide continuing support when the children go home, offering respite to the parents and backup care during periods of stress. Extended families have often worked that way informally, especially in minority cultures where crises are multiple and part of life (Boyd-Franklin, 1989).

But this scenario is too simple. Extended families may be part of the problem as well as, or instead of, part of the solution. Examples come easily to mind: the grandmother who disapproves of her daughter's drug habit and life style, and who makes it difficult for the mother and the man who is her sometime companion and the father of the children to function as parents while the children are in her care, or the extended family of the father, whose members accuse the mother of neglect, take charge of the children via court order, and push out the mother, who is angry, disempowered by rejection, and ineffective with the children in the presence of a more competent sister-in-law.

These patterns are dysfunctional. As in any system with such features, whether the children are officially in foster care or not, family therapy is the intervention of choice. In this respect, kinship foster care is different from the more usual placement. The distinction is important. When children are placed in an unfamiliar family, the operative system has been newly created and the participants have been thrown together by happenstance. They do not carry patterns and shared history developed over the years. The task of professional workers is to encourage the creation of connections, rather than untangling patterns that are established and dysfunctional. It is often true, of course, that some therapeutic intervention with the natural family is necessary. An adolescent girl in foster care may be locked in conflict with her parents, and successful reunification cannot occur unless there is a constructive change in their interactions. By and large, however, the focus of foster care management, in an enlightened system, is the creation of a new cooperative system where none has existed before.

When children are placed with relatives, the situation is different. The extended family has established grooves. They do not need to become acquainted, but they do need to create a structure that will fit the new reality, and that is a difficult task. In traditional foster care systems, it is not generally recognized that it is important to help the family through the transitional period of kinship placement. Placing children with relatives is assumed to be a solution in itself.

In those cases where the extended family is potentially "part of the problem," more intensive help is required in order to resolve the tensions that will block the possibility of reunification. The goals are familiar to family therapists: to establish clear boundaries, clarify hierarchy and generational roles, bring parenting issues to the center, and so forth.

In any foster care situation, it is important to think about systems and to employ some skills that have been developed within the field of family therapy. In kinship foster care, however, long-term family structures and patterns become relevant. Family relationships are at the heart of the contact between the home from which the child has been removed and the home to which he or she has been taken. Here, the skills of the family therapist are directly applicable for assessment of the situation, and, in some cases, for the facilitation of constructive change.

CASE EXAMPLE: THE BAKERS AND THE BARTONS

The following illustration is taken from the Family Studies project described earlier, in which professional staff and the foster and natural families focused on creating a collaborative network and enhancing the possibility of successful reunification. This situation illustrates both the relationship established between the natural and foster families and the need to work with issues in the natural family.[2]

When the project staff first came in contact with Marni Baker and her family, she was 20 years old, engaged to be married, and pregnant. The contact came relatively late in the process. Marni's daughter, Janie, nearly 4 years old, had been in foster care with the Bartons for more than 3 years, and the agency was now working on plans for reunification.

Marni was the oldest of four children in a family that had seen hard times and continued to do so. Her mother, Ada, was a pleasant woman in her late 40s who had been abused by her husband and had been separated for many years. She described being homeless for a period, always poor, and living at times on welfare. Marni was 17 and unmarried when Janie was born. Though the relationship between Ada and Marni was close, they felt it necessary to place Janie in foster care.

The agency placed Janie with the Bartons, a middle-class family, and arranged for visits every 2 weeks at the agency. As time passed, Janie came for weekend visits at Ada's home. Marni had moved out and found a job, but she came to spend time with her daughter during the weekend visits. The family was used to the arrangement and Ada loved her granddaughter, but when Janie came to visit there was constant bickering between Janie and Pam, Ada's youngest daughter, and Ada found them difficult to handle.

As Marni settled into her job, formalized plans to marry James and became pregnant, the agency and family began to plan for reunification. Project staff and participants saw the task as twofold: to create a (belated) relationship between the foster and biological family, focused on getting acquainted and preparing for reunification, and to clarify the natural family's plans for receiving Janie into the family as a permanent member. The map in Figure 11.1 describes the participants and structure at this time.

The foster family, in this case, was clearly more affluent than the natural family—an unusual arrangement in the city system. Marni was somewhat intimidated by the idea of the family and its advantages. She had never visited the home and had met Meg, the foster mother, only in passing during visits with Janie at the agency. After discussion with the staff, Marni made contact with the foster family and, somewhat to her surprise, was invited to visit their home. She came back aglow, proud of

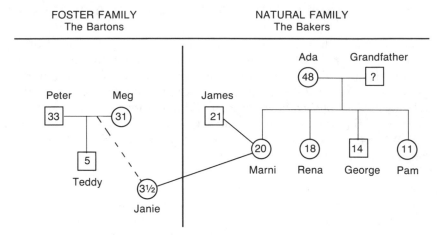

FIGURE 11.1. Map of foster family and natural family structures.

herself for overcoming her nervousness and very pleased with the visit. She and James had gone together. The foster parents had been friendly, Janie had shown them her room and toys, James had played with the children, and they had seen the closeness of Teddy and Janie, who clearly felt like brother and sister. The two families had begun to plan visits for the children after Janie moved. Marni remarked that she was grateful for the way they had cared for Janie and that she wasn't going to say "no" to keeping contact. It was unlikely that Marni understood the sense of loss and disruption that her child and the foster family would feel when Janie "came home," nor did she grasp how helpful it would be to have the foster parents continue as informants, allies, and "extended kin." However, the process of planning together had begun, even if somewhat belatedly, and there was a promising possibility that the natural family could be successfully reunited while keeping contact with people who were very important to the child.

The situation in the biological family had never been explored, and there were unspoken assumptions that this conflict-avoiding family would never have dealt with on their own. Marni and her mother were close and loving, and Ada was a person who shouldered burdens without complaint. But a discussion of their plans, initiated by the staff, opened up a profound difference in expectations. Marni saw them all as "one big family." She expected Janie to return to Ada's home, where she could see her often. She and James would marry and have their child. Marni commented that she had physically left her mother's home long ago but "not in my heart." Ada was surprised. "I thought when you left home, you left home." She adored her granddaughter, but life was a struggle, Pam and Janie didn't get along, and Ada had not expected to be the permanent caretaker for Janie, functioning unofficially as a kinship foster parent.

Therapy was not very difficult or extended. Despite the complexities of the foster care situation, the intervention was similar to the way any family therapist helps parents and their young adult children clarify functions and boundaries. Marni's view that she would be a kind of big sister to Janie, articulated for the first time, implied an unacceptable burden for Ada, and a role for Marni that was not sufficiently mature or responsible. James, fortunately, was helpful and attached to Janie, and the couple began to plan a home for their family of four. On the social worker's instigation, they explored the issue of when to bring Janie home, considering the impending birth of their new baby, and what they might expect from Janie as she adapted to their style of life, their discipline, and the different realities of their family. For all of this, Ada was now an interested but appropriately peripheral observer.

EVALUATING THE APPROACH

In the case of the Bakers and the Bartons, it is clear that the ecological approach had positive results. It enabled the participants to clarify relationships and boundaries and enhanced the possibility of a successful reunification, in which the kinship family would function realistically and the biological and foster families would maintain contact. But it is not easy to establish the "outcome" of the ecological approach in concrete terms. The model is not a package. The goals are many, the approach is complex, and the model must always be applied in a form that is consistent with the context, reflecting the realities and possibilities of the particular agency.

When we examine the model, we see many indications that it is psychologically constructive and that it is apt to reduce the human and economic waste of the foster care situation. It should be reassuring to the child, who has contact with both families, experiences their combined concern for his or her welfare, and is at least partially relieved of deep conflict over mixed loyalties. It mobilizes the biological family, restoring some dignity and combining a demand for their continuing responsibility with a respect for their rights. It endeavors to reduce the mutually negative stereotypes that are formed and fanned when biological and foster families have no contact. It empowers foster families, mobilizing and extending their skills and according them recognition as crucial team members. And it has an important potential for the foster care system and the culture: When this approach is successfully implemented, the necessity for multiple placements should be reduced. The child should adapt more easily to placement, and when problems arise, they can be handled cooperatively in the triadic system that has been established, so that the foster family is better able to cope without requesting the child's transfer.

Since most of these features are not easily measurable, the question of evaluating the model is perplexing. No simple measurement establishes the value or outcome of the approach, but some concrete data can be obtained if it is understood that they do not represent the whole. If the approach is well managed, for instance, foster parents should find it less difficult to manage the child and there should be less movement of children from one home to another than has been typical for a particular agency. Within this approach, also, there should be an increase in the number of biological families that maintain contact with the child and the foster family through the period of placement, and more children should be able to return home. It is also possible that children will feel less abruptly abandoned, in these circumstances, and may show less disturbed behavior in the foster home.

In general, however, the most useful form of evaluation is apt to be the collection, within each agency, of what has been called "formative" data. Formative data are oriented toward direct, practical feedback into the system; they focus on clarifying the procedures that serve the goals, as well as those that do not. That might mean, for instance, a careful documentation of foster parent efforts to reach out and maintain contact with biological families, allowing for an evaluation of the procedures and attitudes that cement relations as well as the practical and interpersonal obstacles to success. Or it might mean a documentation of "troubleshooting" efforts by the network of professional workers, foster parents, and biological family when the child shows disruptive or worrisome behavior in the foster home. In keeping with the model, such issues would be brought to the network for discussion and mutual problem solving, and a record of the process—who participates, in what way, what works, what does not—would become part of an agency's understanding of the usefulness of the approach and, more important, of possible means for improving the process.

Taken as a formal research project across agencies, this kind of evaluation is complex and difficult to carry out. Within an agency, however, formative evaluation is often a matter of capturing events as they occur. Professional staff begin by identifying the goals or procedures they wish to highlight, such as positive contact between foster and biological parents, or frequent contact between the foster child and his or her family, or the developing collaboration between social workers and foster parents. They then document the relevant procedures or events, on a case-by-case basis, tracking the reactions of children, members of both families, and agency staff. The material enables them to discuss, evaluate, and revise, as needed. With this form of evaluation, an agency is best able to solidify the approach, shape procedures to their own setting and population, and, ultimately, to evaluate the relevance and value of the model in their own terms.

LOOKING INTO THE FUTURE

In this chapter, I have presented an ecological model for foster care that focuses on family preservation and reunification and that highlights the relationship between natural and foster families as a means to that goal. The approach emphasizes connections rather than fragmentation, empowerment and involvement of the natural family, and an expansion of roles for professional staff and foster parents. Relevant training must further a broad understanding of families, a change in traditional attitudes, and the development of a cooperative network composed of agency staff and members of the biological and foster families.

It is clear that efforts to implement these ideas can only succeed with administrative support and that this usually requires a review of prevailing concepts and policies. Typically, it is necessary to revise intake procedures so that the natural family is immediately involved in process and planning, introduce more flexibility into the conditions for visiting, coordinate case management, and increase services during periods of crisis and transition.

These are not widely accepted ideas, as yet, and the first moves toward an enlightened foster care system must necessarily focus on basic policies and practices. However, it is useful to note a second level of concerns which must soon be dealt with. They may make the difference between success and failure in applying new models of this nature.

1. An extended foster parent role has implicatons that must be considered. In this approach to foster care, the functions of foster parents include outreach and sustained contact with the natural family, as well as child care. In a sense, foster parents become paraprofessionals. There are issues of status, appropriate pay, and possible overload to be addressed, as well as the clarification of responsibilities and boundaries between foster parents and professional staff. The handling of such matters in specialized or therapeutic foster care may offer a model.

2. Kinship foster care involves specific strengths and pitfalls and should be regarded as a particular subset of foster care. Kinship foster care is generally the preferred solution to placement, minimizing the shock of separation and maximizing the possibility that the extended family can

offer continued support when the children and parents are reunited. But there are special issues in this situation. They range from the kind of long-term family conflict that blocks communication to the simple fact that payment for kinship foster care ceases when children leave the grandmother's house and go home to the mother. People who work with kinship placements must be alert to its special qualities. In these situations, assessment of the extended family is a necessary part of the process, and family therapy may be indicated, in some cases, so that a constructive network can be created and maintained.

3. Optimal foster care requires an integration of developmental and systems knowledge. The basic principle of an ecological model is to form a relationship between foster and natural families, in which the two families focus cooperatively on the well-being of the children. However, the children who come into foster care range from infancy through adolescence, and the issues on which the two families must collaborate will differ in accordance with the developmental stage of the child. With infants, the basic issue is bonding, or attachment—the child's sense of security invested in particular people, and the adult sense of emotional investment in this child. There is a theoretical controversy over the question of whether infants must bond exclusively to one person, for secure development, and that question is particularly relevant in the growing number of cases where it is judged that babies must be placed in care for their safety, as, for example, babies born with positive toxicity, to drug-addicted mothers, or to mothers who are judged to be neglectful or abusive. In those cases where removal is justified, at least temporarily, it is crucial to understand that mother–child bonding will be jeopardized unless contact can be maintained during the period of placement. Babies will inevitably bond to the foster parent(s), and it is important, thus, to deal with the complexities of multiple bonding from the beginning, so that it is possible for the biological family to be reunited in the future.

For young children beyond infancy, the issue is setting limits and working out the balance between autonomy and control. Parents who lose their 2-, 3- and 4-year-old children to foster care may not be adept at control to begin with, but they also miss the subsequent day-by-day contact through which parents and children negotiate, learn from each other, and arrive at workable patterns. When the children come home, after a period, it is possible that the natural parents will not be able to handle challenge, set rules, or carry authority with children who do not recognize their right to do so, and reunification may fail.

For older, middle-years children, one of the major issues is the development of competence in school. For parents, it is a stage that requires involvement in the child's learning and functioning in the classroom. Parents whose children are removed from home are often not skillful in their contact with schools and seldom make an issue of being kept abreast. For its part, the foster care system almost never works with the natural family on questions of the child's schooling. If children are of school age when they are placed, however, the contact between foster and natural parents should include a constant interchange about school-related decisions, reports of the child's progress, discussions about the child's experience in school, and whatever the participants feel is relevant, once they are alert to schooling as a developmental issue.

For adolescents, the developmental issues are familiar and complex, and for urban ghetto children, the risks are great. Parents of adolescents must handle not only the internal challenge to family patterns but the realities of modern society: drugs, sex, gangs, school, and violence. It is neither correct nor productive for the foster family to handle those issues without involving the natural family, and it is unrealistic to expect the family to reunite successfully if they have been out of contact.

Under current circumstances, and for the foreseeable future, children may stay in foster care for months or years, developing, changing, and experiencing the style of handling that characterizes the foster home. If the natural parents are to be effective when the family is reunited — or even in more sporadic contacts, if the child does not return to live at home — they will need relevant skills and credibility. Such skills and credibility do not transfer from didactic courses in parenting; they develop in contact between parents and their own children, and through their negotiation over real issues. An enlightened ecological model for foster care emphasizes the cooperation of the two families, during the placement period, and frequent contact between the child and the natural family. It will need also to provide for an emphasis on the particular issues of the child's developmental stage, fostering the evolution of patterns in the natural family that are viable in the present and can be adapted in the future.

NOTES

1. The project was supported by the Edna McConnell Clark Foundation. The staff of Family Studies, Inc., a New York training center, consisted of Salvador Minuchin, MD, Director; Evan Bellin, MD; Anne Brooks, DSW; Jorge Colapinto, Lic.; Ema Genijovich, Lic.; and Patricia Minuchin, PhD.

2. This case was supervised by Dr. Anne Brooks.

REFERENCES

Boyd-Franklin, N. (1989). *Black families in therapy: A multisystems approach.* New York: Guilford Press.

Fanshel, D., Finch, S. J., & Grundy, J. F. (1990). *Foster children in life course perspective.* New York: Columbia University Press.

Fein, E. (1991). Issues in foster family care: Where do we stand? *American Journal of Orthopsychiatry, 61,* 578–583.

Imber-Black, E. (1988). *Families and larger systems: A family therapist's guide through the labyrinth.* New York: Guilford Press.

Kates, W. G., Johnson, R. L., Rader, M. W., & Strieder, F. H. (1991). Whose child is this? Assessment and treatment of children in foster care. *American Journal of Orthopsychiatry, 61,* 584–591.

Minuchin, P., with Brooks, A., Colapinto, J., Genijovich, E., Minuchin, D., & Minuchin, S. (1990). *Training manual for foster parents.* New York: Family Studies.

Minuchin, S., & Fishman, H. C. (1981). *Family therapy techniques.* Cambridge, MA: Harvard University Press.

Wald, M., Carlsmith, C. M., & Leiderman, P. H. (1988). *Protecting abused and neglected children.* Stanford, CA: Stanford University Press.

12

Foster Family Clusters: Continuum Advocate Home Network

Marcia A. Eckstein

Continuum is one of ten programs operated under the umbrella of New Life Youth Services, Inc., an Ohio-based, not-for-profit organization. Accredited by the Council on Accreditation of Services for Families and Children, New Life offers a range of programs for youth including emergency shelter, residential treatment, family foster care, transitional and independent living, youth corrections, and family outreach services, as shown in Table 12.1.

New Life's mission is threefold: (1) to provide opportunities for troubled youth to become good citizens and to enable them to live productive lives without prolonged dependence on the welfare system and without further involvement in the criminal justice system; (2) to reduce delinquency in the community through direct positive intervention with troubled youth; and (3) to actively engage the local community in the delivery of services to troubled youth and their families.

TABLE 12.1. Range of New Life Programs

Program	Type	Date started	Clients served[a]
Family Outreach Program	In-home services	1989	Not available
Lighthouse Runaway Shelter	Emergency shelter	1974	845
Youth Diversion Center	Temporary shelter	1978	88
Continuum	Family foster care	1978	77
Schott Group Home for Girls	Residential treatment	1969	15
New Beginnings for Sexually Abused Girls	Residential treatment	1987	31
Independent Living Program	Independent living	1980	32
Gateway Apartments	Transitional living	1989	28
Paint Creek Youth Center	Youth corrections	1985	21

[a]Total clients served: 1,137. Third quarter statistics, October 31, 1991.

CONTINUUM BEGINNINGS

New Life's Continuum program started in 1978, about 10 years after the agency was founded. It originated as a peer counseling program offering self-help services to troubled youth. Later, its function was redefined as a community-based residential service to accommodate the growing needs of young people experiencing problems in their natural family environments. The Continuum program was based on the assumption that the majority of troubled youth could be served best in family-home settings within their communities rather than in institutional placements. The program's goal was to develop a variety of temporary living environments in which young people could grow, mature, and eventually return to their natural families or function independently in the community. Continuum evolved over time into a family foster care system called the Advocate Home Network, which provides services to young people with emotional and behavioral difficulties. The network functions as an extended surrogate family under the leadership of professionally trained "advocates" (foster parents) employed by the agency. These advocates provide therapeutic services for the youth and link resources with the network system. Short-term, emergency, and long-term foster care are provided by Continuum.

Youths placed in the Advocate Home Network are in the custody of juvenile courts or departments of human services of Butler, Clermont, and Hamilton counties in Ohio. Advocate Homes are licensed as "family foster homes" by the Ohio Department of Human Services (1991) and are subject to compliance with the Administrative Rules for Public and Private Agencies of the Ohio Administrative Code (5101:2–5). There are five well-established networks, including one in each of the above-mentioned counties, as well as the Long Term Network and the Emergency Network. Currently, services are provided to 55 youths in 28 Advocate Homes in the network system.

NEW DIRECTIONS FOR CONTINUUM

Continuum is and has been a dynamic program, always changing to meet the demands of the constantly changing complexion of the "average client." At its inception, the foster care program was simply that: professional foster care. In response to community need, Continuum has changed in many different ways, several of which are discussed below.

Continuum is a therapeutic foster care program, upgrading and increasing the training hours an advocate must have in order to be able to accept the more difficult and challenging behaviors of the youth. Continuum meets the criteria for a treatment foster care program as described in a survey done by Hudson, Nutter, and Galway (1992). These criteria are as follows:

1. The program is explicitly identified as a specialist or treatment foster care program with an identifiable name and budget.
2. Payments are made to foster parents at rates above those provided for regular foster care.
3. Training and support services are provided to the treatment foster caregivers.
4. A formally stated goal or objective of the program is to serve clients who would otherwise be admitted to or retained in a nonfamily institutional setting.
5. Care is provided in a residence owned or rented by the individual or family providing the treatment services.
6. The treatment foster caregivers are viewed as members of a service or treatment team.

Continuum was originally developed as a program for troubled teens. There are much younger children in the program today. In a program of approximately 50 children, almost 25% are under 11 years of age, the youngest of whom entered the program at age 2 after having spent his entire short life in a hospital.

The presenting behaviors are much more difficult and require more highly trained foster parents than in years past. Violent youths are seen more frequently. In the past, we worried about where little Johnny was hiding the marijuana; now, the concern is whether or not Johnny is violent enough to rape, physically harm someone, or commit arson. At least 85% of Continuum's children have been physically, emotionally, or sexually abused.

The training schedule and structure are evolving. Effective in 1992, all foster parents are required to take Therapeutic Crisis Intervention (TCI) which teaches physical restraint techniques. According to Ohio State law, if this procedure is used, the foster parent must be retrained at least once a year. The State of Ohio requires foster parents and spouses to have 12 hours of training per year, an increase of 4 hours per year from 1991. Continuum advocates are currently required to have a minimum of 40 hours of training per year, and spouses and coparents are required to have a minimum of 12 hours. This is expected to increase.

A contract counselor was added to Continuum's staff in 1990. The youths are able to see this counselor when they are on a waiting list for outside counseling. The agency plans for this position to become full time in the near future.

Funding

New Life Youth Services, Inc., is partially funded by the United Way. Most of Continuum's income is provided through Purchase of Service contracts with local child welfare agencies and juvenile courts. United Way

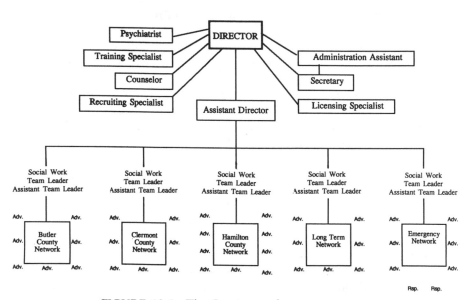

FIGURE 12.1. The Continuum foster care program.

and other contributors provide financial support for four of the networks, and the Long-Term Network obtains financial support from The Casey Family Program.

NETWORKS AND TEAMS

There are three types of networks within the Continuum framework: the three Classic Networks, the Long-Term Network, and the Emergency Network. All three types of network provide therapeutic foster care. Advocates are members of a team (network) who meet once a week to train, problem solve, and report on the progress of the children in their home.

The Classic Network is the oldest model and most closely represents what Continuum was at its inception. There are three networks within the Classic Network model: the Butler County Network, the Hamilton County Network, and the Clermont County Network. These networks of foster parents are grouped geographically not only to encourage a strong sense of community, but also to enable the network members to be available for each other in an emergency. This proximity is vital in making the network concept work. Network members who call the same location "home" share similar concerns regarding the youth in their community and have more in common in other ways, making it easier to collaborate. A sense of pride is fostered, and each network considers its home county to be the best location in which to raise a child. The Classic Network Model is the backbone of Continuum's program and serves as the springboard from which other networks have evolved.

The Long-Term Network is a joint research project initiated in January 1991 by The Casey Family Program of Seattle, Washington, and New Life Youth Services, Inc. The Long-Term Network differs from the Classic Network in that it accepts children only between the ages of 6 and 15 years of age who are in need of long-term foster care as determined by the juvenile courts and departments of human services in Ohio. Hearing of Continuum, the Casey Family Foundation has sponsored research to identify and measure the various service aspects of the Continuum program.

The Emergency Network evolved when The Hamilton County Department of Human Services requested a specialized network for youth who would otherwise have been served in a group shelter. Recruitment of advocates is especially challenging for this network; these children are in crisis at the time of referral. This network began operations in 1992.

The services available to the Emergency Network are more intensified than those of the Classic Network. There is a Behavior Management Specialist, a contract psychiatrist, and two youth workers available to help the advocates. No more than one child is placed in the home at any time. (The only exception to this would be two siblings.) These are short-term placements with a maximum of 90 days. The Emergency Network provides substantial support for the youths and foster parents in an attempt to stabilize the children enough so that they can move to a more permanent setting, such as home, residential, or foster care. In contrast to the Classic and Long-Term Networks, the Emergency Network will accept all children. The Emergency Network does no preplacement visits. If there is a home available when a child is referred, placement occurs immediately.

CONTINUUM PHILOSOPHY AND VALUES

Continuum is a long-term, therapeutic, community-based family foster care program providing services to troubled youth. Some of Continuum's values and beliefs are as follows:

1. Youths are better served in their communities in family-type settings when out-of-home placements are necessary due to breakdown in the family unit.
2. Many youths in substitute care benefit more from a network of extended families than from the traditional family foster care method of service delivery.
3. Foster caregivers can be prepared for professional roles to provide therapeutic services to youths with more complex emotional and behavioral problems.
4. Professionally trained foster caregivers can effectively advocate for the needs of youth in placement.
5. A network of emotional and concrete supports can reduce stress for foster caregivers, helping them to be more effective in therapeutic interventions with youth in placement.
6. Networks of family foster caregivers can help to normalize substitute family care and reduce the stigma for youth in placement.

CONTINUUM GOALS AND OBJECTIVES

The goal of Continuum is to provide an environment in which young people can grow, mature, and eventually return to their natural families or function in the community as independent young adults. Continuum objectives are as follows: (1) to increase the level of youths' functioning in home, school, and the community at age-specific developmental stages; and (2) to empower foster parents in their service provider roles through the Advocate networking system.

TARGET POPULATION

Continuum accepts youths who are adjudicated or otherwise deemed dependent and/or neglected by the juvenile courts and departments of human services in Ohio. These youngsters range in age from newborn to 18 and may be male or female, and any culture, religion, or ethnicity.

How Youths Enter the System

Youths enter the child welfare system when their natural families can no longer provide appropriate supervision. The removal of a youth from his or her natural home is an action of last resort, initiated only after efforts have been made to resolve the problem. When all intervention efforts have been unsuccessful in resolving conflicts while the family is intact, it is preferable to remove the youth for a temporary period of time until the situation is rectified. In some instances, it is necessary to remove the youth from the home for an indefinite period.

Youths who are removed from the home fall into two categories:

1. *Dependent, neglected, and abused.* These youngsters have been exposed to a variety of unhealthy family situations, including an unsuitable home environment, abusive and inappropriate parenting, and households without parents (due to illness, death, or abandonment).
2. *Juvenile offenders.* These are youngsters who have violated the law. Juvenile offenses are divided into two categories: status offenses (e.g., running away, truancy) which are offenses unique to children, and delinquency offenses (e.g., stealing, assault) which would be considered criminal offenses if committed by an adult.

THE ADVOCATE HOME NETWORK MODEL

Continuum is a family-centered systems approach to advocacy and problem solving for youth in foster care. Its underlying assumption is that youth in placement are served best in home settings that replicate a natural family environment. The environment supports the youths' physical, social, emotional, intellectual, and spiritual development.

The model operates between four interdependent levels: the youth, advocate, advocate network, and community. The advocate home ("foster family") helps the youth to cope with developmental issues, peer and family relationships, school, work, and other community demands. The advocate network ("extended family") supports the primary nurturing system in coping with the demands and stresses of foster parenting. The advocate network system utilizes therapeutic resources to support, problem solve, educate, consult, and intervene in order to maintain an adaptive balance between the youth, foster family, and community systems.

RECRUITMENT, LICENSING, TRAINING

Advocates in the program are employees of the agency. A rigorous interviewing and screening procedure is followed in selecting candidates for advocate positions. The foster parent must meet the standards of New Life Youth Services and the Ohio Department of Human Services (ODHS) for foster home certification and foster caregiver authorization (Ohio Revised Code: 5101). These are the "General requirements to be certified as a foster caregiver" set forth by the State of Ohio. Very generally speaking, a potential foster caregiver must meet the following conditions:

- be 21 years of age,
- able to support his or her own household (financially),
- in good physical health,
- a resident of the State of Ohio for a minimum of 1 year,
- not a convicted felon,
- have his or her home inspected by a state-certified fire inspector, and
- have room in the home for a foster child.

In addition to ODHS requirements, New Life Youth Services requires the following of their foster caregivers:

- police checks (city and county),
- fingerprinting (state),
- experience in child care or supervision,
- a bed and private space available for the belongings of a child,
- the capacity to work as part of a team,
- community awareness,
- openness of value system, and
- a sense of willingness to understand and learn from life experience.

The orientation and training of advocates for professional roles is based on the requirements of the ODHS (1991) for authorized caregivers prescribed in the Ohio Administrative Code. Potential foster caregivers (and their spouses or coparents, if applicable) are required to participate in 18 hours of orientation. Topics addressed during orientation include the following:

- ODHS Administrative Code Chapter 5101:2-7, "Administrative Rules for Family Foster Homes";
- New Life Youth Services personnel policies;
- advocate job description;
- description of Continuum and other New Life programs;
- history of the program;
- philosophy of the program;
- program policies and procedures;
- summary of network concept (treatment team);
- brief summary of referral agencies and specific procedures;
- emergency procedures;
- confidentiality;
- paperwork requirements;
- home study, certification, and recertification process;
- briefings on types of children in the program; and
- referral and intake process.

Training is given very high priority. The first agenda item at every weekly team meeting is training by the contract counselor or behavior management specialist. New Life Youth Services requires at least 40 hours of training per year for advocates-which exceeds the 12-hour minimum set by the ODHS. Incentives to attend training sessions include pay increases and an annual award given to the advocate who has accumulated the most workshop/training hours. Most training sessions are arranged in-house with guest speakers who cover various topics, some of which are listed below:

- working with the sexually abused child,
- STD/AIDS communication,
- childhood developmental stages,
- teamwork/working within a group,
- parenting,
- TCI,
- allegations of abuse and how to handle them,
- drugs and alcohol,
- eating disorders, and
- cultural differences and similarities.

Advocates are encouraged to attend workshops within their own communities that pertain to children or parenting issues.

Advocates receive an hourly wage, fringe benefits, and per diem for each youth in foster care. They are paid for full- or part-time professional services provided to the Advocate Home Network according to their specif-

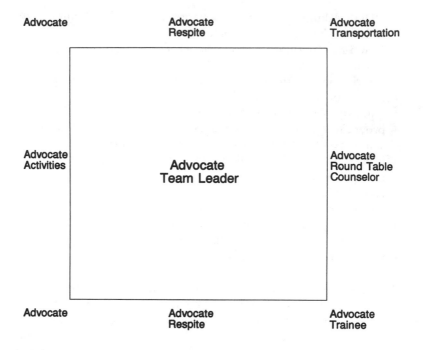

Advocate   Advocate   Advocate
                 Respite   Transportation

Advocate   **Advocate**   Advocate
Activities   **Team Leader**   Round Table
                                             Counselor

Advocate   Advocate   Advocate
                 Respite   Trainee

FIGURE 12.2. Network jobs.

ic job assignment: team leader, round table counselor, activities coordinator, transportation coordinator, respite provider, or trainee (see Figure 12.2). The advocates average from 5 to 40 hours per week. Advocates are evaluated annually by New Life Youth Services and receive wage increases based on job performance. Family foster homes are recertified yearly by the ODHS.

Good advocates are incredibly hard to find, and there is no magic formula of qualities that a person possesses that makes for a good advocate. Perhaps 1 recruit in 50 actually completes the entire process and becomes a licensed foster caregiver. Of those, some will drop out within the first year. High priority status is placed on recruitment and retention. New Life Youth Services is a member of the Foster Care Cooperative (FCC), a group of Greater Cincinnati and Northern Kentucky custodial and noncustodial agencies that provide foster care. This group meets approximately once a month to plan activities for foster parents and to share ideas on recruitment and retention. The FCC is very unique in that its members, some of whom would otherwise be competitors drawing from the same geographic pool to recruit foster parents, work together to improve the public's image of foster parenting in an effort to develop an interest in it as a profession.

One focus of the Continuum program is to meet the need for out-of-home placements for African American youth. In 1991, a full-time recruiter was hired, and one of her goals is to increase ethnic diversity among the service providers in the Advocate Home Network. This goal was reached in 1992, when 50% of all Continuum foster parents were African American.

The recruitment process has changed dramatically since a full-time recruiter was hired. Early screening is now possible, wherein the recruiter visits the home of the recruit to deliver the application, explain the program, and get a sense of the depth of commitment on the part of the recruit. This initial visit enables the recruit to ask questions about the agency and the program.

THERAPEUTIC INTERVENTION

Continuum uses seven primary intervention methods in its therapeutic work with youth:

- *Behavior modification:* The advocate and the social worker use time outs, positive reinforcement, and daily and weekly school report cards.
- *Crisis intervention:* The advocate and social worker restabilize situations such as those involving runaway behavior, truancy, parent–adolescent conflicts, and natural family crises.
- *Case management:* The advocate and social worker coordinate services with the referring agencies, county courts, and natural families.
- *Social supports:* The advocates and youths use a variety of resources: county caseworker, probation officer, therapist, family members, clergy, other advocates, and the social worker.
- *Advocacy:* The social worker and the advocate obtain entitled services for youths from schools, counties, courts, and probation officers.
- *Mediation:* The advocate and social worker resolve disputes with the county worker and probation officer concerning goals and treatment plans for the youths.
- *Education and process group:* The social worker and other agency staff conduct a range of informational groups. Some topics include study skills, sex education, problem-solving skills, family issues, and foster sibling relationships.

SERVICES

The following is a list of the core services provided to youths in the program:

- therapeutic foster care counseling,
- vocational/educational planning,
- school liaison,
- court liaison,
- recreation activities,
- transportation,
- health care,
- daily living/independent living skills training, and
- continuing job education training.

These are only core services. Additional and more specific services are added to/included in each child's program plan. Some of these could include: (1) participation of foster parent in counseling with the youth, (2) hygiene training, (3) sex education and birth control, (4) administration of medication, (5) anger management, and (6) parenting skills.

CASE EXAMPLE: TERESA

The following story of "Teresa" is a composite one, with the majority of the facts being derived from the incidents in the life of the model for Teresa. Names, of course, have been changed. Incidents that further illustrate the program have been taken from experiences with other foster children and inserted into this story. For simplicity, we have used only one child's name, Teresa, for all examples and illustrations.

Family Background

When Teresa was 13 years old, her mother "gave" her to Tom to be his wife. At that time her father was incarcerated for murder. Teresa and Tom (a convicted felon in his mid-30s) lived together as man and wife for 1 year, until he violated his probation and was sent to jail. This event precipitated an investigation by the local county Department of Human Services, and Teresa was referred as a foster care placement to Continuum. During her year with Tom, Teresa had not attended school because he did not "make" her do so.

The dysfunction of Teresa's family went back at least one generation, as Teresa's mother, Sabrina, had been prostituted at a very early age by her own parents. Sabrina showed concern for her daughters, but also allowed them to be used by her various husbands, boyfriends, and "johns" for sex in exchange for money or groceries. At least one of the men physically abused Teresa. Teresa reported that the sexual abuse began at age 4 and continued over a period of several years.

It is interesting to note that, upon entering Continuum, Teresa did not consider herself to be a victim of sexual abuse but only of physical abuse. She saw her sex-for-money (or groceries) activities as a way of making a living, a job, one which she could perform at a level equal to or better than her mother. Had she not chosen this profession, she would have considered herself sexually abused. Teresa insisted, however, that even though her skills were taught her by her mother, the decision to use those skills was her own.

Teresa and her mother were virtual peers while she grew up, sharing not only sexual partners but also the parenting responsibilities of the younger sisters, Gail and Gerri. While the younger girls were sexually abused by at least one stepfather, Teresa remained the primary victim. In this environment, Teresa learned that she was responsible for the safety of her younger siblings — that if she satisfied the sexual needs of her mother's associates, her younger sisters would not have to do so. She also learned that she was one of the family's main breadwinners, selling sexual favors for money and groceries. When Continuum received the referral, Teresa was 14 years of age, acted much older, dressed much older, and had no friends her own age. She also smoked, drank, used excessive profanity, had used illegal drugs, and treated adults as peers. One of the main goals identified in Teresa's program plan was to help her to simply be a teenager — a role she had never assumed.

Referral, Preplacement, Program Plan

Teresa was referred by telephone from a local Department of Human Services. Identifying information on Teresa was given (name, age, gender, etc.) as well as historical information, family history, school information, and presenting behaviors.

After the referral was taken, the Continuum social worker called an advocate who had adequate space and the skills needed to help Teresa. The Continuum social worker informed the advocate of all the data which had been given to her by the county. After they discussed the case, the advocate agreed to meet Teresa during a preplacement visit.

Teresa spent two weekend preplacements at the foster home prior to official placement in the home. Four preplacement days are offered to referring agencies by Continuum at no cost. This gives the child and the advocate an opportunity to get acquainted before placement is finalized. Teresa and her advocate had reservations about each other. The advocate was concerned that Teresa might be too worldwise for her family. Teresa, always independent and headstrong, was concerned about the family structure, its rules, and how they would affect her life and freedom. Despite these reservations, Teresa and her advocate agreed to give the placement a try.

It is Continuum's policy that within 3 weeks of placement, a program plan meeting is arranged and a program plan developed for the child. In attendance at Teresa's program plan were Teresa, her county caseworker, the advocate, and the Continuum social worker assigned to supervise the advocate's network. During this meeting, Teresa was asked what goals she wished to achieve during her placement and how she hoped to achieve them. Her advocate was asked to express how she would be able to assist Teresa in achieving her goals. The county caseworker and Continuum social worker described other services available to Teresa by the county, Continuum, or other community resources (i.e., Alcoholics Anonymous). Every Continuum child is involved in his or her own program plan and goal setting to the extent they are able. Teresa proved extremely goal oriented, even stubborn, and set out to achieve her goals, in some instances, just to prove that she could.

Network Jobs and Teamwork

Youth Advocate Family

Teresa's advocate was young, energetic, and very open-minded regarding behavior management techniques. Because of her youthful countenance and Teresa's "much-more-mature-than-her-age" air, one of the advocate's most challenging jobs was establishing lines of authority. This was done through consistent limit setting and enforcement with immediate confrontation when problems arose.

The advocate's family consisted of herself, her husband, two younger sons, ages 4 and 5, and one other foster daughter. This other foster daughter was Teresa's age but very different from Teresa. She and Teresa displayed the normal amount of sibling rivalry and tension during their 4-year placement; however, they developed a strong bond that still exists today. One year after their emancipation, Teresa was asked by her foster sister to be a bridesmaid in her wedding.

During Teresa's placement, her advocate gave birth to a baby girl. Teresa proved helpful during the pregnancy and became very devoted to the newborn, who happily returned her affections. This was a very natural, unstructured way for Teresa to learn parenting skills, and she seemed hungry for this type of guidance and knowledge.

At the time of Teresa's placement, Sabrina's home was under investigation by the Department of Human Services because of allegations made by Teresa. One of the first crises Teresa and her advocate faced together was Teresa testifying against her mother on charges of sexual abuse and child endangerment. The trial was terribly painful for Teresa. Her mother accused Teresa of destroying the family and telling the whole world their secret. Sabrina was sentenced to 18 months in prison. Consequently, Teresa's younger sisters, Gail and Gerri, were referred to Continuum. The custodial agency specifically requested that the two younger sisters not be placed in the same home with Teresa, as Gail and Gerri were furious with Teresa for "telling." Gail and Gerri were placed with a Continuum advocate who was part of Teresa's network. This was done deliberately, in an effort to keep the sisters as close to each other as possible in order that the family bonds would not be further weakened or traumatized.

The contrasts between Teresa's biological family and her foster family were great. Her advocate strove to teach Teresa "life skills," such as how to do well in school, cook, clean, and find and keep a job. Sabrina taught Teresa that "life skills" meant getting yourself and your client high, pleasing men sexually, and collecting enough money to pay the rent and feed the family. The advocate's family attended church together; Teresa's family watched pornographic films together. The advocate's family had definite "heads of the household" (she and her husband); Teresa's mother had been in competition with Teresa for "clients" and pay, and whoever made the most money claimed leadership responsibility.

The competition between Teresa and Sabrina impacted on Teresa's relationship with her advocate. Teresa saw her advocate as threatening to her own sense of independency, and power struggles ensued. The advocate was just as stubborn as Teresa, and she was very determined not to give up on her. The advocate contacted every member of her network to help with Teresa.

Team Leader

The complexion of the networks has changed over time. Team leaders have a minimum of 5 years' experience at Continuum. The advocates range from 1 to 9 years of experience. In the beginning, all the advocates had approximately the same amount of experience. Teresa's advocate soon discovered that Teresa's case would be particularly challenging, and she relied heavily upon her team leader and her network for help. The team leader, who is also Continuum's educational liaison, monitored Teresa's progress in school and ran interference when any problems arose. Teresa's grades indicated that she was capable of college preparatory work, and she chose this course of study with the guidance of the team leader. The team leader became Teresa's trusted confidant and perhaps the first male in her life with whom she could have a nonexploitative relationship. He visited the foster home at least once a month to check her progress and to provide encouragement. Teresa also saw the team leader at Continuum social functions, including roller skating parties, Halloween parties,

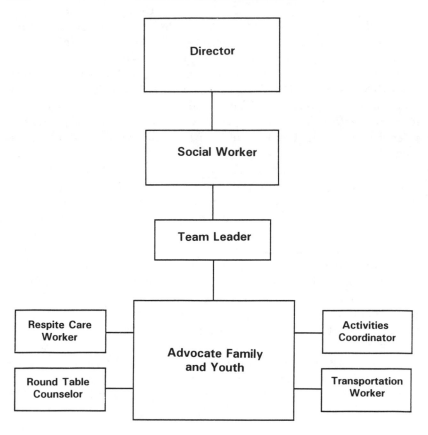

FIGURE 12.3. Network support for the advocate family.

and Christmas gatherings. He became a person she could call if she were angry or frustrated, or just needed a sympathetic ear.

The advocate and Teresa responded well to the team leader and depended on him for advice and consolation when needed. Because of their shared respect for him, he was extremely effective at diffusing crises between Teresa and her advocate.

Activities Coordinator

The activities coordinator took Teresa to church every Sunday, and afterwards brought Teresa to her (the activities coordinator's) home. Often, on these Sundays, several Continuum foster children and several of the activities coordinator's grandchildren were there playing records, visiting, and having dinner. During these Sunday outings, Teresa was able to socialize with peers and learn more age-appropriate behavior. It was from exposure to this group of peers and the other teenager in the home that Teresa gradually learned how to dress and act more in accordance with her age.

One youth, who often spent Sunday afternoons at the home of the activities coordinator, was Jay, a biracial, severely behaviorally disturbed teen who was prescribed psychotropic medications for depression and aggression. Jay's background was very troubled but very different from Teresa's.

Jay's mother and stepfather had been abandoned by their parents and had grown up in a state school where they met. Jay's mother is retarded, and both mother and stepfather are described as having explosive, violent personalities. Jay's mother was committed once to a psychiatric institution. During her inpatient stay there she had sexual contact with Jay's father, who was also a patient. When she became pregnant, she said nothing to her husband (Jay's stepfather) and, even after Jay's birth, tried to convince Jay's stepfather that he was the father of the child. Jay's mother and stepfather are Caucasian, however, and Jay is biracial. When the stepfather confronted Jay's mother, she changed her story to one of being raped while at the institution and claimed that Jay's biological father was deceased. This explanation allowed baby Jay to remain in the home, but it was the beginning of a very troubled childhood for Jay. He was physically abused by his stepfather and neglected by his mother, who was still struggling with her psychiatric and physical frailties.

Jay has three sisters, all of whom share the same father and Caucasian physical characteristics. Jay was acutely aware of the differences between him and his sisters and became a loner and the family scapegoat. As if to confirm his sense of not fitting in, Jay was the only child placed outside the home. This occurred when Jay was 7 years old. Prior to his placement at Continuum, Jay spent time in five different placements. These included institutions, group homes, and foster homes. During these years, Jay had no contact with his mother and stepfather.

When Teresa met Jay, he was extremely shy and angry. He responded to harmless teasing from another youth by becoming overwhelmed and then violent. During these outbursts, he often attempted to intimidate others with his size, further isolating himself from the peers he so desperately wanted to befriend. His aggression manifested itself in verbal abuse, crying, pounding walls and floors, breaking furniture or other items—even if they belonged to him—throwing objects, and even assaulting a foster parent's dog. When this happened, the other youngsters would get out of his way. Teresa, however, was not so easily intimidated. Being a large, strong girl (she and Jay shared a tendency to overeat), and given her background, she did not consider Jay's aggressive acting out to be a threat.

Teresa felt sorry for Jay and listened to his complaints of teasing at the hands of the other youth. She helped him with his homework and proved instrumental in encouraging Jay to develop his socialization skills, particularly with peers. She was an experienced guide in this particular area as she, too, had found it difficult at first to interact with peers.

A major dilemma occurred in Jay's life when he was 17, a year after he entered the program. The child welfare laws changed, and Jay's commitment status went from one of permanent custody to long-term foster care. After 10 years of no contact, his mother and stepfather requested visitation. Jay had strong, mixed feelings about this event. He was elated to have his family back in his life and terrified of what the future might hold. His mother and stepfather put considerable pressure on him to return home upon emancipation from the county at age 18. However, Jay worked very hard preparing to enter New Life's Independent Living Program. He reported to his Continuum social worker that his parents are still violent, his mother abuses his stepfather, and that living conditions are extremely crowded. (Jay's 16-year-old sister had a baby, which contributed to the chaos and crowded conditions in the home.)

Teresa was patient listening to Jay's problems and encouraged him to take his time in making the decision whether to go into Independent Living or home. The pull of natural family proved to be the stronger of the two options. Jay felt especially responsible to go home when his mother asked him for financial aid—which he gave her out of his earnings from his job as an assistant janitor.

Jay rejoined his family shortly after he turned 18. Follow-up information is scant, but it is known that he and his family found it difficult to survive in poverty and overcrowded conditions. They eventually moved out of the state; Jay ceased taking his medication and became involved with legal difficulties.

During Jay's placement at Continuum, Teresa was his friend, probably the only one he had who was in his age group.

The Transportation Worker: Gail and Gerri's Advocate

Teresa's sisters were referred to Continuum after they spoke to the school counselor about events in their mother's home. Teresa pressed charges against her mother and the man who physically abused her while she lived at her mother's. They were prosecuted and sent to prison while the girls were in foster care. The breaking up of the family angered the younger girls and they, along with Teresa, were referred to counseling. Teresa visited them often at their foster home, initially to make sure that they were being treated properly. Once she developed a relationship with that advocate and learned to trust her, she was able to let go of the role of being their caretaker. However, she continued in her big sister role, for example, admonishing the girls to behave if they wanted to remain in the safety of this home.

Teresa's advocate and the younger girls' advocate worked very closely together in an attempt to maintain the family attachments. Phone calls and visits were encouraged and overnights were commonplace. Gail and Gerri's advocate held the role of transportation worker for the network. If Teresa needed transportation to school, counseling, doctor's appointment, or other place when her advocate was not available, the transportation worker drove Teresa to her destination. This provided Teresa and the transportation coordinator with an opportunity to get to know one another, and it gave Teresa a chance to check on the progress of "the kids."

Roundtable Counselor

As young as she was, Teresa considered herself very much the adult. As a result, she and her advocate did not always agree on what privileges should be allowed for Teresa. An example of this occurred when Tom (Teresa's "husband") was released from prison. Teresa did not understand why she was not allowed to date him. She claimed they were "in love." Because of the difference in their ages, his prior living arrangement with Teresa, that he had been a sexual partner of Sabrina prior to living with Teresa, and that he was a felon, the county banned him from seeing her. Tom frequently broke the restraining order and was seen waiting for Teresa at school. Teresa did not approve of the ban and tried to make contact with Tom. When she lost privileges as a result, she because furious and hurled insults at her advocate, social worker, school authorities, and county caseworker.

Teresa did not always act out in such an obvious fashion when she perceived that someone was trying to keep her from getting what she wanted. She was very good at keeping quiet and making plans for herself without the consent or knowledge of her advocate, Continuum social worker, or county case worker. At one point, for example, Teresa told her advocate that she wanted to visit her father in prison. Her advocate said she would call the Continuum social worker to get this request approved by the county. When the social worker called Teresa to verify the request, Teresa informed her that she already called the prison (a long-distance call), received permission from prison officials to visit on a specific date, and arranged for transportation (her boyfriend) to take her to the prison. It was a roundtable counselor who explained to Teresa that, while what she did was not wrong, it would have been more thoughtful of her if she had gone through the proper channels with her advocate and social

worker. The roundtable counselor informed Teresa that she was responsible for paying the long-distance call to the prison.

The roundtable counselor was often contacted to help resolve conflicts. Present at roundtable discussions were Teresa, her advocate, Continuum social worker, and the roundtable counselor. The network team
leader and other advocate family members (including other foster siblings)
involved in the conflict were often present in these meetings. On occasion
and as circumstances permitted, Teresa's county caseworker participated
in a roundtable discussion.

The roundtable counselor's role is that of objective observer who
listens to all sides of the story before making a recommendation. The activity of the roundtable counselor increased during Teresa's second year
in placement, when Sabrina was released from prison on parole. Teresa's
grades decreased, her defiant behaviors in school and at home increased,
and her substance abuse resurfaced. After multiple roundtables and consistent support from her primary and secondary advocates, Teresa began
to calm down and resumed her more constructive behaviors. Positive and
negative feelings emerged from this process. Teresa admitted that she was
proud to have "made it" in foster care placement for 2 years, but she was
frightened and angry that her mother was free to become a part of her
life again.

Respite Care Worker

At the time of Teresa's placement, respite care was provided by any network member willing and able. Respite can occur at the request of the
advocate, the child, or both. Sometimes respite is as simple as removing
the child from the home for a "cooling down" period, during which time
the respite care worker takes the child for a soda, a walk, or just a long
drive. Longer respite includes overnights, weekend visits, or caring for
the child while the advocate attends to a personal problem such as illness.

While it is still true that respite care is done by an advocate who is
willing and able, Continuum recently changed by assigning a respite care
worker for each network. Continuum aggressively searches (from within
and outside the program) for families who are willing to assume this
responsibility. There is an entirely different dynamic at work in the home
of someone who does only respite care. The time is shorter and the honey-
moons are more frequent, until such time as the child becomes more accustomed to the home, and its rules and rhythms. Once the child is
familiarized with one respite home, there is potential for growth in the
relationship with the respite worker. There is also the risk that the child
will learn to play upon the sympathy of one advocate to the detriment
of the other. To avoid this trap, networking and team support are essential.

Teresa used respite well and was not shy to ask for it before an incident became inflated or more complex. During her placement she spent time at the homes of the team leader, the transportation worker, and the roundtable coordinator.

As more issues were addressed in counseling, Teresa's anger would surface and she would become verbally abusive to her foster sister or advocate. In these tense times, Teresa often found respite at the homes of other advocates who lived nearby.

The geographic clustering of network homes is critical to the effectiveness of the respite care worker. Crises are more easily dissipated if the parties involved are separated quickly, leaving less time for verbal tension to give way to more extreme, even physical, aggression on the part of the child. When the respite care worker is able to distract the child from the situation before more threatening behavior presents itself, the advocate has a better chance of regrouping, stepping back, and considering options.

The foster parent who provides respite is always informed of the child's history and problems. This information is shared during weekly team meetings. Interestingly, it is often the other team advocates who convince the primary advocate that respite is needed. Indeed, the primary advocate's closeness to the child plays a major part in the situation. It often clouds an advocate's judgment and blinds him or her to the subtle signs of stress that secondary advocates easily pinpoint—because they have experienced it themselves.

Program Director

Continuum's program director became personally involved with Teresa early in her placement. Recognizing Teresa's academic and leadership ability, she encouraged Teresa to become a Buddy/Tutor. In this subprogram, students who are doing well in one subject tutor a "buddy" who is struggling. This is a great self-esteem tool for both tutor and buddy, giving each the opportunity to experience goal setting and goal achievement. Tutors are paid minimum wage to help another child. Teresa took her responsibilities in this Buddy/Tutor program seriously and, as a result, made a success of it for herself and her buddy. Jay was one of the "buddies" who benefited from Teresa's tutoring.

The Team as a Whole

Once the team has had a chance to meld, the team meetings are extraordinary. Advocates know more about their team members, often, than they do about their own siblings. In fact, they often act like siblings—bickering and supporting each other in the same breath. The old sibling rule, "I can say what I want about my family—but don't you try it," applies here.

The team meets once a week to discuss the most sensitive issues. They are very familiar with each other's problems, and they expect help when they need it. They counsel each other and make jokes; they all hurt when one hurts.

We call it a team, but it is really a family. When one cannot devote as much time and energy to the network because of personal problems, the others cover for him or her. The phone procedures illustrate how, when one has trouble in the home, everyone gets a call. For instance, if a child refuses to go to school, the advocate calls the buddy. If the buddy can't get the child to go to school, the assistant team leader is called. After that, the whole incident is reported to the team leader, who calls the network social worker, who tells the program director. Then the whole matter is discussed at the next team meeting, and everyone brainstorms about what to do in case of recurrence. The team members operate on the principle, "If you don't tell us, how can we help you?"

The beauty of this network team is that all the roles can be switched. The advocates know what everyone else does because they fill in for each other. When the transportation person is ill, someone else takes over. When a network grows large enough that there are more advocates than jobs, the jobs are shared. Every roundtable counselor needs a roundtable counselor, sooner or later.

Natural Parent Interaction

As mentioned earlier, Sabrina was convicted and sent to prison on charges of sexual abuse and child endangerment. She remained there for 18 months, during which time she and Teresa exchanged occasional letters and telephone calls. Sabrina expressed hostility toward Teresa at first, condemning her for "ruining the family name."

One of the conditions set for Sabrina upon her release from prison was that she enter into family and individual counseling. The court made it clear that there would be no unsupervised visits with her daughters, and no chance of reunification without counseling and parenting classes. Sabrina genuinely desired her family's reunification. She had trouble breaking from her past, however, and experienced many setbacks along the way.

Sabrina had a very difficult time dealing with the jealousy she felt toward Teresa's advocate. She encouraged Teresa to be defiant, telling her, "She can't tell you what to do." Teresa's advocate had contact with Sabrina for most home visits and at every court hearing over the years. To ease the tension between them, the advocate assured Sabrina that it was not her intention to steal her child's love from her. The advocate explained that she would always act in Teresa's best interest, and that included accepting Sabrina as a person and as the mother of Teresa. The communication between Sabrina and the advocate was always straightforward and honest despite their differences.

Sabrina was responsible for transportation to home visits, but Sabrina often had car trouble. When Sabrina's car was not running and the county was unable to provide a case aide to transport the girls to their visit, the advocate often provided transportation. Sometimes the county staged the visit at a shopping mall or other neutral setting for a couple of hours so they could at least have a short visit with their mother.

When visits became unsupervised, Sabrina's behavior changed. The girls were often late returning from visits, with no prior warning. Sometimes they were not returned at all and, when the advocate called, the excuse was the car was not running and they would return the next day. Teresa reported smoking marijuana and drinking alcohol while at her mother's home. After one of these visits, Teresa returned with a picture of a naked woman. When confronted, Teresa became hostile, not wishing to turn over the item to authorities as evidence because it had been a gift from Sabrina. Teresa saw it only as a harmless prank on her mother's part.

Another time, Gerri (Teresa's youngest sister), wore a revealing blouse to school, which forced school authorities to send her home. (She hid the blouse from her foster mother and changed at school). The blouse was a gift from Sabrina.

Sabrina was not aggressive but manipulative, a feature she taught her daughters well. Her attempts to undermine the advocate's authority were always reported and dealt with promptly, with consequences for Sabrina issued by the court.

After many rocky starts, Sabrina began to understand that Teresa was mature enough to recognize her attempts at manipulation and resolute enough to refuse to let it thwart her progress. Teresa declared that Sabrina would never be a mother to her, but would always be a friend. From that time forward, Sabrina seemed less anxious about being in competition with Teresa's advocate. It was also at this time that Teresa verbalized that she would never again live with her mother but, instead, would become a frequent visitor to check on the safety of her younger sisters.

Throughout placement, the advocate consistently advised Teresa that she could always love her mother even if she rejected her behavior.

A mutual respect developed between Sabrina and the two advocates involved in the care of her daughters. The level of respect on Sabrina's part is best illustrated by the fact that, after the two younger girls were sent home, Sabrina called their (former) advocate to ask for help in disciplining them, complaining that they just "wouldn't listen" to her.

Epilogue

After 4 years of placement in the same foster home, Teresa was emancipated by the county upon her graduation from high school, which occurred shortly after her eighteenth birthday. At that time she had been rejected by two branches of the armed services because of her weight. She worked at a fast-food restaurant, saved her money, and rented an apartment with her long-term boyfriend.

Teresa kept in contact with her foster family, and she often earned extra money baby-sitting for her advocate's children. Teresa's younger sisters were returned to the custody of their mother shortly before Teresa's emancipation. Teresa kept her word on checking on them and called her Continuum social worker to report any progress or setbacks.

Today, Teresa is no longer with her boyfriend and lives with her grandparents who are the original perpetrators of sexual abuse against Teresa's mother. She remains in contact with her former advocate, shows up on occasion at program social events and even brings her mother with her. The success of Teresa's story lies not only in the fact that she broke her family's cycle of abuse, but that she made peace with her family. She was able to return home and live among them without being victimized.

REFERENCES

Hudson, J., Nutter, R., Galway, R. (1992). A survey of North American specialist foster family care programs. *Social Service Review, 66,* 50–63.

New Life Youth Services. (1989). *Continuum program youth advocate manual.* Cincinnati, OH: Author.

New Life Youth Services. (1990). *A report to the community 1969–1989.* Cincinnati, OH: Author.

New Life Youth Services. (1991). *The Long-Term Network interim report.* Cincinnati, OH: Author.

Ohio Department of Human Services. (1991). *Administrative rules for public and private agencies: Ohio administrative code.* Columbus, OH: Author.

V

REUNIFICATION

With the 1980 Child Welfare Adoption Assistance Act (PL96-272) all welfare agencies were compelled to return children to their own families from placement as quickly as possible. The positive side of this may have been the reduction in the long separations that often became permanent, but more attention has been directed to the negative outcome—children returned prematurely, only to be placed out of the home again, at best, or, too often, to be injured or killed by parents utterly unprepared to care for them. Reunification, as each of the chapters in this part suggests, is a good thing, but must be carefully prepared.

Karen Gail Lewis, who has written about working with siblings in the welfare system, describes how their connectedness can facilitate the reunification process. Please note that very often these siblings are separated in their placements, so that reunification involves their reattachment to each other as well as to their parent(s).

Lindsay Bicknell-Hentges outlines particular stages that need to be worked through in the reunification process, noting the ambivalence and lack of confidence that underlies even the most eager of participants.

Finally, Rocco Cimmarusti, who designed a curriculum to train welfare workers throughout Illinois in a multisystems approach to reunification, writes about how to convert workers to an appropriately cautious, positive view of families.

299

13

Sibling Therapy: One Step in Breaking the Cycle of Recidivism in Foster Care

Karen Gail Lewis

Children are removed from their homes when the courts ascertain that the parents are not adequately caring for them. They may be placed in foster or group homes with the hope that the parents will solve their own problems. The ultimate goal, when possible, is for the children to be returned home. Unfortunately, once they are home, the tension often increases and the original problems resurface; hence, the number of children who return home only to be placed again is very high (American Public Welfare Association, 1992; Block & Liebowitz, 1983). Over the years, there have been many ideas about the cause of foster care recidivism and the means for assuring a successful family reunification. Most often, though, the focus for change is on the mother. The roles of the father, the children, and even society are overlooked as possible sources for intervention.

To do justice to the topic of foster care, there needs to be consideration of the broader social and economic issues within the country and of the possible racist underpinnings that account for the high percentage of African American children in foster care (American Public Welfare Association, 1992; Eastman, 1985; Gurak, Smith, & Goldson, 1982). Although these issues are poignant to the topic of foster care, this chapter will isolate one aspect of recidivism—the siblings' role. The cyclical pattern of recidivism is presented followed by a description of a three-step plan for breaking this pattern (Lewis, 1991). Emphasis here is on step one — sibling therapy, including the structure of the sessions, interventions, and the role of the therapist. The main premise is that improving the siblings' behaviors and their relationship will help decrease the tension once they are reunited at home. This approach is not intended to blame the children for the placement, but, rather, to help them make a conscious connection between their behavior and their parents' ability to deal with them. The issues of applicability of this treatment approach for therapists working in agencies and in private practice is also discussed.

THE CYCLICAL PATTERN OF RECIDIVISM

There is a cyclical pattern for many families involved in foster care. It goes like this: A children's protective service (hereafter called the Agency) decides the parents are neglecting or abusing their children; the children are placed together or separately in a temporary home; parents are supposed to solve the problems that caused the placement (e.g., drugs, alcohol, depression, self-abuse, mental illness) before the Agency will consider returning the children. Too often, the Agency does not provide parents with the needed services, such as substance abuse treatment, homemaker services, job training, or individual or couples therapy. While parents may have periodic visitation, if the children are in different foster homes they may have to see them separately, which decreases the frequency of being with each child. This also means the children may not get to see each other, for the court seldom mandates sibling visitation (Hegar, 1988).

The content and quality of the visits are limited by the artificiality of the setting, such as in the social worker's office, a foster home, a park. This presents at least two major glitches. Even when parents get to visit their children, the excitement may lead to the children's vying for parental attention, with escalating friction. Under the best of conditions, even "model" parents might feel incompetent to give quality attention to demanding children. The second glitch is that parents' behaviors and responses are bound to be shaped by the awkwardness of having a judgmental spectator — for the social service worker's responsibility *is* to judge parents' ability to deal with their children.

If the visits go smoothly and the children are returned home, the prior issues and family dysfunctional structure may still persist: parents' emotional problems; financial, social, and environmental problems; problems between the parents; each child's individual and social problems; as well as problems among the siblings. In addition, the children must face the stress of returning to their former schools, readjusting to their peers, teachers, and classwork. Not having skills for verbally expressing their anger, confusion, and sadness, they may explode in their most familiar language—fighting and screaming (Minuchin, Montalvo, Guerney, Rosman, & Schumer, 1967). As conflict among the siblings increases, parents resort to their typical behavior for dealing with stress, which may, of course, lead back to the beginning of this cycle, with the children being placed in foster care because of parents' abuse or neglect.

While simplistically described here, in reality this cycle is usually far more complex. For example, frequently, only some of the children are returned, which increases the tension and blame during visitation. Those children returned may behaviorally express their guilt, while those remaining in placement may behaviorally express their hurt and abandonment. Also complicating the cycle are all the other relationships parents have with extended family and friends and their residual shame about having had their children removed.

Thinking systemically, this cycle can be punctuated at any point, that is, by identifying the problem from different perspectives. The Agency's typical punctuation is parents' (usually mother's) inadequacy, as described above. However, punctuating the cycle with the children's behavior offers another entrance into helping the family. That cycle would look very different: If the children's behavior becomes more manageable, the mother may feel less threatened and out of control, which will allow her to function better, which leaves the children less deprived, and which decreases the need for their removal.

THE CHILDREN'S ROLE IN RECIDIVISM

The children's role in recidivism, specifically as it relates to the parents' functioning, has been a neglected subject. Since children often internalize and reflect parental turmoil, their behavior may become more out of control, making it more difficult to discipline them. Ignoring the children's role in this feedback loop inevitably gives them more power than anyone intends. Certainly no social worker would willingly give children the responsibility for such a major decision as to whether they should be returned to their parents, yet, in fact, that is what often happens. Some children, so angry that they want to punish their parents, misbehave, proving parents are not capable of handling them. This is probably an unconscious decision, but they may only be able to show their pain through aggression. Their-out-of control behavior may reflect how out of control they feel about their whole life.

On the other hand, some children are so solicitous of their parents, especially single mothers, that they are on their very best behavior during the visits but cannot sustain that once they are returned home. Either way, children have more *indirect power* in the decision about returning home than may be recognized. Instead, they should have more *direct input.* They need to understand the connection between their behavior and the possibility of their returning home, so they can make conscious decisions about their behavior.

CHILDREN FROM CHAOTIC HOMES

Children from disadvantaged, underorganized (Aponte, 1976), low socioeconomic families—the largest percentage of children in foster care (American Public Welfare Association, 1992)—tend to be action oriented with unfocused behavior. According to Minuchin et al. (1967), they do not expect to be heard, and if heard, they do not expect a response; the volume of their voice is more important than the content; they have no negotiating skills, so they do not expect a resolution to conflict; fighting with siblings is a primary means of relating. Although there is much apparent conflict among these children, the meaning of the fighting is not always clear. Since they may communicate through fighting, deciphering the messages is crucial. Some of the more common meanings include the following:

- *Predictability:* In their chaotic, uncertain world, there is safety and familiarity in the predictability of the fights. Siblings know how a fight will begin, who will initiate it, how the other will respond, who will do what next, and how it will end.
- *Sense of competence:* Regardless of who wins the fight, there is satisfaction in initiation. Starting the fight is a way to take charge of something in their lives. "The competence comes not from the winning but from the attack" (Minuchin et al., 1967, p. 294).
- *Safe deflection of anger:* In these families, open expression of anger is not safe. Parents are bigger, stronger, and potentially dangerous. It is not an equal battle. Deflecting the anger toward a sibling is safer; the retaliation may not be so brutal. An angry parent can eject a child from the home, whereas a sibling cannot. Further, siblings are familiar with the typical alternation between fighting and playing.
- *Expression of affect:* In their world, open expression of affect is often not valued. Fighting, though, is a socially acceptable means of making contact. Also, since these children externalize their feelings, fighting can diffuse their tension, fear, anger, and hopelessness.

- *Avoidance of silence:* Noise and movement are a reassurance of their own presence and that of others. Silence can be experienced as abandonment, plus it leaves too much room for unacceptable affect to surface.

Fighting, then, is a way to stay connected (Bank & Kahn, 1982; Lewis, 1986b). Siblings are emotionally engaged as long as they hit and shout, which reinforces their presence in each other's lives. At some point, though, the fighting can move beyond connection and become abusive or incestuous.

At the other extreme are the children from chaotic homes who have not developed connections; they pull away from each other. While there is no fighting, there is also no sense of relatedness. Their isolation may be their self-protection, without recognizing that they share the same pain. They can not imagine they have anything to learn from or give to each other. In fact, in families with multiple comings and going, the siblings may not even know each others' names or ages.

THREE-STEP PLAN TO REDUCE
FOSTER CARE RECIDIVISM

The three-step model consists of sibling therapy, mothers' group therapy, and family therapy. In sibling therapy, the children learn to recognize their role in returning home and to express their feelings in less destructive ways. In the mothers' group therapy, mothers learn to feel more competent as parents and become better connected to their extended family, peer group, and community. In family therapy, mother and children meet together, focusing on issues specifically related to improving the chance of a successful reunification. This three-step plan is aimed at families with children under 14 years of age.

STEP ONE: SIBLING THERAPY

In order to break the cyclical pattern from the children's perspective, it is necessary to help them deal with each other and their emotions in more constructive ways. Sibling therapy is one way to help them do this. Sibling therapy is a forum for bringing brothers and sisters together in the same room to deal with mutual problems. A relatively new concept, sibling therapy has been used with children and adults with a wide range of problems (Kahn & Lewis, 1988). To offer this type of treatment, therapists need to consider the goals of the therapy, the role of the therapist, the structure of the sessions, and interventions.

Goals

It is likely that many of the children have multiple problems—intrapsychic, interpersonal, social, academic. These, together with the effects of economic deprivation, parental problems, extended family problems, current family adjustment, prior family crises, and overt and covert racism and classism, leave children burdened beyond any reasonable comprehension. With their having so many massive problems, the therapist may feel as overwhelmed as the children, and therapy may seem to be a mission impossible.

Therefore, the goals need to be focused and circumscribed. Goals need to be set for individual children and for the sibling unit. As a general guideline, here are some possible goals that can help the siblings improve their interactions while emphasizing their mutuality:

- understand why they were removed from their parents;
- express their feelings about being removed;
- alleviate their guilt for causing the breakup of their home; assess what was their fault and what was not;
- express and then alleviate their blame of each other for the breakup;
- talk about their feelings of being separated from each other (if in different foster homes);
- talk about their adjustment to the new home, neighborhood, school, friends;
- discuss the visitations—what goes well and what they believe needs to be changed;
- express their feelings about returning home and what changes they can make to help the family run smoother if they do return;
- express things they like about each other;
- learn to play and talk together; and
- learn to translate their feelings into words so they can say what they really mean or ask directly for what they need.

While there are many other important issues, they can wait. Some therapists believe it is important for these children to work immediately on solving their intrapsychic problems; however, these issues are not even reachable until their daily life settles down. Dealing with prior sexual abuse may also need to wait. However, current or recently discovered sexual abuse needs immediate attention.

This list seems long and very complicated for young children, yet it is not impossible to make some inroads in all of the above within a few months. Clearly, none of the topics can be dealt with completely, given the uncertainty of the children's continuation of the treatment and the other crises that arise, often out of their control. Sometimes, the similarities between the daily crises and the issues involved in their returning home can be discussed. For example, when 8-year-old Josh is removed from one foster home because of beating his sister, the therapist can say,

> "Josh, you must have been feeling real hateful to have hit her so hard. Were you really so angry at her or was hitting her a way to hit back at all the people who have hurt you so much? You have never talked about how you felt when your dad hit you and your mother. I wonder if you put these feelings into your fists, when you can't put them into words; I also wonder if you are angry that only Jake moved back home last week. Do you think there is a connection between these things?"

If Josh says no, the therapist needs to makes the connection very clear, adding,

> "You didn't have any control over your father beating you or your mother; you didn't have any control over the grownups behaving in ways that were harmful to you and that caused you all to be removed. However, you do have control over your hitting. Hurting your sister does not help your parents hear how angry you are and, in fact, when you let your feelings out with your hands, you end up getting punished—but you don't deserve to be punished. You are not bad."

This may not be said all at one time, but pieces of it need to be repeated over and over in each session and each time Josh does something that gets him in trouble. He needs to hear the direct connection between, "When you do bad things, you cannot go home" and "You are doing bad things because you feel you are so bad for not stopping your daddy from hitting your mommy." When children understand the connection between their behavior and the events in their lives, they have a chance to gain some control over their otherwise powerless position in the family. Beyond the age of 3 or 4, children can understand that if two of them fight, mother might walk out, or if one child feels lonely, perhaps another is feeling the same way. They may or may not be able to make changes in their behavior, but seeing the connection between the issues and the advantage of their working together as a unit may help them become more readily available to learn how to make the changes. At the same time, they need to understand that they are only one part of the family. Regardless what they do, mother and father may not be able to do their part. When that happens, they need much reassurance that if they do not return home, it is not their fault.

Role of the Therapist

Many therapists are hesitant to see siblings together, especially if there are more than two. However, when the children are seen together, therapists can gain more appreciation for how overwhelmed even the best of parents can be in trying to handle four or six or eight active children at one time. While seeing them all together is important, with large families it can sometimes be helpful to also see them in subgroups, divided by age, sex, living situation, or type of problems.

In meeting with the children, the therapist must be directive and focus the play and the discussion to the relevant topics. For example,

> "I hear from your foster mother that some of y'all had a tough week. Lori, you burned Carol's dress; Carol, you were hitting Carlos; and Carlos, you hid in your room and refused to go to school all week. I know your mother didn't show up for her promised visit last week. Do you think maybe this was a way to show how angry you each were at her? Let's try something. Let's do last Sunday over again, and see if we can understand how each of you was feeling. This time, Lori, you pretend to be your mother; Carol, you can be Lori. Carlos, you be Carol, and I'll try to be you, Carlos. Let's start with your mother, you Lori, coming to the door."

These children need more than just a reflection of their feelings, as is done in traditional play therapy (Axline, 1969). They need direct confrontation with the vital issues of their lives. For children too young for the preceding conversation, the same idea can be played out with dolls: The therapist enacts a scene with the dolls that demonstrates their feelings about mother's not showing up and their behavior toward each other (see example in Lewis, 1986c). Young children will let you know through their comments or participation in the play if your comments are accurate. If so, then the next play scene can follow up on the alternative ways the children could have expressed their feelings. For instance, the sibling dolls can wonder to each other whether mother is going to visit; they can talk about how angry or sad they are that she has again let them down and their worry they will never be able to go back home.

If there is any chance the children will live together—with their parents or in a foster home—or stay in touch if living separately, a prime task for the therapist is to connect them with each other. In order to do this, Andolfi's five stages of the therapist's role (Andolfi, Angelo, Menghi, & Nicolo-Corigliano, 1983) has been modified for working with these children (Lewis, 1986a).

In Stage 1, the therapist is an invisible member of the group. This can last from a few minutes to a few sessions. The children know each other, whether they live together or have not seen each other for a while, so the therapist is the "stranger." The therapist's role is to monitor their level of anxiety and activity, which is usually high in the beginning.

In Stage 2, which may start during the first session, the therapist becomes the central figure, organizing the activity, intervening in conflicts, and dealing with each child directly. While remaining central, in Stage 3, the therapist becomes the matchmaker, helping the children relate to each other. She may bring two siblings together around a game or activity or direct them to have a specific discussion. For example, "Olin, Shyrl is playing by himself; Why don't you join him."

In Stage 4, as the siblings relate more to each other, the therapist moves out of the center, becoming a coach. If a leader is needed, the parental child becomes central, with the therapist available as a coach.[1] For example, the therapist might add, "Hey gang, your brother Bryon said to begin cleaning up," or "Would you like an idea for getting more order, Bryon? Why don't you suggest the twins clear the table while the rest work on the floor." For many families, treatment may not last long enough to reach this stage.

Stage 5 is the ideal posttherapy relationship. The therapist becomes the former therapist and is no longer needed. The siblings can support, nurture, and assist each other. This stage may never be reached while the siblings are young, but it is a model of what they can achieve as they grow older.

In addition to the direct work with the siblings, the therapist needs to be in contact with the children's new and old schools. During the sibling therapy, it is helpful to encourage the children to talk to each other about their adjustment to the changed schools, their new classmates, and the classwork. The sharing and mutual problem solving serve to strengthen their concern for and availability to each other.

Structure for the Sessions

Activities during the sessions can be structured or unstructured, depending on how the children deal with their anxiety. If their anxiety becomes too overwhelming and they become wild, free play is counterproductive. They would do better with a structured activity where there are rules, guidelines for behavior, and instructions. The structured activities can be unrelated to the children's issues, such as arts and crafts, board games, or sports. They also can be specifically focused on the issues, such as drawing a picture of the worst and best thing that happened during the visitation last week or a role play re-enacting a bad scene at breakfast. It is important not to underestimate young children's capacity to talk or to do things as complex as role plays and even reversal role plays, where they take someone else's part.

For those children who become constricted with anxiety, structured activity may further inhibit their expression; they may do better with free play. Unstructured activity allows the children to do what they want with whatever material is in the room, without directions from the therapist. This might take the form of one child playing alone with the dollhouse while two others flip through picture books and a fourth makes clay figures.

Conversations during the Activity

Whether the activity is structured or not, the conversation during each session must be focused on the specific theme(s) chosen by the therapist. For example, in the structured activity of making Christmas tree decorations, the therapist directs the conversation to what has happened during the week and relates that to their problems in the placement or in returning home. When one sibling won't share the paste or criticizes the other's decoration, the therapist relates that to the problems the child is having with siblings or friends and includes the siblings in understanding and helping solve the problems.

> "Tommy, you get in trouble all the time for this very thing, don't you, taking things that don't belong to you without asking first. You know that gets grownups mad at you, and you have heard your foster parents talking about having you move out because of it. Let me ask each of you guys: Why do you think Tommy does that? How do you think he feels inside when he grabs something without bothering to ask?"

During an unstructured activity, the therapist must work harder to get the children to talk about the issues. The therapist must find creative ways to tie issues together and to get the children's attention, since they may not be paying attention to each other or whoever is speaking.

> Five young siblings, ages 5 to 12, living in three separate foster homes, meet for the third time the week after Thanksgiving. They enter the room and begin running around, playfully punching and pushing. The therapist (in a voice loud enough to be heard over their screaming or shouting) compliments them on how well they are playing together, on not leaving anyone out, and on knowing the difference between play fighting and real fighting. They are burning off energy and renewing contact, since they have not seen each other for 2 weeks. In a few minutes they settle down with two at the doll house, one with paints, and two boys roughhousing. The therapist loudly asks, "What did you have for Thanksgiving?" Two boys, between swings, call out, "pumpkin pie" and "turkey." The therapist keeps asking, "And what else?" After listing

all their foods on the board, the therapist says, "I know something you didn't have for Thanksgiving." The oldest girl, with a chip solidly on her shoulder, challenges, "Yea? What?" Since the boys are now making such a noisy ruckus, the therapist lowers her voice (to attract their attention) and says, "Each other." The younger boy dashes to the therapist and begins punching her stomach. She quickly cradles him (see below) and says, "That makes you real mad, doesn't it? You were really hoping to be together. It's hard enough not being with your mom, but not to be with each other makes you really mad *and* sad, doesn't it?" While the boy is being cradled, the oldest two talk about what happened to prevent their seeing each other. The therapist says to them, "Do you think your brothers and sister know you were disappointed you didn't see them? Maybe you could tell them how upset you were." This leads to the group circling close together on the floor and talking about former Thanksgivings when they were all together; they make plans to be together next year.

Clinical Interventions

The interventions for these children must connect the children's behavior, the feelings underlying their behavior, and the effect of their behavior on others. Interventions can be grouped into three categories: those that focus on development of their mutual caring, on the containment of their out-of-control behavior, and on their connections between the behavior and their central dramas. The term "brother" and "sister" are frequently used to remind them of and reinforce their special mutual relationship. The language used in the following examples needs to be adapted to the age and ability of the child, and not all of the comments are necessarily made at one time.

Mutual Caring

These children often have few models for showing affection and interest in each other. Some useful techniques for teaching siblings to listen to and care about each other include prodding, distinguishing, and singing.

Prodding coaxes the children to go beyond their typical responses to each other. There are many variations. It can be used for teaching siblings to notice each other: "Have y'all noticed how excited your sister is about her school project? See if you can ask her to tell you about it." Or, "Do you notice anything different about how your brother Bob looks today?" Donny punches Bob, saying, "Hey, you got a cool hair cut there."

When one child is more quiet or rowdy than usual, the others can be prodded to notice, as in the following illustration:

THERAPIST: Glen, have you noticed Blannie is acting different today? Why don't you ask her what's going on, how she's feeling?"

GLEN: Naw, she's always like that.

THERAPIST: I don't think you are being as sharp an observer as I know you can be. But, the only way to find out for sure is to ask. Go ahead, ask her how she feels.

GLEN: (*Ignores therapist.*)

THERAPIST: Does it make you feel funny, talking real nice to her? But, let me ask you, when you are real sad, don't you ever feel lonely and wish someone would be nice to you?

GLEN: Yea. (*He gives an example from the prior week.*)

THERAPIST: So, you do understand how nice it is that someone cares enough to think about you. So, don't you think Blannie might also like to feel that you care, like you did with your foster mother?

GLEN: What's wrong, Blannie?

BLANNIE: Nothing.

THERAPIST: Do you believe that, Glen?

GLEN: (*He drops his drawing and goes over to her.*) Come on, you can tell me. I bet you [*sic*] feeling real sad.

(*Blannie looks away, then bursts into tears. Glen looks uncomfortable and starts to turn away.*)

THERAPIST: Glen, why don't you put your arm around her. You said you really liked it when your foster mother did that for you.

(*Awkwardly he does, and Blannie turns toward him and hugs him real tight, crying harder. In a few minutes, she begins to tell him what she is so sad about.*)

Another version of prodding can be used with getting them to give each other positive feedback. When Jerry lets Darcie share the puppets he is using, the therapist says, "Darcie, can you tell Jerry how nice it was for him to let you use the puppets, too?" This can open up a discussion of why they sometimes don't share with each other. Such a prod allows Darcie to recognize Jerry's positive behavior (not to take it for granted), and it teaches her how to respond. If done repetitively, it may begin a new format for their playing with each other.

Distinguishing is a technique to combat children's exaggeration in lumping all people together. When Charlie screams at his siblings, "You all always pick on me," the therapist can say:

THERAPIST: Think about this for a moment. Think real carefully. Do all of them pick on you?

CHARLIE: Well no, Janie doesn't, but that's because she is only 2.

THERAPIST: What about Nana? Marty? Pete?

CHARLIE: Pete does all the time.

THERAPIST: Does Nana?

CHARLIE: Not really, well sometimes, but not that much.

THERAPIST: Now, with Pete. Does he pick on you all the time—every single moment of every single day?

CHARLIE: No, stupid, but (*turning to Pete*) I can't stand it when you call me names.

THERAPIST: OK, now you're getting specific. That's great. You are angry at Pete when he calls you names—not all the time, but every time he calls you names. Can you tell Pete that? Just tell him how you hate the name calling.

Singing is a wonderful joining technique that diminishes age and personality differences. Singing can be used instead of talking to each other. The therapist can start a conversation in "sing-song" (e.g., operatic, rap, rock): "Josh, Do you see Janie's drawing a real nice picture there. Can you tell her something you like about it" (going very high or very low to catch their attention and engage their senses of humor). "Maybe you could tell her you like the colors or the little dog?" "Janie," he screeches, "I like your pikkkkture. You draw oh so verrrry prettttty." The therapist then sings to Janie to sing something nice to her sister sitting across from her, and the "nice songs" get passed around.

Certain songs, such as Sly and the Family Stone's "We are Family," can be used as a fun way to emphasize the "we-ness" of their special relationship. The repetitive lines of "We are fam-i-ly; I've got my brother and sister with me" can be adapted to each family's sibling configuration (e.g., "I've got my four brothers with me" or "I've got my sisters and brother with me"). The rhythm and the words can be soothing. Used as an end of the session ritual, the message of the song coincides with one of the messages of the session: however bad everything else is, you've always got your siblings.

Containment of Behavior

Some useful techniques for controlling the children's behavior include redirecting, reframing, cradling, and sokka-bopping.

Redirecting is a way to refocus the misbehavior without drawing attention to it. Three brothers are physically fighting. The therapist rings a bell and says, "If you're going to fight, let's do this right. Let's mark out a boxing ring" (which they eagerly do), "and two of you go to the corners. The third will be the timer. How long should each round be? Two minutes? What rules should we have?" (Discussion follows.) The plan is enacted and the timer is helped to enforce the rules and ring the bell after 2 minutes. They then switch roles.

Reframing is a way to verbally change a negative behavior into a positive and caring interaction. When 12-year-old Bonny is pushing or pinching her 8-year-old brother, the therapist says, "Bonny, you really love Boyce a lot, don't you? I can tell. You look real tough, but I can tell pinching is your way to show you like him." Bonny's reaction is typical to such a comment. "Ugh! Hell no. I can't stand the m.f." "Well," I respond, "that's what you say, but Boyce, you watch closely, and you, too, will be able to see that she is trying to get close to you." This is repeated whenever she hurts him. Bonny is faced with a win–win situation: Either she stops hurting him or she acknowledges affection for her brother.

Cradling is a technique for physically protecting the siblings and the therapist. It is useful when a child is exhibiting harmful behavior. Seven-year-old Amy screams and bites her brother. The therapist lifts her in her arms and cradles her like a child, slowing rocking, while tightly hugging-in Amy's arms so she can't move them. She softly sings, "Rock-a-bye baby on the tree top. . . . " Amy screams, "Let me down; I'm not a baby, I'll bite you." The therapist calmly says, "You are hurting so much inside and, like a baby, biting and screaming is your only way to let us know. Like a little baby, you can't talk with words. Amy wiggles and screams, trying to get down. "You see, that's just what babies do, so I must be right. When you no longer want to be babied, you will stop screaming and biting, and then I'll know to put you down." Amy lowers her voice and tells the therapist in a firm, 7-year-old voice, "Put me down; I'm not a baby." "You see, when you no longer need to be a baby, you know how to talk as a very grown-up 7-year-old." When she gets down, she pulls away and immediately runs to bite her brother. The therapist grabs her quickly and cradles her again, repeating the cradling. This time, Amy relaxes her body and allows herself to be held and rocked for a short time. The therapist speaks softly about how hurting others is the only way she knows to show how she hurts inside. The cradling turns to fun baby time, with Amy and the therapist goo-gooing and laughing together. Her little brother joins in babying her, enjoying the changed birth-order role.

Sokka-bopping[2] is a technique of using rubber bats to express anger. Paul, age 16, is the oldest of six children. He alternates between ignoring, hitting, and playing with his siblings. In one session, 10-year-old Zina is bothering him, and he goes to smack her. The therapist says, "You really get mad when she pesters you, but does hitting get her to stop? No, so let's try this instead." She hands them each a sokka-boppa. "Paul, you are much bigger than Zina, so let's make this a bit fairer. Since you are right-handed, you use your left hand. Now, each of you try to hit it out of the other's hand." If that still gives Paul too much of an edge, they both can be blindfolded, have their feet tied together, or use some other playful means for equaling the odds. After a few minutes of warm-up hitting, the therapist says, "Zina, hold your bat out straight. Now Paul, I want you to try to hit it out of her hand. Hit real hard, and with each hit, tell her how mad you feel when she pesters you."

Paul starts, one sentence with each hit. "I hate you bugging me. It makes me so angry and want to just smack you." The therapist offers some other sentences for him to try, such as, "It makes me just as angry as when dad hits me. I want to hurt you as much as he hurts me." Paul continues on his own, "I hate having to be responsible for you kids. I'd rather be with my friends." After a while, he stops, sweating from the exertion. Zina is still holding her bat tightly with both hands. Paul says, "I really do love you, Zina, it's just that sometimes you really get me mad." Zina starts to cry and Paul hugs her. The other siblings, having quietly watched, gather around Paul and tell him they love him.

This leads to a discussion of how Paul gets in trouble with Mom if they don't obey him. They talk about what they can do to make it easier for Paul with mother, and for themselves with him.

Central Drama

There is often one central trauma in each child's life that gets repetitively reenacted (Rosenberg, 1980). Siblings become wedded to the roles they played at the time of the trauma. While the main trauma for each child may be different, the roles can intertwine, so that one is locked into a self-abusing position and the other into an abusing one. Sibling therapy, like individual play therapy, can provide a corrective emotional experience, but with the siblings all present, there is an opportunity to readjust their relational responses to the trauma, as well.

Once the children understand how their roles were created, they can see ways to untangle them and come to some resolution with each other and around the trauma.

Six months ago, Danny and Eddie, ages 9 and 8, respectively, were placed in a foster home after a teacher reported that Eddie had not eaten for several days. Although placed together, Danny's constant attack on Eddie was causing the Agency to consider separating them. As a temporary stopgap, Danny was referred for individual therapy; the therapist chose to see the brothers together.

The therapist surmised the major crisis for this family had occurred about 4 years before, when Eddie woke up in time to see his father stab his mother. Danny, who slept through it, responded to the trauma by becoming protective of mother, often skipping school to be with her, especially when she was drinking heavily; placement prevented him from continuing his self-imposed watch. During a drawing project in the first session, when Danny hit Eddie, the therapist separated them and asked,

THERAPIST: Why are you so angry with Eddie, Danny?

(*Danny lists a bunch of minor incidents.*)

THERAPIST: OK, but I wonder if you are also angry at him for causing you to be taken from your mother. You did a pretty good job of trying to always be there with her.

(*Danny ignores the therapist and Eddie.*)

THERAPIST: You blame Eddie, don't you, for y'all being with the Smiths?

DANNY: Yea. If he hadn't been such a baby, we wouldn't have to be there. He always cried and bothered Mom.

THERAPIST: That's not why you aren't with your mother, Danny. You both know that. You are not living with your mother now because she has her own personal problems that made it difficult for her to take good care of you two. It was not Eddie's fault.

EDDIE: You see! It's your fault. You always pick on me.

THERAPIST: (*interrupting them*) It's neither of your fault. But Danny, I have a feeling that each time you hit Eddie or call him names you are getting back at him for telling his teacher he was hungry.

DANNY: He didn't have to do that.

EDDIE: But I was hungry.

THERAPIST: Hitting Eddie is easier for you than getting angry at your mother for not feeding you. You were hungry, too. You really feel bad for her, don't you?

DANNY: She tried hard. She didn't mean to drink and she wanted us to eat more, she told me so. But she didn't have no [*sic*] money.

THERAPIST: (*Later*) Eddie, I wonder why you don't stand up to Danny when he is so mean to you?

EDDIE: I can't. He always hits me.

THERAPIST: I know, but you could tell him to stop or even hit back.

EDDIE: No I can't. (*He cries.*)

DANNY: What a crybaby.

THERAPIST: Eddie, I have a thought. I wonder if when Danny hits you, it reminds you of how you watched your father stab your mother. You felt helpless to stop it then, and now you again feel helpless. You were too little to help your mother, but you aren't too little to stop Danny from picking on you. (*Later*) You know, Danny, when you pick on Eddie, that causes the Smiths to be very upset, and you know they are thinking about moving you to another home. It doesn't make sense that you should keep on hurting your brother Eddie—the one family member who is still with you—out of your anger at both of your parents. (*To Eddie*) It doesn't make any sense, Eddie, that you set yourself up for Danny to hurt you. That won't make your mother any stronger; it won't bring her back, and it won't make your father visit you more often or be any nicer to any of you when he does visit.

This conversation takes place throughout the rest of the session, while the boys work on several structured tasks. After this session, each time Danny hits Eddie, the therapist says, "Danny, it is not Eddie's fault you are at the Smiths," or "It is easier to be mad at Eddie than at your mother, isn't it?" That always stops Danny, even though he pretends he doesn't hear or he argues it isn't true. (Sometimes he is willing to use the sokka-boppas against "mother.")

Each time Eddie eggs on the fight or refuses to protect himself, the therapist says, "It wasn't your fault you couldn't protect your mother," or "You couldn't protect your mother from your father, but you can protect yourself against Danny." Disconnecting the earlier crises from their current behavior provides a basis for new ways to relate. After a few weeks, the hurtful behavior continued in the therapy sessions but ceased in the foster home. That allowed them an appropriate place to deal with the anger without risking their living situation.

STEP TWO:
MOTHERS' GROUP THERAPY

Helping only the children would be no more effective in breaking the cycle of recidivism than helping only the mother. Therefore, it is also crucial to help mother (and father, if involved) with her issues and then to help the family work together on reunification.

Group therapy may be a more effective treatment for these women than individual therapy. Many of them struggle against a fourfold prejudice: being female, a single parent, poor, and non-White. In addition, too often, they are emotionally cut off from their extended families and social communities. Having their children in placement is one more sign of their inadequacy, their failure; it broadcasts to all that they have lost total control over their lives.

Group can become a haven for them to feel understood by their peers. For many, the group is the first time they have talked to others about their feelings of losing their children. The group encourages self-empowerment and mutual aid (Gitterman & Shulman, 1986; Lee, 1988; Parsons, 1991; Pinderhughes, 1983), allowing the women to experiment with new behaviors, to learn interpersonal social skills, and to gain some control over at least some parts of their lives (Lewis & Ford, 1990; Shapiro, 1990). Through learning that others value what they have to offer, they may develop a sense of their own worthiness and competence. As they solve specific problems within their daily lives, they feel better about themselves as women and as mothers. The camaraderie that develops in the group chips away at their isolation, so that they learn to turn to others for support, such as extended family, neighborhood, church. (For more information about the mother's group therapy component, see Lewis, 1991.)

Since one goal of the separation is to give mothers a chance to become better and more caring parents, they can begin working on this while in group. Even though their children are not living with them, they can practice and then carry out ways to appropriately keep in touch with their children, the foster parents, and their children's teachers.

STEP THREE: FAMILY THERAPY

As the children and mother make progress in their respective group therapies—while still living apart—they meet together weekly for family therapy. The goals for mother should include learning how to play and have fun with her children and how to appropriately discipline. The goals for the children should include being able to talk more easily about their feelings, to ask for what they want from the others without fighting or screaming, and to share their mother. (For more information about the family therapy component, see Lewis, 1991.)

When the children misbehave during the sessions, the therapist may coach, but the mother should be the one to directly respond to the children. If the children do not listen, the therapist can reinforce their mother's message, as, for example, "Arlene, your mother told you not to do that," or the therapist can encourage the mother to restate her expectations and enforce them. But it is important that the therapist not take over the mother's role.

To help the family members deal with specific problems that interfere with possible reunification, the therapist can direct them in role plays and reversal role plays. Re-enacting family situations that cause the most difficulty can be fun as well as effective in stretching each person's options for new behaviors.

Seven of Mrs. Kay's eight children, ages 4 to 14, had been placed throughout the previous 5 years. Only the 4-year-old was with her and her alcoholic husband at the time of the fire. She had been struggling to get her life in order, end the marriage, and ask for her children to be returned. The fire threw her into a serious depression with reverberating effects for the children who were planning to come home.

Referrals were made for individual therapy for several of the children, at two different clinics. When it was discovered they were siblings, a decision was made to see all eight of them together. The first few sessions were devoted to introducing them to each other (the youngest had only met the oldest once); they talked about their feelings of having to remain in placement because Mother had no home yet, and about their jealousy of the youngest. Then the children were seen in subsets of boys and girls, older and younger, and those living together (they were in five different homes).

Simultaneously, Mrs. Kay participated in a mothers' group, where the other women understood her trying to keep her marriage together in order to get the children back. They understood her financial double-bind: She needed a large enough apartment so they could live with her, yet without her children, she was not eligible for medical assistance. After the fire, they encouraged her not to give up, kill herself, or flee.

Because the children had been spread out, living in areas outside of public transportation lines, her visitations were infrequent. Therefore, the family therapy became their only regular visitations. The children were thrilled, some of them not having seen her for months. It is overwhelming being with eight excited children, and it took mother and two therapists to help provide appropriate boundaries and enough arms for the needed control and hugs. The therapists primarily focused attention on helping mother figure a way to play with each of the children at different times. There were adult "powwows," so she could decide which children she could play with together, which could wait, and how to stay connected with those who had to wait. Sometimes during these moments, the children were told to "hold it a second; Mom's thinking."

Mrs. Kay was coached to think about different ways to relate to the 4-year-old and the 14-year-old. She was coached to ask one of the older children to watch the younger ones while she talked with the 10-,

11-, and 12-year-olds about school. She tried out different discipline methods. During each visit, she was encouraged to talk with all of the children together about how much she wanted to be with them, but that they would have to take turns. "I'll try to be fair, but you have to cooperate." Occasionally, when two of them would be fighting, she told them she would not take them back. She was encouraged to turn this from a threat into a discussion of her fear of not being able to handle their fighting when there were so many things going on at one time with eight children. With the therapists' help, she came up with an alternative sentence, "You have to do your part to help out if we're going to all get back together."

Within a few months, the children were returned home—two at a time, causing more hurt and jealousy for those returned last. Mrs. Kay continued with her group, getting ideas from the other women in using the social service system more effectively, such as obtaining, homemaker assistance, day care, and an afterschool job for the 14-year-old. The children were occasionally seen together or in subgroups, dealing with their individual problems and their feelings about being home. What allowed this treatment plan to go so well was the full cooperation of the Agency in paying for transportation and each of the three weekly therapies. Unfortunately, as with so many families, when she was evicted because her children were making too much noise, Mrs. Kay took them and left the state. No further follow-up was possible. The good news, though, was that prior to their departure, the children were doing adequately in school, when evicted she did not become dysfunctionally depressed but took action, and when she left, she kept her children together.

ISSUES FOR AGENCIES AND THERAPISTS

Does it work? Does meeting with the children together teach them to see their part in making the reunification work better? Do they learn to care more for each other and to see how their actions affect each other? Does having mothers in a mothers' group help them develop a sense of personal worth and gain inner strength to be more functional parents? Does seeing the children and mother together circumvent problems that may occur once they are reunited? There are no research data to answer these questions, but even if there were, these three components—sibling therapy, mothers' group therapy, and family therapy—are only part of the picture. There are at least two other important elements essential to the success of this treatment approach: the social service agency and its workers, and the therapists (Itzkowitz, 1989). For this chapter, the discussion of applicability is directed only to therapists and to the sibling therapy component.

I have done a good deal of professional training on sibling therapy, and the responses I receive are fairly similar: "What a wonderful idea." "It makes a lot of sense." "I love the opportunity to be able to do something different." In many of the follow-up conversations, professionals mention the benefits of seeing the siblings together. Social service workers say there is more disruption in sibling placements than in individual child placements, which forces them to place siblings separately. Therefore, they like knowing they can refer the children for sibling therapy that may help them remain together.

Therapists note how the complementary roles of "trouble-maker" and "goody-two-shoes," for example, are reinforced when only one child becomes the focus of individual therapy. Further, they note how parental children are often seen in individual therapy to "rescue" them from the responsibility of supervising their siblings. This ignores how integrally related is the caretaker role to their self-esteem. Sibling therapy, on the other hand, can teach parental children to delegate power to the other siblings as well as take time to be with their friends.

Therapists also comment on the benefit of the children learning to know their siblings, to be able to turn to them for support. Even if they never return home, they will at least know there are other family members around who care.

Given these benefits and given the excitement therapists express about sibling therapy, how are we to understand that even after specialized training, the ideas are not incorporated into their practice? Their explanations can be divided into three areas: logistics, lack of agency support, and therapists' anxiety.

Logistics

There is a general consensus that the logistics of seeing the siblings together become too overwhelming. For instance, therapists do not provide (and social workers do not request) sibling therapy because it may require coordination between several sets of foster parents, workers from different foster agencies, group homes, schools, and so forth. If transportation must be provided for each child, then taxis must be paid for travel and waiting time, or social workers are tied up waiting for them. Further, therapists are already too overwhelmed with ongoing cases and paperwork to see the siblings together. As one woman said, "I'd like to just forget the paperwork, but if you do that, it all falls apart and that really hurts the children."

Lack of Agency Support

Most agencies are struggling to stay financially solvent, which means innovations that require money usually are not well received. Sibling therapy can be seen as a financial drain for the logistical reasons mentioned above. Some agencies are overtly supportive as long as therapists add these groups to their already full schedule; however, therapists need extra time to plan and then run the group. Money is needed for group supplies and supervision and training. In addition, many agencies offer little encouragement to undertake any new programs.

Therapists' Anxiety

One primary concern that is rarely mentioned aloud is therapists' hesitation to face the chaos of seeing more than one child at a time. As one social worker said, "I take siblings to visit with each other in pairs, but it is too chaotic to have more than two at a time. It is hard enough to keep the six children in my own family connected. With these kids, it'd drive me crazy."

Therapists have numerous psychological explanations for not seeing the children together, such as that the oldest child needs to be helped out of his or her parental role, or the aggressive child may hurt the quiet one. However, as the social worker quoted above said, seeing so many kids together can be anxiety provoking. Since few mental health graduate schools offer more than cursory training in any type of group therapy, they may not have had special training in running children's groups. In addition, the anxiety could increase at the thought of seeing several out-of-control children together, especially if there is no group supervision. But most therapists who discussed this said, "I just don't think about it."

SUGGESTIONS FOR OFFERING SIBLING THERAPY

What is needed to make it happen? An agency may be more responsive to the request to run a comprehensive treatment involving the children and the parents if it comes from within the agency, by someone willing to undertake the venture. The agencies where I provide ongoing consultation are more likely to offer this than places where I have done a one-time training. For therapists committed to the idea, it takes marketing skills to sell agencies sibling therapy or the three-step approach and to avert the anticipated objections based on time and money. Many therapists do not have these entrepreneurial skills. With the current excitement about home preservation, though, there is a chance that the three-step program can be incorporated into these programs already offering challenging and new treatment options.

What would make it more sellable, of course, is proof of its success in cutting short- and long-term costs. Unfortunately, there is no systematic follow-up research. Long-term follow-up is difficult for the obvious logistical factors of families' mobility and multiple agency involvement. Research on short-term follow-up on individual families is do-able. From the families I have been able to track, even if the children have continued to have difficulties (which most have), there has been a notable difference in their use of and relationship with each other.

CONCLUSION

The cyclical pattern of recidivism in foster care suggests there are missing links in understanding the phenomenon. Using a systemic framework and changing the punctuation of perspective may open new options for creating change. The traditional perspective is to see the mother (or parents, if the father is involved) as the sole focus of intervention; the mother is the problem and the children are placed for their protection. This, though, overlooks the reality of the feedback loop; that is, when one part of the family is experiencing difficulty, the rest will be affected and react in ways that reinforce the difficulty of the first. This means that the mother's problems can cause problems for her children as well as her children's problems causing an overwhelmed mother even more difficulty as she attempts to deal with them.

Breaking the cycle requires, at a minimum, a three-step intervention involving the children, the mother (parents), and then the family together. The focus of this chapter has been primarily on the first component—sibling therapy. Seeing the children together and in subgroups gives them a safe forum for understanding the connections between the difficulties they are having in their daily lives and anticipated problems in returning home. It also provides them the occasion to express their distress and helplessness with others who share their situation. Rather than physically vent their feelings on each other, they learn alternative ways of dealing with them, such as talking together, which can break their emotional isolation. While the type of interactions between the children may not change dramatically, the quality can. For example, the fighting may change from being nasty, with the intent of hurting each other, to play-fighting, as a way of sharing their mutual anger.

Seeing the children together opens the possibility of creating a sense of family and positive connection between the siblings, of helping the children recognize the consequences of their behaviors with each other and with mother, and of learning to enjoy playing and problem solving together. Whether they eventually return home or remain together in the foster home, they will have a smoother relationship and the special awareness of at least some family ties.

NOTES

1. Therapists tend to overlook the necessity in large, single-parent-headed or working parent families of having at least one child who assumes leadership and responsibility for managing the other children. This is sometimes referred to as a parental child. The role of parental child is not in itself bad; it is only detrimental if it is a rigidified role, and the child has no opportunity to also be with peers.

2. Sokka-boppers are handmade versions of the Batakkas. They can be handmade from pillow scraps donated by upholsterers.

ACKNOWLEDGMENT

An earlier version of this chapter was published in Lewis (1991).

REFERENCES

American Public Welfare Association. (1992). *Characteristics of children in substitute and adoptive care*. Washington, DC: Author.

Andolfi, M., Angelo, C., Menghi, P., & Nicolo-Corigliano, M. (1983). *Behind the family mask: Therapeutic change in rigid family systems*. New York: Brunner/Mazel.

Aponte, H. (1976). Underorganization in the poor family. In P. Guerin (Ed.), *Family therapy: Theory and practice* (pp. 432–438). New York: Gardner Press.

Axline, V. (1969). *Play therapy*. New York: Ballantine Books.

Bank, S., & Kahn, M. (1982). *The sibling bond*. New York: Basic Books.

Block, N., & Liebowitz, A. (1983). *Recidivism in foster care*. New York: Child Welfare League of America.

Eastman, K. S. (1985). Foster families: A comprehensive bibliography. *Child Welfare, 64*, 565–585.

Gitterman, A., & Shulman, L. (Eds.). (1986). *Mutual aid groups and the life cycle*. Itasca, IL: Peacock.

Gurak, D. T., Smith, D. A., & Goldson, M. F. (1982). *The minority foster child: A comparative study of Hispanic, Black and White children*. New York: Fordham University, Hispanic Research Center.

Hegar, R. (1988). Legal and social work approaches to sibling separation in foster care. *Child Welfare, 67*, 113–121.

Itzkowitz, A. (1989). Children in placement: A place for family therapy. In L. Combrinck-Graham (Ed.), *Children in family contexts: Perspectives on treatment* (pp. 391–412). New York: Guilford Press.

Kahn, M., & Lewis, K. G. (1988). *Siblings in therapy: Life stages and clinical issues*. New York: Norton.

Lee, J. (Ed.). (1988). *Group work with the poor and oppressed*. New York: Haworth Press.

Lewis, E., & Ford, B. (1990). The network utilization project: Incorporating traditional strengths of African-American families into Group work practice. In K. Chau (Ed.), Ethnicity and biculturalism: Emerging perspectives of social group work [Special Issue]. *Social Work with Groups, 13,* 7–22.

Lewis, K. G. (1986a). Sibling therapy with children in foster homes. In L. Combrinck-Graham (Ed.), *Treating young children in family therapy* (pp. 52–61). Rockville, MD: Aspen.

Lewis, K. G. (1986b). Sibling therapy with multiproblem families. *Journal of Marital and Family Therapy, 12,* 291–300.

Lewis, K. G. (1986c). Systemic play therapy: A tool for social work consultation to inner-city community mental health centers. *Journal of Independent Social Work, 1,* 33–43.

Lewis, K. G. (1991). A three step plan for African-American families involved with foster care: Sibling therapy, mothers' group therapy, family therapy. In K.G. Lewis (Ed.), *Family systems application to social work: Training and clinical practice* (pp. 135–147). New York: Haworth Press.

Minuchin, S., Montalvo, B., Guerney, B. G., Jr., Rosman, B., & Schumer, F. (1967). *Families of the slums: An exploration of their structure and treatment.* New York: Basic Books.

Parsons, R. (1991). Empowerment: Purpose and practice principle in social work. *Social Work with Groups, 14,* 7–22.

Pinderhughes, E. (1983). Empowerment: For our clients and for ourselves. *Social Casework, 64,* 312–314.

Rosenberg, E. (1980). Therapy with siblings in reorganizing families. *International Journal of Family Therapy, 2,* 139–150.

Shapiro, B. Z. (1990). The social work group as social microcosm: "Frames of reference" revisited. *Social Work with Groups, 13,* 5–21.

14

The Stages of the Reunification Process and the Tasks of the Therapist

Lindsay Bicknell-Hentges

In recent years there has been an increasing trend to remove children from their parents' care (Gershenson, Rosewater, & Massinga, 1990). Some estimate the child welfare system alone places over 200,000 children in an out-of-home placement each year (Knitzer, 1989). Whether these children are placed in foster homes, group homes, residential treatment centers, or inpatient settings, they have joined the growing number of children who are spending parts of their childhood and adolescence in the care of someone other than their natural parents.

The tendency to remove a child from an apparently dangerous situation is an understandable result of a natural desire to protect the vulnerable. Those charged with the responsibility for protecting children's welfare must balance often conflicting goals, including protecting children, safeguarding the rights of parents, and preserving families. In many situations, the caseworkers who work directly with the children have impossibly large caseloads, and this makes it difficult to get to know the children and families for whom they make decisions. Gershenson et al. (1990) reported that child welfare workers often have no training to deal with the complex family issues present in their caseloads. Consequently, the deciding balance becomes tipped in the direction of immediate "remedy" to a crisis: The child is removed from the home. Lloyd and Bryce (1985) have identified several specific groups of children who are at risk of going into substitute care: children at risk of abuse and neglect; children whose parents have conditions that limit parental functioning; status offenders and minors adjudicated delinquent; emotionally disturbed children; developmentally disabled children; and children from multiproblem families.

Despite the recognition that children in out-of-home placements are frequently cut off from their families as well as being "abandoned psychologically and sometimes literally by the public system that assumes responsibility for them" (Knitzer, Allen, & McGowan, 1978, p. 5), there still exists pervasive antiparent bias, proresidential bias, and fiscal barriers that hamper the provision of adequate services to families in trouble (Knitzer, 1989). These barriers contribute to children remaining in out-of-home care for extended periods of time, moving from place to place, and losing the chance to develop a stable, caring relationship with an adult. Fanshel (1971) reported that the longer children are in foster care, the greater are their chances of becoming emotionally disturbed. Other authors (Maas & Engler, 1959; Solnit, 1973) have also stated that children need the promise of continuity of environment and permanent relationships to grow emotionally. Since examinations have shown that foster parents often ask for the removal of their foster children when a crisis arises, and the turnover rate of institutional child care workers is extremely high (Sarata & Behrman, 1982), the goal of stability is problematic for foster care as well as for institutions.

Lloyd and Bryce (1985) have concluded that the decision to remove a child from his or her home is a drastic one that should only be made with great deliberation and care. This decision disrupts whatever continuity a child has been able to experience and introduces additional emotional risks. They concur with Gershenson et al. (1990) that the awesome responsibility of these decisions is often left to workers who do not understand the power and dynamics of family relationships and who have limited access to resources for family assessment.

Once a child is placed out of his or her home, the child's family shares the impact of this extreme strategy. The child's right to a family often becomes a low priority in placement systems where parents are rarely explicitly encouraged to maintain frequent contact with their children and are either actively discouraged from maintaining contact or even forbidden to see, call, or correspond with their biological children in some instances (Knitzer et al., 1978). Agency practices have been shown to significantly impact maintenance of family contact with the placed child. Proch and Howard (1986) found that parental visits with children in foster care were more likely to be scheduled and in the parents' home when the plan specified family reunification as a goal. Furthermore, they also discovered that parents typically complied with visitation schedules, not visiting unless regular visits were scheduled. Parents are not always entitled to information on their children's progress and sometimes are not even informed when their children are moved (Knitzer et al., 1978). Unfortunately, a family's lack of contact can be read as disinterest by a caseworker or child care worker, who may respond by even further reducing efforts to maintain parent–child contact.

The loss of contact with a child in placement compounds the initial impact of removing a child from his or her parents' care. The message sent to the parent of a placed child is a strong one. Moss and Moss (1984) described the guilt a parent can experience from failing in the culturally defined role of parent as well as the shame of not living up to one's ideal as parents. They pointed out the difficulty parents can face when answering questions like the following: "Where is your child? Why isn't he living with you? Will he come back?" (p. 171). Gershenson et al. (1990) confirmed the drastic effect that placement has on families: Parents with children in substitute care describe feeling intense sadness, anger, guilt, despair, and humiliation. These parents know that they have failed as parents, and they are left essentially powerless with a host of strangers making most of the decisions about their own children.

The child in placement and his or her family are placed at certain risks. Consequently, the current challenge by child and family advocates is to avoid and reduce placement stays whenever possible. To date, the most promising strategy that acknowledges the need to protect the child and preserve the family is the provision of family-centered placement prevention and reunification services. These services represent a rapidly growing portion of child welfare services (Nelson, Landsman, & Deutelbaum, 1990). However, despite the enactment of the Adoption Assistance and Child Welfare Act (PL 96-272), that mandated that public child welfare agencies provide services to avoid out-of-home placement and to reunite families as quickly as possible, once placement has occurred, a shift toward the goals of family preservation and reunification must still attack the pervasive antiparent bias and fiscal barriers that have compromised the provision of comprehensive services to families (Knitzer, 1989).

Several models committed to preserving families and reunifying whenever possible have been developed. Nelson et al. (1990) identified three distinct models (crisis-intervention, home-based, and family treatment) for family-centered placement prevention programs that attempt to provide a range of services that meet the concrete, supportive, and therapeutic needs of families. But no clinician can adequately provide therapeutic services within any model without fully understanding the dynamics of family systems.

For optimal success, any reunification strategy must be implemented by clinicians who are cognizant of the ebbs and flows in the process of reunification and who have experience managing the resistance that naturally occurs in such an intense process. Reunifying a family splintered through placement ignites a range of emotions within children and parents. The therapist can act as a resource for understanding, predicting, and normalizing the fears and frustrations that frequently arise during this process.

The present chapter offers a road map of the reunification process, describing the stages of the process as well as the tasks of the therapist at each stage. The model and the accompanying case study demonstrate typical transitions and practical strategies that can be applied to enhance the reunification process.

REUNIFICATION: THE MODEL AND ITS ASSUMPTIONS

This model was developed through experience as a therapist and clinical supervisor in a group home within metropolitan Chicago. Cases identified as appropriate for reunification were referred by staff members within the institution. Thorough implementation of this model requires education of referral sources regarding the characteristics associated with successful reunification. This education must address the proresidential bias that is often evident among residential staff members and child welfare case managers.

As in other types of therapy, referrals tend to increase when the reunification therapist takes the time to personally connect with the referral sources. In a residential setting it is critical that support for reunification is garnered among the residential staff involved in each case. The staff has extensive contact with youths and their families and can unknowingly sabotage the best-laid plans for reunification. Reunification therapists need to meet with these staff in an attempt to develop common goals. This time is well spent in avoiding some of the potential systemic roadblocks that may arise in the reunification process.

This approach to family reunification is based upon several basic tenets. The *first*, most important tenet is that a child has a right to a family. A *second* fundamental assumption is that it is easier to remove a child from his or her family than it is to reunite a family. A *third* essential assumption is that several factors both inside and outside the family inhibit family reunification. Finally, the model is based upon the *fourth* assumption, that successful reunification strategies identify and overcome the obstacles that inhibit reunification.

Operating from these assumptions, the therapist who is assisting in the reunification process functions as an advocate/consultant, as well as a therapist for the family. The therapist must operate from an understanding of the complexity and intensity of the dynamics of the reunifying family. As any family therapist has discovered, the dynamics of families can be very powerful. The reunification therapist must also consider the systems outside of the family that impact the reunification process. The family in the process of reunification is not functioning as a separate, self-determined entity. Input from judicial, child welfare, education, and mental health professionals are usually involved in the decision process that governs family reunification. The powerful systems to which these professionals report impose an equally powerful influence on the reunifying family. Consequently, the therapist must deal artfully with the dynamics and resistance arising within these larger systems as well as within the reunifying family.

For the sake of simplicity, the reunification process will be discussed in discrete, sequential stages, providing a process-level road map for navigation in family reunification. I am aware of the limitations of applying a stage model to dynamic systems such as families interacting with social systems. Each family is a living entity that reacts to each planned and unplanned intervention in its own way. Thus, the idea of a road map is more useful if one remembers that this road is under construction and delays and detours are to be expected. Furthermore, in families with more than one child in placement, each child can be rejoining the family at a different rate, so several stages may be ongoing and interacting simultaneously. Despite its limitations, the road map in such a situation can be useful, if not rigidly applied. The map does provide some information concerning the beginning and ending of a journey, as well as landmarks in between.

Having accepted the assumptions of this road map, the reunification therapist can begin to project the journey ahead. Table 14.1 outlines the stages in the reunification process. Each stage lasts 2 to 4 months, though this varies widely across families.

First, the therapist must define the "family" that will be reunited. "Family" can mean parents and siblings, grandparents, other relatives, and even foster parents, in certain cases. Once the family has been defined and reunification has been initiated, many families enter a second stage during which family members fear and distrust each other, the reunification process, and the involved service providers. Frequently, distrust and fear are followed by the third stage, that of idealism, once there is some belief that both the parents and children are committed to the reunification process. As the idealism begins to break down following extended interaction and contact between parent and child, the family enters the fourth stage, the reality stage, in which the real parent–child conflicts be-

TABLE 14.1. Stages of the Reunification Process

1. Defining the family	Identifying who will and will not be considered "family" in the reunification process
2. Fear and distrust	Identifying the aspects of reunification that are frightening and diffusing of resistance
3. Idealism	Idealizing of reunification by the family and exploration of potential problems by the therapist
4. Reality	Resurfacing of conflicts and dysfunctional patterns within the family and implementation of new styles of interaction by therapist
5. Second phase of fear	Open expression of fears concerning reunification and realistic assessment of the viability of reunification
6. Return	Return of the youth, grieving, structural reorganization of the family, linkage to community-level support services, and termination

gin to resurface. Predictably, these renewed conflicts lead to the fifth stage, a second fear phase, in which old issues arise, but now in the context of commitment to the reunification process. The sixth and final stage involves the actual physical return of the child home and restructuring of the family as the child is integrated back into the family system.

DEFINING THE FAMILY

For many children, the task of defining their family is relatively simple: There are parents, the siblings, and the extended family. For a growing number of children who have seen their nuclear family break up, defining their family has become more complex: There can be parents, stepparents, brothers and sisters, stepsiblings, half-siblings, and the extended families of each of these. In addition, many children grow up in a network of close friends of the family who may be given "relative" status, rendering them "aunts," "uncles," and "cousins."

> Defining the family of a child who has been in out-of-home placements for an extended period of time can be very difficult. For example, Bruce is 14 years old. He has had no contact with his biological parents since he was 3. He lived in four foster homes for varying lengths of time, but

still maintains contact with his last foster mother, with whom he lived for 5 years, until he was ten. He has also had sporadic contact with a maternal great aunt over the last 6 years. To complicate matters more, Bruce has been living in a group home for the last 4 years, where he has seen a myriad of child care workers come and go. One set of house parents, however, seriously considered taking Bruce into foster care. The task of defining Bruce's family remains extremely difficult even though the complexity of his case is minor compared to many.

Several issues typically arise when identifying who will and will not be considered "family" in the reunification process. As pointed out before, these children and families are living under constraints of mandates from child welfare and judicial systems. As a result of the termination of parental rights, some parents are no longer "parents" in the legal sense. Others may not have lost full rights, but may not be allowed to have any contact with their child(ren).

Another relevant consideration involves the degree of interest that the child and "parents" show for the reunification process. But analysis of interest is not a simple process. Families may not have been explicitly encouraged to maintain contact with their children, and their lack of contact may indicate either a lack of interest or an attempt to comply with agency practices and regulations. The parent labeled "unfit" may simply be waiting for the caseworker or child care worker to initiate a regular schedule of visitation (Proch & Howard, 1986), while the workers may interpret such a lack of contact as lack of interest in the child.

After a child has been in placement for an extended period of time, the child's family begins to reorganize into a structure without the child. This further complicates the analysis of interest in reunification. The child may sense his or her loss of a "place" in the family (that often includes physical changes in a household in which there is no longer a room or bed kept empty for the child). The family may have reorganized to try to maintain and protect the remaining family members from the systems that "take away children," but a placed child perceiving this change may have difficulty admitting his or her interest in returning home. The self-protective stance of the family and child trying to avoid further disappointment and rejection impedes the process of identifying the interest in reunification. Neither the child nor parents who feel hurt by the placement process can be expected to readily admit interest in reunification. In the confines of the therapy room, children have stated it so clearly: "I really want to go back to my parents, but I don't think they will want me, so I'm not going to ask them. I don't want to be hurt again."

A final issue arises in defining the family who will be reunited. The potential success of reunification must be considered. In some cases, both the parents and child report to be highly motivated toward reunification, yet other constraints impair the viability of this option. In one particularly disappointing case, a mother and her 15-year-old son were both totally committed to the reunification process, but the chronic mental illness of the mother and intermittent explosive behavior of the son presented major roadblocks to the process. Although the goal of reunification seriously motivated each to actively pursue treatment for these individual problems, the mother's repeated episodes of psychosis (during which she would become paranoid and abusive to the son) and the lack of adequate substitute resources for the son during her hospitalizations disrupted the reunification process. Eventually, the son shifted his goal from reunification, which required his mother's stabilization, to an independent living program that depended on his own stability and maturity. Such shifts in goals need not be viewed as failures but as appropriate revisions of goals as the reunification process uncovers new information.

Case Example: Sam

Defining and redefining the family of Sam was essentially the stickiest issue to arise in his reunification case. Sam's therapist had to remain flexible in determining the goals of the reunification process. Sam was a 10-year-old White youth with two older sisters, Judy (age 16) and Nancy (age 17). Judy had been sexually abused by her father when she was 6. Subsequently, the father was imprisoned and the family moved to another state. At puberty, Judy began sexually acting out and severe conflicts started with her mother. After several months Sam also developed behavior problems. Both Sam and Judy were removed from the mother's home when Sam was 10, after several violent episodes between the mother and her children.

Sam's mother was rather high functioning, and the family appeared to be a good candidate for reunification. However, as the reunification process was initiated, it became evident that the mother was more invested in the return of Sam and more ambivalent about the return of Judy. The therapist worked with individual family members and the family as a whole in the process of defining the family. Judy's positive adaptation to the residential environment exacerbated the tendency for her to withdraw from the family.

The therapist resisted the family's efforts to return Sam home without Judy because the tendency to reorganize the family without Judy was so strong. However, conflict was increasing between Judy and her mother as Judy began to work through issues related to her sexual abuse. Ultimately, 2 months after the removal of the children from their home, a family court judge ordered that Sam be returned home immediately without Judy. Following this decision, the family quickly reorganized into adversarial camps: Judy against the rest of the family.

Judy continued her positive adjustment at the group home, whereas Sam's return to the family went very smoothly. After Sam's return, the family became more resistant to the return of Judy. Two months later, Judy and her family agreed that she would remain in the group home until she graduated from high school the following year. Consequently, the task of defining this family lasted about 4 months and led to a definition of "family" that did not include the reunification of Judy. Judy remained in the group home until graduation, as planned, and Sam continued to live with his family without significant problems.

Clearly, defining the family stands as a critical, yet difficult process. The therapist must help both children and parents explore their desire to reunite and fears of failure and rejection, while considering the viability of reunification in each instance. Taking a neutral position, the therapist must also try not to be blinded by other's perceptions of the viability of reunification. Caseworkers and child care workers may understandably present an antiparent bias that must be weighed carefully against the strengths of the individual family in consideration.

FEAR AND DISTRUST

Once the family to be reunited is defined and its members identified, and once reunification is accepted as a tentative goal, the actual reunification process is underway. The official declaration of reunification as a goal tends to propel the family into a stage of fear and distrust. Although these feelings may not be expressed overtly, both the child and parent(s) fear and distrust each other. Frequently, the family has failed in at least some significant way that has led to the removal of the child. Now the thought of attempting to repeat the failed process encourages all to examine why the family blew apart. The tendency to cast blame is a natural protective measure to avoid repeating the same mistakes. The blame can be directed toward the parents, the child, the larger systems, or some other target.

In the face of this distrust, the therapist can bring the fears out into the open and diffuse defensive reactions to blaming by defining ambivalence as a universal experience in this process. The therapist can help each member of the family to identify the aspects of reunification that are both frightening and appealing. With some families, individuals need to be alone with the therapist at first, to free up this line of conversation. Through normalizing the ambivalence, the therapist gives permission to distrust while also highlighting the desire to reunite. Some of the resistance that begins to appear can also be diffused by active therapeutic restraining: The therapist can take the position of encouraging the family members to pay attention to their fears and move slowly through the reunification process, emphasizing the validity of concerns.

Case Example: Joan

The fears that arose in the case of Joan were very serious. Joan was a 16-year-old who was removed from her mother's care after she received several serious beatings by her stepfather. Joan was completely sold on the idea of reunification until the process was underway and she faced the actuality of returning to an environment in which she had been repeatedly hit, closed-fist, in the face. Her fear and her mother's unwillingness to separate from her stepfather immediately became the focus of therapy for several months after the reunification process was initiated.

As the therapist actively maneuvers to confront and negotiate around resistance, he or she may need to clarify the role of the therapist in relationship to the larger systems involved with the family. Some families conclude or are even told that the family therapist will determine when a child can return home. If this view is maintained, then the therapist is effectively limited from full access to information about the family. What family would tell a therapist something they believe would impair their ability to reach a desired goal? The therapist must provide an alternate model for his or her role in the reunification process.

One way to shift the therapist out of the judge-and-jury position is to clearly outline the steps that have been identified by the governing system (e.g., judicial or child welfare) as necessary prior to reunification. The family can review with the therapist what they have been told must be accomplished to facilitate reunification. Ideally, this can be reduced to stages with typical time frames:

1. The family must attend therapy weekly.
2. Day visits will be set up initially.
3. If these visits go well, then overnight visits will be considered at the next case review.
4. Parents must remain in any required treatment programs.
5. The child must meet the required behavior standard at the placement site, and so forth.

By specifically delineating the task of each participant, the responsibility of determining the success of reunification is shifted from the therapist to each person in the family. Reunification must be linked to objective criteria that the family can strive for, or the process can become very undefined and confusing for the family.

A necessary facet of identifying such criteria is outlining the resources available to the family and the constraints that can impede the reunification process. Frequently, it is left to the therapist to be able to recognize the strengths and resources of the family. Fears of parental incompetence may be heightened after placement of a child has occurred and overshadow the inherent strengths that exist. Within sessions devoted to strengthening the parental subsystem, the therapist can address fears and force the acknowledgment and identification of strengths as well.

During this stage, the relationship of the family to larger service systems must be discussed. Feelings about the initial removal of the child and the ensuing events can be voiced. In addition, any misconceptions concerning the rights of the family in relationship to the larger systems should be cleared up. The therapist can position himself or herself as an advocate for the family, encouraging optimal utilization of available resources. Many families need assistance in establishing a nonadversarial relationship with judicial and child welfare professionals. Learning to work with instead of against the same service systems that have been related to such disappointment and pain can be a difficult shift for many families.

In addition to the family's ideas about the involved service systems, the therapist must also deal with the reality of the involved systems. Some professionals involved with the family may be overtly or covertly against reunification. Caseworkers, foster parents, and child care workers may fear reunification. They may not think that returning the child home is in the best interest of the child. Too often, however, this decision may be based upon false, outdated notions about the parents of the child. As the therapist begins to get to know the family, he or she should be prepared to deal with resistance that is arising outside the family as well as within. The therapist should keep an open mind while speaking to other professionals, not blindly accepting either an anti- or pro-reunification stance.

Neutrality is an essential position to operate from in order to accurately assess all of what is known about a child and family in determining the viability of reunification. From this position, the therapist can also best accurately communicate with other professionals in other roles, diffusing extrafamilial resistance while remaining receptive to the viewpoints of others who are interacting with the parents and child. The therapist must never forget that an inappropriate reunification can have drastic and even fatal results.

IDEALISM

The idealistic stage in the reunification process can be marked by a shift that occurs once there is some belief by the family that both parents and children are committed to the reunification process. At this point the family usually enters the honeymoon phase in which all members collude to make each other look good. The parents and the children generally make an unusual effort to please each other and avoid conflict.

Case Example: Johnny

In Johnny's family the idealism was particularly extreme. Despite Johnny's frequent violent outbursts and his mother's chronic mental illness, the family attempted to sell the therapist on the notion that all of their problems would be solved by reunification. The therapist simply challenged the family to examine the problems that still existed within the family and to more realistically consider the impact of reunification.

The position of the therapist must change when the family begins to report that all problems would be solved by reunification. The therapist can counter the growing tendency of the family to join together in a coalition against the placement staff, renewing the adversarial position that was softened in the prior stage. Typically, during this stage children will repeatedly complain about treatment at their placement site, encouraging parents to complain about their children's care.

When the pendulum swings in the direction of idealizing the family, the therapist can both normalize the need to idealize while challenging the ideal beliefs. By predicting future potential problems, the therapist can challenge the family to explore the negative consequences of change: the negative things that can happen if the family is to reunite. Discussions can be initiated that will address how things will change for the child and the family if the child returns home. At this point, the therapist must remind the family that there were reasons for the initial removal of the child and that the patterns that were laid down prior to placement have not really been dealt with and could easily resurface. For a while, at least some family members will probably deny that problems could arise. By gently keeping the possibility of problems alive, the therapist paves the way to the reality stage.

REALITY STAGE

Though the length of the honeymoon varies depending on the amount of family contact and denial, eventually the real parent–child conflicts resurface. The children and parents begin to act more naturally and the old interactional patterns and wounds become apparent.

Frequently during this stage, the children start vacillating between complaining about their parents and about their placement environment. There seems to be an almost irresistible tendency for the children to compare home and the placement site as places to live. Particularly children who have been out of their home for an extended period of time will have trouble with the fact that there are almost always some good things about each option that will be lost if they choose the other option. Not unlike the conflict that children of divorced parents may experience, this conflict is particularly confusing to children who have had so little control in their lives. Given a sense of control, they want to utilize it, yet the vacillation between their options keeps them without specific goals and homeless. In order to have a home, they must choose an option that necessarily is not ideal and includes some loss of advantages and relationships. Choosing more losses is difficult for children who have already experienced so many, so they tend to vacillate to avoid consciously choosing another loss. The therapist can frame these vacillations not as a sign of rejection, but as a test of parental loyalty as actual reunification nears.

One of the dangers of this stage is that mutual fear and distrust will ignite the old destructive interactional and/or abusive sequences. The therapist needs to block old negative sequences and use conflict as an opportunity to introduce strategies for conflict resolution. At the same time, the therapist must reassure the family that the conflict that they are experiencing is better than a denial of problems. The familiarity of the conflict can be very frightening to a family that has been out of control. To combat this fear and to decrease the chance of escalation, the therapist can encourage the family to limit the discussion of particularly intense conflicts to therapy sessions where they can have additional support in blocking old sequences.

As new styles of interaction are practiced, opportunities arise to introduce strategies for positive communication and effective parenting. Some of the families have very limited tools for dealing with negative behaviors. During this stage, parents and children become more open to discussing different strategies for discipline. Children can be encouraged to offer feedback on rewards and punishments that they feel would be effective and appropriate.

At this point as well as throughout the reunification process, the therapist must be vigilant for any signs of regression toward dangerous behaviors on the part of the parent or child. Although committed to the reunification process, the therapist needs to step out of that role and repeatedly assess the risks that are present, remembering that not all families will be honest about incidents that could disrupt the reunification process or lead to charges or re involvement in the investigation process. This delicate balancing of roles by the therapist is essential to monitor the safety of the reunification process.

Case Example: Joan

During the attempt to reunite her family, Joan came in for therapy after her return from a weekend visit to her home. Since Joan was attractive and always immaculately groomed, her therapist noticed immediately that her hair was covering half of her face, which she kept carefully turned away. Glimpsing a discoloration around Joan's eye, the therapist confronted her about the shiner she was attempting to hide. Although Joan never admitted to being hit again by her stepfather, the therapist spoke to her about the implications of such behavior recurring and within weeks Joan reported that she would not return home unless her stepfather was no longer in the home. Sometimes the therapist must resort to speaking "as if" certain behaviors are occurring, because the family colludes in silence in an attempt to control their own destiny (i.e., reunification). However, the therapist can still strongly impact the family system and must report such occurrences to the child welfare department.

THE SECOND FEAR STAGE

The re-emergence of conflict precipitates renewed fears concerning reunification. The fears are similar to those experienced before, but exist in the presence of a stronger commitment to the reunification process. Parents and children can more openly express their ambivalence about reunification and realistically identify the remaining concerns.

On the other hand, new forms of resistance to change and sabotage may occur during this stage. Children may act out or strengthen vacillations between coalitions against parents and placement staff as the reality of reunification gains strength.

The role of the therapist is very critical at this point in reunification. The stakes have become high for the child and the parents. They have allowed themselves to believe that reunification is possible and have invested themselves in the process. The vulnerability can be terrifying as they imagine rejection or a return of negative sequences. The therapist can help the family not repeat past actions as well as hold onto old meanings. Through the therapist's eyes, the family can get a new view of each other. They can break old patterns by consciously considering what old behaviors and beliefs they want to keep and what they want to discard. As they gain some confidence, they can begin to predict and, thus, circumvent new problems that may invite old negative responses.

One very fruitful line of discussion at this point is to begin to talk about the actual day-to-day routine that will occur when the child returns home. The parents can offer what they view as expected and acceptable behaviors, and the family can plan the consequences of behaviors. Returning children can describe their expectations about their own and their parent's behavior. Hopes for the future as well as fears about abuse must be openly discussed so potential problems can be explored before they arise.

As noted above, success does not always mean reunification. The decision not to reunite does not necessarily end the role of the therapist or the involvement of the family. It is important that both the parent and child are told that the effort each made was worthwhile and that they can consider how they want their relationship structured in the future. Families need to see that they can play an important role in their children's lives even if reunification does not occur. In one case described earlier, moves toward reunification led to a mutual decision that Judy, a 16-year-old girl, not return home. This decision was ultimately viewed as positive by the girl and her family. Furthermore, she continued to visit her family every weekend and holidays, remaining an active part of their lives while completing high school and making a transition into an independent living program. This option appeared to be the best for the child and her family and was framed in such a way that no one felt like they had failed.

THE RETURNING PHASE

In some cases, the process of reunification will lead to the return of a child or children to the family. Adequate preparation will ease the transition of the child returning home, but the process of parents resuming full parenting while children adjust to the new rules and structure remains difficult. In addition, children who are leaving a placement site can also be grieving for relationships they have made away from home.

The therapist can help the family adjust to the structural reorganization as a new member is integrated into the family system. In addition to the physical changes that may be necessary to provide a permanent bed for the returning child, family members will experience shifts in relationships when a new person is added to interactions. Jealousies and conflicts can be discussed in therapy sessions while the family is reorganizing. Each family member can discuss his or her own experience as he or she establishes a place within the reunited family.

Another important task of the therapist in this final stage involves the assessment of family support services, as the family is prepared for the transition from the reunification therapist to community resources. It is critical that linkages to necessary support services are firmly in place prior to termination with the reunification therapist. Before the termination, the therapist needs to predict future crises and help the family plan for specific actions to be taken during conflict. The family is best prepared when a clear plan of action is established prior to the onset of any crises.

Case Example: Lisa

Prior to reunification of the family of Lisa, a 15-year-old, the family and therapist carefully explored potential problems and solutions. The family left the final session with an arsenal of strategies to avoid replication of the problems that had led to Lisa's placement.

As the therapist prepares the family for the future, the family can be reminded of the changes they have made. The role of the therapist as consultant can be re-emphasized to highlight the active role the family has played in adapting to reunification. It is important that the family leave the reunification process feeling personally empowered rather than dependent on the therapist. The therapist can encourage this feeling of independence by reviewing past changes in behavior and perceptions as well as strategies the family has developed for future problems. Careful linkage to community resources completes the provision of the tools needed by the family to increase the success of reunification.

Beyond the family interventions, the therapist must work closely with any other involved professionals during the returning stage. In many instances, judicial and other systems must approve the return home. The therapist's active advocacy for the family in these larger systems throughout the reunification process can help assure that no larger system surprises arise at the time when the child is returning home. One of the therapist's final tasks is to inform the family of the procedures that will be utilized by professionals to monitor reunification and ways to cooperate in this process.

As with any therapeutic termination, grieving and loss are usually experienced as the family says good-bye to their reunification therapist. This loss can reopen old wounds created in earlier losses. The therapist can explore the strategies that each family member utilizes to cope with this and other losses. Framing this loss as a positive result of growth can also help the family in managing their pain at separation. Finally, the therapist can predict that some families will develop problems soon after termination as a way of blocking termination. By giving the family some control over the sequencing of the final sessions with the therapist, the impetus to block termination can often be avoided. Families can be given the choice of a "weaning" process in which sessions are scheduled with decreasing frequency (once a week, then biweekly, then monthly) or ending sessions with the promise that they can call for one or two "booster" sessions during the next 6 months. Some families prefer to terminate knowing they will definitely see the therapist one more time while others prefer to feel free to call for a session or simply reassurance when they want it. Giving the family the option eases termination fears and decreases the chance of an immediate crisis following termination with the therapist.

The family leaves reunification therapy with a new view of themselves and practical strategies for dealing with problems. Successful termination aids the family in self-monitoring and use of community resources. All families should be able to identify the warning signs that assistance is needed and know where appropriate assistance can be obtained.

THE RETURN OF A PLACED ADOLESCENT

When Lisa Jones first walked into my office, it was immediately apparent that she was comfortable in the client role. She said she was so glad to have a therapist and dove right in to reporting the sequence of events that brought her to a group home. My immediate reflex was to slow her down, but she had been well programmed in previous psychiatric hospitalizations to openly disclose to strangers the intimate and embarrassing details of her life.

As she talked at length about the first 15 years of her life, I observed the adolescent before me. She was attractive and socially skilled, with an incredible desire to please, yet her irresistible smile and active attempts to connect did not conceal the cloud of depression and self-doubt that burdened this young lady. After our first hour, I reviewed the salient points of her story. Lisa was a middle child in a family with twelve children. She reported that she had always been independent-minded and could never remember being close to her parents, as some of her siblings seemed to be.

Although Lisa said she could not identify a specific time when her relationship with her parents had soured, her eyes teared up when she spoke of being sexually assaulted in the third grade. When asked about her parents' response to this incident, she said they did not believe her when she told them. Lisa reported that her mother got angry with her for making up such a story and that trust was never renewed between them.

Despite increasing conflict with her parents, Lisa led a rather unremarkable life until she entered middle school, where she began hanging out with the "wrong crowd" by her report. The next 2 years that led up to her first hospitalization were a blur of chronic alcohol and drug abuse, promiscuous sex, and escalating truancy. Lisa admitted that her parents became completely unable to impact her behavior. Consequently, they signed her into an adolescent drug treatment unit when she was 13, after a string of nights when she did not return home.

After 6 months of individual and group therapy bolstered by immersion in a 12-step AA program, Lisa returned home. Over the next 6 months, her behavior gradually deteriorated to a self-destructive cycle, and her parents had her rehospitalized in a different program. During the next 9 months, Lisa actively participated in an inpatient drug treatment program. She said that she realized her own responsibility for her behavior and decided to change her life.

The staff of the unit bolstered Lisa's self-esteem and challenged her to confront her parents in order to verbalize her anger rather than acting it out. Lisa described very intense "family therapy" sessions in which she screamed at her parents for not giving her enough attention and not believing her story about the assault. Her parents responded by attacking her impossible behavior and total disrespect for their authority. As reported, the content of these sessions appeared to be fairly limited to mutual blaming. Although the hospital staff praised Lisa for letting out her feelings, Lisa found these sessions so traumatic that she vehemently refused to ever participate in family therapy again. She also made it very clear that her parents completely shared her sentiment for family therapy.

Not only did Lisa's parents refuse to attend further family therapy sessions, they had also refused to let Lisa return home after release from the hospital. Consequently, when the family's hospitalization insurance was depleted, Lisa was placed in a group home. Lisa and her parents were so polarized that the parents made no attempts to contact her after she entered the group home. As a result, Lisa came to me feeling totally abandoned by her parents and idealizing the staff of the psychiatric unit she had just left. She wanted her parents to trust and appreciate her, as the staff had, and she felt angry and betrayed at being placed out of her home.

Defining the family was a relatively easy task from Lisa's position. She had no other parental figures besides her biological parents, and she wanted to return to her family. From her parents' perspective, however, they had unsuccessfully parented Lisa, and now she was in a setting where adequate structure was provided to prohibit her from self-destructing. Furthermore, they had eleven other children making constant demands that easily filled any void left in Lisa's absence. Given how difficult it was to provide for so many and that several of these had serious problems in their own right, Lisa's parents' lives were full to overflowing without even thinking about her.

Considering the extreme disaffection between Lisa and her parents, I opted to build a solid relationship with Lisa prior to attempting any family sessions. When the theme of these individual sessions repeatedly focused on her parents' not initiating contact, I reminded Lisa that I really could do nothing with her parents until I began to talk with them. Respecting her resistance to such contact, I waited to contact them until she asked me to, then I further hesitated, asking her if she was surely ready to have me hear their side of the story. Despite an obvious fear of such contact, she asked me to call them about 6 months after she arrived at the group home.

I knew the initial contact with Lisa's parents was extremely critical.

Their experience with therapists was very negative. Their expectation was that any therapist would blame them for Lisa's problems and castigate them for abandoning her. The reticence in Mrs. Jones's voice was very obvious when I told her who I was. As I spoke with her, I worked very hard to join with her and positively frame her concern for Lisa. I addressed how painful her conflict with Lisa must have been and how upsetting it must have been for her to have a child living in a group home after such obvious sacrifices to try and help her.

The joining was effective, and Mrs. Jones spoke of her own depression and utter loss of any idea of how to even relate to Lisa, much less parent her. During the entire conversation, I did not suggest having family therapy sessions, but rather asked if I could consult with Mr. and Mrs. Jones as a resource, since they so intimately knew of Lisa's tendencies and history. As we said goodbye, the relief felt by Mrs. Jones that I seemed to understand her was evident.

Even after the initiation of one phone call to the parents, the repercussions were immediately apparent in my next session with Lisa. The alienation from her parents was so strong that she felt completely betrayed because I did not represent her parents as villains, but reported that her mother seemed to care about her. "They tricked you. They lied to you and you fell for it," she sobbed. And I began the ever-so-delicate dance of rebalancing alliances across a completely polarized family.

Luckily, I had known that my relationship with Lisa was very solid. Although she would always have an immediate, betrayed response when I neared her parents, our relationship was strong enough to endure. When I reassured her that I had her interests at heart and believed her experience of the world was true for her, she renewed her trust in me. I constantly reminded her that I would have to get close to her parents in order to help her go home.

After several phone contacts and the necessary rebalancing following each, I had positioned myself sufficiently to convene a family session 3 months after initiating contact with the parents. I reassured all that I would not let this be a blaming session, but a focus on future goals. I informed both Lisa and her parents that I would spend an hour with her parents first, so they could know me better, and then I would bring Lisa into the session. Everyone, myself included, was nervous.

When the parents came in, I told them that Lisa had had many opportunities to tell me her story, but they had not. I encouraged them to vent their true feelings, negative and positive, before she entered the room so I could get an accurate view of their perspective. They spoke of all the scenes and disappointments, while I listened and showed them I understood. Then I brought Lisa into the room, and I did most of the talking.

I traced the painful history, normalizing the distrust all of them felt.

I assured them that extensive blame casting was not helpful or necessary since it had been accomplished in prior therapy. Finally, I asked each of them what were the most important things they wanted to happen concerning Lisa's life and her relationship with her parents, knowing well that parents and child ultimately wanted similar things.

Lisa agreed that she wanted to remain drug-free, but said she wanted a relationship with her parents. Both Lisa and her parents admitted that relating was very difficult, but I reassured them that rebuilding trust takes time. I told them that only through new, positive experiences could trust be rebuilt, that words alone could never do it, on either side. I encouraged their skepticism while encouraging them to slowly provide opportunities for new experiences that could test trust in the present. I took a definite stand that I could not predict whether returning Lisa home would work or not.

The session ended by defining what the parents and Lisa needed to happen before they could fully commit to reunification. In addition, we outlined the constraints that impeded reunification, such as the potential use of drugs by Lisa and the limited parental energy left over for Lisa after meeting their other demands. The session ended with a review of the available resources, highlighting the deep feelings and concern obviously existing between Lisa and her parents. Lisa and her parents left the session pleased by the lack of blaming, but still very cautious about future family work.

Since Lisa's parents lived far from her placement site, family therapy was scheduled only once a month. Although this constraint slowed the reunification process somewhat, the time lapse also allowed a complete reaction and integration between sessions. Whereas, prior to the first family session, Lisa had established a strong collusion with her child care workers against her parents, this shifted after the first family session. Lisa changed from complaining to the staff about her parents to complaining to her parents about the placement. Lisa began to idealize her parents and family.

The parents were trying hard in the next session. When Lisa reported how unhappy she was at the placement, they were obviously distressed. They stated that they were pleased with her success in school and wanted her to start coming home for visits, something they had consistently refused to do in the past. Although her parents were still afraid that Lisa would regress if she returned home, they were definitely viewing her more positively and expressing more commitment to her returning home.

While framing the new parent–child unity as a very positive sign, I also explored the negative consequences of change. I helped the family consider what negative things could happen if Lisa were to return home. This time I encouraged Lisa and her parents to gently express their fear of future problems in the context of their concern for each other and their desire to be reunited. I normalized Lisa's need to idealize home while reminding her of the problems that continued to exist there for her, such as the negative peer influence and her parents' chronic unavailability. During this session I did less blocking of negative affect, but I did focus the dialogue in a particular direction, aimed at moving the family into a more realistic view of each other and their present situation.

Three months after the reunification process had begun, Lisa began making weekend visits home twice a month. Parent–child conflicts began to resurface, but these were not around all of the same issues of previous conflicts. On home passes, Lisa obeyed curfews and did not use drugs or alcohol, yet her sense of not having a place in the family was very strong. Her complaints centered around the lack of a close, intimate relationship with her parents and siblings. She reported feeling unneeded and unnoticed and, in reciprocal fashion, her parents complained that she acted like a guest when home and did not pull her weight in family chores. Some of her visits ended in overt arguments with a parent around one of these issues. In the next session, Lisa and her parents spoke freely about this new, overt conflict. It was frightening to all and made everyone question the viability of reunification. Lisa expressed doubts about returning home. She considered remaining in placement until she graduated from high school.

As she expressed clear confusion over which situation would work best for her, her parents changed from reluctance for reunification to letting Lisa decide where she needed to be. I positively framed this conflict and confusion as a more realistic view of a complex situation. I pointed out the differences between the old and new styles of conflict. For the first time, I encouraged them to fully express their real feelings through positive communication. By this time, my relationship with both Lisa and her parents was very strong. They had learned that family therapy could be difficult without being destructive. Communication in the sessions became freer and freer as everyone felt the safety of the therapeutic situation.

The realism of the new interactions with her parents was frightening to Lisa. She had to learn to work toward returning home in the face of the drawbacks and limitations. At one point, she fell back into her old role and lied to her parents about where she was going. Her parents' immediate response was also fear: "Is this the old Lisa finally showing her true colors?"

However, the past sequence of parent–child interaction was not repeated. Before Lisa had an extended discussion with her parents about dishonesty, I confronted her on the fact that such an action could sabotage her plans to return home. We discussed her reasons for lying and what her parents' understandable reaction, a loss of trust, would be. When she discussed the lie with her parents, she was able to apologize, not defend her actions, and ask them what they felt would be an appropriate punishment. Her parents were totally shocked when she accepted the punishment without argument.

This interaction turned out to be very pivotal, propelling the family into quick reunification. Both parents and child gained new hope by replaying an old scene with such a new ending. At the next session, 6 months into the family therapy, Lisa and her parents agreed that it was time for her to return home. We reviewed Lisa's role and responsibilities as a family member. Both she and her parents outlined their needs, expectations, and fears concerning reunification. The parents re-established their parenting by clearly defining the rules and consequences of broken rules that they had decided upon for Lisa. Lisa clearly articulated her own needs while accepting their demands.

Before the session ended, each participant predicted potential crises and how they could be successfully negotiated. We set up a schedule of future sessions to deal with any problems that might occur. Seven months after the start of family therapy, Lisa returned home soon after this session.

Although Lisa was very afraid of returning to her old peer group at school, she quickly discovered that she had different interests than before and fit in with a more positive group. She and her mother reported at later sessions that their relationship was surprisingly close. As Lisa renewed her interest in positive activities, such as sports, her mother's fear for Lisa began to lessen and their interactions became freer and more natural. Both were very pleased when they discovered that they enjoyed talking for extended periods.

Lisa also maintained a closer relationship with her father and several siblings. She found a new responsible role watching over younger siblings. This helped her self-esteem and gave her a positive function in her family.

With stronger family relationships, Lisa reported that she had no urges to return to substance abuse. She had other positive peer activities and had no desire to self-destruct or show her parents her pain. I reminded her that she may always remain at risk for substance abuse and to watch any growing tendencies in that direction that she may want to deny.

Termination was frightening for Lisa and her family. Each feared that old patterns would recur. I gave them a choice of gradual weaning or ending our sessions with two "booster" sessions in reserve to deal with future problems. The family chose to end family sessions, but have Lisa return to see me as needed during the next few months. I saw Lisa three additional times before final termination. I also made several phone calls to both parents to assess their view of reunification and reinforce the changes made during therapy.

By our last contacts, Lisa and her parents had lost most of their fears concerning reunification. The parents reported disappointment that Lisa did not do more around the home, but they were very pleased with her school performance and lack of involvement with drugs or alcohol. Lisa had reciprocal minor complaints about her parents, but overall the issues that arose tended to be typical parent–teen concerns that were dealt with in an appropriate fashion. Both Lisa and her parents said that they were glad that Lisa was home and that they felt equipped to deal with any problems that arose. On our last contact, I congratulated them on their success and reminded them of the availability of local services if they should be needed.

By carefully dealing with resistance, I was able to help the family successfully negotiate the impasses that could have stopped the reunification process. Maintaining a neutral stance, I realistically presented the hopes and fears about reunification without getting trapped in a position of idealization or pessimism. This balancing allowed the family to participate in the reunification process in a well planned manner with their eyes open wide, preparing carefully for each next step along the journey. This preparation enabled them to consider and succeed at something that had seemed impossible, allowing Lisa to complete her adolescence in her own home under the care of her own parents.

REFERENCES

Fanshel, D. (1971). The exit of children from foster care: An interim research report. *Child Welfare, 51,* 344–354.

Gershenson, C., Rosewater, A., & Massinga, R. (1990, January). *The crisis in foster care: New directions in the 1990s.* Family Impact Seminar, American Association for Marriage and Family Therapy, Research and Education Foundation, Washington, DC.

Knitzer, J. (1989). *Collaborations between child welfare and mental health: Emerging patterns and challenges.* New York: Bank Street College of Education.

Knitzer, J., Allen, M., & McGowan, B. (1978). *Children without homes: An examination of public responsibility to children in out-of-home care.* Washington, DC: Children's Defense Fund.

Lloyd, J., & Bryce, M. (1985). *Placement Prevention and family reunification for the family-centered service practitioner.* Iowa City, IA: University of Iowa, The National Resource Center on Family Based Service.

Maas, H., & Engler, R. (1959). *Children in need of parents.* New York: Columbia University Press.

Moss, S. Z., & Moss, M. S. (1984). Threat to place a child. *American Journal of Orthopsychiatry, 54*(1), 168–171.

Nelson, K., Landsman, M., & Deutelbaum, W. (1990). Three models of family-centered prevention services. *Child Welfare, 69*(1), 3–21.

Proch, K., & Howard, J. (1986). Parental visiting of children in foster care. *Social Work, 31,* 178–181.

Sarata, B., & Behrman, J. (1982). Group home parenting: An examination of the role. *Community Mental Health Journal, 18,* 274–285.

Solnit, A. J. (1973). Child placement—on whose time? *Journal of the American Academy of Child Psychiatry, 12,* 385–392.

15

Preparing Child Welfare Agencies for Family Preservation and Reunification Programs

Rocco A. Cimmarusti

Over the last decade or so, child welfare services have been subjected to a radical change in the focus and nature of service delivery because of the family preservation movement (Norman, 1985). Family preservation and reunification programs appear nationwide (Frankel, 1988; Samantrai, 1992) and have been given government support through Public Law 96-272, the Adoption Assistance and Child Welfare Act of 1980 (McGowan, 1983; Pine, 1986). While there has been recent controversy surrounding the philosophy of preserving families and the effectiveness of such programs (Ingrassia & McCormick, 1994), several studies have reported positive outcomes (Barth & Berry, 1987; Berry, 1992; Frankel, 1988). Controversies and trepidation notwithstanding, the focus of the child welfare system nationwide has shifted to a concentration on the family and on permanency planning (Bribitzer & Verdieck, 1988; Emlen, 1981; Maluccio, Fein, & Olmstead, 1986; Seaberg, 1986; Stein & Gambrill, 1985). As a consequence, the need for training direct service providers in family preservation and reunification models has increased (Gleeson, Smith, & Dubois, 1993; Miller & Dore, 1991).

This chapter, which is based upon my experience, examines the challenge of preparing agency administrators and staff for family preservation and reunification programs. I will begin by describing the context for our work and then examining the theory that underlies this multisystems approach to family preservation and reunification. From there, I will explore the concomitant challenges and opportunities afforded by the various points of entry into agency programs and illustrate their experience through examples.

THE CONTEXT

In 1989, while at the Institute for Juvenile Research, I was awarded a contract by the Illinois Department of Children and Family Services (DCFS) to develop a curriculum for working with families needing family preservation services (Cimmarusti, 1989). DCFS used this curriculum as part of its statewide mandatory training. As the theoretical basis for the family preservation effort in Illinois, the curriculum emphasizes a multisystems approach and is based upon the contributions of the structural and strategic schools of family therapy (Cimmarusti, 1989).

Upon completion of that contract, I was asked by administrators at DCFS to develop a curriculum for the family reunification initiative. Also based upon a multisystems approach, this curriculum particularly examines the impact of placement on the "reunification system" as well as the unique challenges involved in a systems approach to reunification. The reunification system is described as composed of several levels, including the child, the family, the extended family, and the foster family (Cimmarusti, 1990). This curriculum was also used as statewide mandatory training for agencies who contract with DCFS.

As a result of implementing these curricula, DCFS administrators requested that I consult to private agencies whose family preservation or reunification programs were at risk of losing their funding because of programmatic or clinical problems. As of this writing, I have done this type of troubleshooting consultation over ten times throughout the state. Other requests for consultation to family preservation and reunification programs have been accepted as well. I and my staff combined have offered program or clinical consultation to almost one-third of the family preservation and reunification programs in Illinois. Thus, through these training and consultation experiences we have developed an ability to articulate the particular issues involved in preparing an agency staff for such programs.

I have discovered, for example, that many caseworkers do not provide family preservation or reunification services in a balanced fashion;

there is either too much emphasis on protecting children from harm or not nearly enough. Family preservation and reunification efforts that focus only on narrow units of intervention risk having limited scope and applicability for the caseworker and the family. In order to assess and intervene effectively to meet the mandate for "reasonable efforts," family preservation and reunification workers must address a variety of issues, on multiple levels.

Later in this chapter I will examine my preferred approach to the task of employing reasonable efforts. Though the reasonable efforts mandate has become national policy in child welfare, the actual practice of involving the family in a coherent and consistent fashion is, by some indications, lagging behind. In my experience across the state, I have observed family preservation efforts practiced in ways that fall woefully short of an approach that is thorough and sufficiently encompassing. Each of these inadequate ways does not allow the caseworker to fully appreciate and manage the enormously complex issues involved in most family preservation and reunification cases. For the purpose of explanation and illustration, I have arbitrarily categorized these approaches below, and though the illustrations may appear to be outlandish, they are based on actual observations. Sometimes casework falls into a category because of the program's philosophy or the supervisor's orientation. At other times, category membership is representative of the caseworker's own orientation to casework.

In one category of approaches to family preservation and reunification, caseworkers narrowly focus their intervention efforts on the mother and mistreated child while ignoring extended family members, partners, or others. In fact, the research data, reported by The Chapin Hall Center for Children from their massive study of family preservation services in Illinois, indicate that virtually no family preservation program involves the extended family at the point of initial planning and goal setting (Schuerman & Rzepnicki, 1991).

Caseworkers in this category usually fail to consider the impact of the larger system, including their own efforts, as an important component of the very problem they are trying to alleviate. They often conceptualize their work as "treating the dysfunctional maternal–child dyad" without recognizing the need to consider if the relationship between mother and child is strained by the relationship of another party to both, or by the negative effects of the child protection investigation conducted by the state, and so on. In the exclusively meaning-oriented version of this category, caseworkers might first explore with mother the meaning of providing money before providing any money, occasionally leaving the family strapped for cash while mother "works through" her "dependency needs" and the worker works through any countertransference issues.

A second category of family preservation or reunification casework employs a strict family therapy approach that unintentionally neglects to work with larger systems outside the family. Caseworkers so inclined usually see the value of a systems approach but often do not conceptualize the need for their intervention into larger systems or minimize their own role in protecting children. These caseworkers will be quite focused on family dynamics, but underfocused on concrete needs (cash assistance, housing) or on the child protection issues. Caseworkers within this category may view working with a number of interlocking systems as too difficult, too time consuming, and possibly as usurping the responsibility of others. In my experience, the root of this view is often an underestimation of their ability to manage the multileveled system. They may not feel empowered to assume the task, which, ironically, is how their client families often feel.

A third category of casework regards the focus of the work as providing only "hard" services or parent education to the family. Here, caseworkers often fail to recognize the complex nature of family preservation and reunification cases. Within this approach, services are often provided in a stereotyped fashion: For example, birth parents need parenting classes, most birth mothers will need drug counseling, and so on. Consequently, caseworkers will routinely begin their involvement with a client family by informing the family of the available services from their program and request that the family choose those services that seem most useful. This may seem to be a respectful approach to the family, since the caseworker does not tell the family what to do, but there may not be enough importance placed on building a therapeutic relationship or on the identification and resolution of problems. Further, there is some evidence that an exclusive concrete services approach is more useful with families who physically abuse their child(ren) than with families who neglect children (Berry, 1992).

Recently there has been considerable public attention cast on the deaths of some children who were involved with the child welfare system. Sadly, such tragedies may have uncovered yet a fourth, all too prevalent, category of approach to family preservation and reunification, one that causes caseworkers to leave children in the home for no other reason than because it is agency policy. As I will discuss below, family preservation and reunification work should be a process wherein the caseworkers use skill and thought. Blindly leaving children in homes where there is ample evidence of potential harm is not only bad family preservation, it is malpractice. Returning children to homes where there is prior evidence that the caregiver is dangerous to the child is not just an oversight—it is malfeasance. In part, it is because caseworkers do not look past their own limiting orientations or consider the family system within the larger system that such offensive casework occurs. Consequently, a conceptual model that directs the caseworker to gather information from a myriad of sources, take a broad, yet optimistic, view; consider history and previous behavior, coordinate services with other providers; and, finally, to use common sense, is all the more urgently needed.

THE MULTISYSTEMS APPROACH

My preferred approach to family preservation and reunification casework focuses on a multileveled system that is relevant to high-risk, multiproblem families and that includes the child or children, the other biological family members, extended family members, significant members from the community, and members of the group of professionals serving the family.

Family preservation and reunification efforts are more manageable if caseworkers have a conceptual framework that allows them to observe the whole picture or enables the worker to move from level to level when needed.

The multisystems approach, therefore, offers family preservation and reunification caseworkers a flexible, internally consistent conceptual model for working with difficult, high-risk families. It is based upon concepts from the family therapy field and specifically informed by the work of Breunlin, Schwartz, and MacKune-Karrer (1992) and others (Aponte & Van Deusen, 1981; Boyd-Franklin, 1989; Hartman & Laird, 1983; Imber-Black, 1988; Minuchin, 1974; Minuchin & Fishman, 1981). It allows the caseworker to combine the varied perspectives of a large number of people involved with the identified family into a unified conceptual whole. Additionally, it empowers the caseworker to utilize his or her professional competencies while also empowering the other members of the multileveled system to be competent to provide their own perspectives.

It is not so much that other approaches are incorrect or bad as it is that they tend to emphasize only one perspective for understanding and intervening into the system or are unclear as to their perspective. Fundamental to the multisystems approach is the notion that the members of each level of the multileveled system have a view about what is occurring in the system that is valid in its own right and hence is considered a part of the truth regarding the system. Together, these "partial truths" about the system combine to depict a more accurate view or understanding of the system, even though the system cannot be known in its entirety (Keeney, 1983). Consequently, approaches that make it difficult for the caseworker to access an optimal number of partial truths from a variety of levels or that lead the caseworker to believe that the entire truth lies at only one level or with only one or two members are unduly restricting and constraining of the caseworker and therefore less effective.

The multisystems approach draws an arbitrary boundary of what constitutes the relevant system of intervention around the family, extended family, community, and other service providers. Therefore, it requires coordinating the demands and services of the systems affecting the family (e.g., extended family, juvenile court, social service agencies, school). It concentrates on constraints at any and all of the levels of the system and regards the caseworker's role as intervening to remove them. By focusing on constraints, it goes beyond the traditional ecological approaches, which focus on fit with the environment (De Hoyos & Jensen, 1985) or intervene to teach the family to better negotiate with its environment (Germain & Gitterman, 1987).

The focus on constraints, which is discussed further below, is novel in that it helps shift the caseworker's thinking about families as resistant and unmotivated to thinking about them as somehow being kept as they are. Consequently, the casework tasks become, first, identifying with the family the constraints that keep the family from developing better problem-solving skills, more effective coping styles, and greater flexibility, and second, working with the family members to obviate the identified constraints.

The multisystems approach offers strategies for balancing the seemingly conflicting goals of child protection and family empowerment. It equips child welfare workers with a way of thinking about families that is more amenable to managing these demands and that stems from the family therapy field, which results in examining competence rather than pathology and finding positive connotations rather than pejorative labels. This contribution is a hallmark of the multisystems approach and underlies the premise that families are good for, rather than bad for, children. Assuming this premise from the outset of services leads the caseworker to manage cooperatively with the family, rather than to serve as an authority figure who only monitors the child's protection. This subtle shift in attitude has profound implications to family preservation and reunification practice: The family is seen as competent but constrained instead of incompetent and pathological.

The process of family preservation and reunification is best served if the family as a whole develops a sense of mastery, self-determination, self-efficacy, and self-evaluation. Development in such areas empowers families and increases their ability to establish a healthy sense of control. Therefore, the caseworker's initial efforts to obtain the family's approval of the goals of family preservation or reunification are a key element in achieving child protection through family empowerment. The caseworker seeks the family's approval from the perspective of collaborator and even includes asking the adult caregivers if the referred child is indeed considered a part of the family. Caseworkers, who begin with the notion that the group of adults and children in front of them constitute a family without first asking every member questions such as "Who is in your family?" or "Is he (or she) a member of your family?" miss an opportunity for self-definition by the members and for identifying who among the adults are possible appropriate resources for caring for the abused or neglected child. In addition, caseworkers who fail to empower families risk intruding a set of values about families that may lead to confusion and difficulties later.

A further word of caution about this approach is necessary. While it is of great benefit that families not be given pejorative labels, the emphasis on strengths should never underestimate real problems. My experience has shown that all too often caseworkers fail to recognize real deficits within individuals that constrain change within the system. Some caseworkers lack a base of knowledge about normal child, adult, or family physical and psychological development that is a prerequisite to working effectively within a multisystems approach.

What follows is a brief examination of various aspects of the multisystems approach. First, specific theoretical components of the approach are identified, which include the notion of interacting levels, a focus on strengths, and a focus on the identification and removal of constraints. Second, the issue of assessing the multileveled system's functioning is described. Last, the issues of collaboration and reading feedback are considered as the processes upon which the entire multisystems approach is driven. A comparable examination of the approach is described elsewhere (Cimmarusti, 1992).

Interacting Levels

The multisystems approach stresses the importance of a multileveled perspective. Identifying a multileveled set of interacting entities and their attributes is an arbitrary way of drawing a boundary around the forces that influence a child-welfare-involved family. More importantly, engaging the family in this process of identifying who is significant to them at the various levels simultaneously empowers the family, elicits important assessment information, and develops the caseworker–client relationship in a collaborative rather than authoritarian fashion.

Once identified, the family preservation and reunification worker then assesses: (1) the ordering of the organization in the multileveled system, (2) the quality of the relationships contained within, and (3) the patterns of interaction within and between the various levels. Constraints in these three dimensions are considered central to the treatment of families in need of preservation or reunification.

The levels that are important in each family preservation and reunifi-

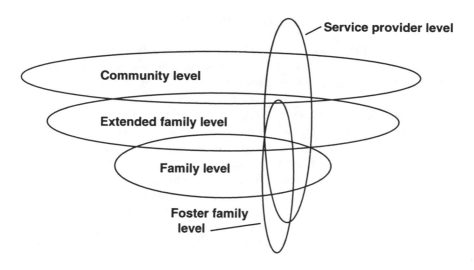

FIGURE 15.1. The interacting levels of family preservation and reunification.

cation case are illustrated in Figure 15.1. The particulars of who is represented in each level, however, should be primarily driven by the particular family being served and secondarily by the caseworker's sense of who is significant in these levels: (1) The *family* level includes all members of the nuclear family: mother, father, children; (2) The *extended family* level includes any significant relatives, grandparents, aunts, and play parents; (3) The *community* level includes peers and significant people from the neighborhood, church, work, or school; and (4) the *service provider* level includes the caseworker, his or her supervisor and agency of employment, the public child welfare agency, the legal system, and other service providers (e.g., homemaker, case aide, etc.). Notice how the service provider level is seen as transecting the other levels. This is meant to illustrate the need for the caseworker to exert his or her efforts across the multi-leveled system.

The first four levels remain the same in family reunification efforts, but are joined by (5) the *foster family* level, which includes the significant caretakers of the child in placement. It may not be relevant to family preservation efforts unless the child has been placed outside the home. Notice in Figure 15.1 that the foster family level is depicted as transecting the other levels. This is done to illustrate the concept that the foster family's actions have impact across a broader perspective than just the family.

Focus on Strengths

The approach embraces an optimistic view of people. It regards all systems (individuals, families, etc.) as possessing unique competence. Competence at one level, however, may not be effective or even demonstrated at another level. Nonetheless, there is always potential competence, and significant change can occur when it is developed. The crack-addicted mother, for example, may have what we would assess as a very constrained life: social support from other addicts only, estrangement from her family, intense poverty and the consequent desperation it can foster, poor judgment, and an inadequate education and few work skills—an unfortunate picture all too common in urban settings. Yet there is more to this woman than just these constraints. There are strengths present, and if they can be harnessed they may begin to help this woman help herself. Perhaps she has, for example, a sense of humor and resolve that helps her survive against all odds. She may have pride—even though it appears to be misplaced in relationship to her addiction. She may have an ability to evaluate her own situation and may often know better than the caseworker that she is in trouble. She has wishes and dreams, like the rest of us. And while these strengths may seem relatively insignificant in comparison to the power of the constraints in her life, this is where the multisystems model must begin if it is to respect the dignity of human beings.

It would be naive, however, to suggest that caseworkers emphasize strengths blindly or close their eyes to deficits. Assessment should be approached from the perspective that competencies and deficits probably both exist. Caseworkers should make a comprehensive assessment of the individual in the family in order to minimize risks. The competent caseworker should be someone who is highly skilled in assessing a variety of ills (e.g., addictions, mental illness or retardation, and physical signs of abuse and neglect), yet does not have a pessimistic view of people.

As difficult as it sometimes is, maintaining an optimistic attitude toward people helps the caseworker and benefits the intervention process. People who feel valued and respected are more likely to change than those who feel belittled and blamed. The competency-based emphasis of the approach, therefore, not only helps the caseworker empower the family system, but also helps communicate and build a supportive, empowering, and positive treatment environment. Emphasizing strengths is not only applicable at the level of the family, but also with people from the other levels as well.

Within the service provider level, for example, caseworkers sometimes overlook the invaluable amount of information that is available from the homemaker who is working with the family. Homemakers often have a candid, common sense view of the family that is free of theory biases.

They have also often witnessed family interactions that are kept to a minimum when the caseworker visits. The strengths-oriented caseworker would never allow preconceived notions about homemakers to stop him or her from finding out what valuable information the homemaker might possess.

Removal of Constraints

The concept of constraints implies that living systems are the way they are because they are kept from being otherwise by a variety of factors (Bateson, 1972). Some of these factors might be constitutional properties; the presuppositions, beliefs, or life scripts of the members of the system; the repeating patterns of behavior within the systems; and the presuppositions, beliefs, and scripts of the larger environment in which the system resides. The implication of this notion of constraints for family preservation and reunification caseworkers is that abusive and neglectful family systems are regarded as behaving as they do because they are constrained from behaving some other way.

The nature of dysfunction is therefore understood from the perspective of constraints. Dysfunction can be briefly described as the narrowing of behavioral options, the loss of trial-and-error behavior, decreased styles of coping, and/or maintaining intractable beliefs (Walsh, 1982). Constraints that increase the likelihood of such forms of rigidity are the target of intervention. In family preservation or reunification work such constraints may be embedded at any or all points of the multilevel system: the very biology of people; the beliefs and presuppositions of individuals; the rules and patterns of interaction among people within a family; the nature and availability of the resources in a family, community, and among service providers; the nature of the relationship between family members and other service providers; and the mandates and policies governing child welfare institutions.

Rarely in working with today's families will the caseworker find that constraints only exist at one level. More likely there are constraints at many levels. In one family, for example, the child may suffer from Fetal Alcohol Syndrome (FAS) and the mother may suffer from alcoholism; extended family members and the mother may have been in conflict for years and therefore maintain little contact; the school may have failed to put the child in the appropriate educational placement; the family preservation caseworker may know little about assessing FAS; and the public child welfare agency may be facing fiscal cutbacks that limit funding for alcohol treatment or special children's programs. There is a recursiveness (interaction effect) among these constraints such that each not only creates limitations in the particular level that it occurs in but also impacts and constrains the other levels as well. For example, on the one hand, the child's physical and emotional problems add idiosyncratic challenges to the child's development as well as to the requisite skills needed to raise such a child. On the other hand, the mother's alcoholism most likely challenges her child-rearing skills.

If the caseworker and client can form an alliance that identifies the significant constraints and makes efforts to address them, then the multisystems approach is functioning optimally. When, however, the constraints are so pervasive or have such a lock on the client's functioning that the client is not able to cooperate with preserving placement of the child(ren) in the home, or the alliance between caseworker and caregiver is insufficient, then the caseworker can and should shift focus toward having the child placed out the home for the purposes of safety. Within the multisystems model, this moment is handled so caseworker and members of the multileveled system (especially including the family) will agree that placement is the only logical decision, and they will work together to determine the most appropriate placement.

Assessment

As I have indicated, the issue of conducting a thorough assessment is considered vital to a multisystems approach. It is important to be able to assess the individual functioning of the significant members of the family, particularly the children and their caretakers because deficiencies in these individuals' functioning produce constraints that limit the alternatives within the system. Caseworkers, therefore, need to be well trained in both individual growth and development as well as the dynamics of systems. They should be adroit at assessing physical and psychological development, mental illness, substance abuse, attachment and bonding, and intellectual functioning. The time-limited nature of family preservation and reunification efforts necessitates that the caseworker be very efficient at assessment.

Two dimensions are salient in assessing the dynamics of systems — organization and sequences. Through a focus on *organization,* the caseworker is able to consider the operation of the multileveled system as a whole, that is, the arrangement of the various members of the system and the function each member serves in the life of the whole. Of importance here is the issue of leadership. Does the multileveled system operate under the aegis of any agreed-upon leader? Are there several leaders in competition? Do the leaders instill harmony and balance in the system or do they promote disruption?

The notion of *sequences,* or patterns of interaction, is the second salient dimension of the caseworker's assessment of the system. Sequences occur both within and between the various levels (Breunlin & Schwartz,

1986). It is important to remember that sequences repeat over time, yet constantly undergo slight changes as they reflect the dynamics of everyday demands and unrelenting individual and family development. Therefore, from the perspective of sequences, the family that appears so rigid and resistant may alternatively be viewed as having an internal oscillation between stability and change, which must be utilized for the sake of change. Since neglectful and abusive families are often thought of as unchanging, it is useful to remind workers of this point.

Collaboration

For a multisystems approach to work optimally, the caseworker should establish collaborative relationships with the various significant parties in the multileveled system; this may include extended family members, people from the community, and other service providers. In order to establish such a relationship, the caseworker must first engage members from all parts of the various levels in a manner that allows him or her to advocate for all parties without becoming an advocate for only one. I think of collaboration as composed of mutual respect between caseworker and other, an agreement at all levels for the caseworker to perform his or her job, and the capacity of each party to add to the conceptualization about and goals for the family.

The multisystems model works best if there is someone facilitating the process. In my opinion, the caseworker should be the one who leads the facilitation, coordination, and management of the case because of his or her responsibility for permanency planning. Yet, sometimes, caseworkers are too quick to validate the opinion of other service providers at the expense of their own opinions. While some in the service provider level may be threatened by the suggestion that the caseworker have the facilitator role, it is clear that everyone else in the service provider level has more narrowed interests than the caseworker, such as the family therapist's goal to improve functioning or the guardian *ad litem*'s goal of protecting the rights of the child. These more narrow agendas necessarily constrain the other providers from taking the broad view and cooperative stance that is the hallmark of the multisystems approach.

Reading Feedback

Reading feedback is essential for testing assessment hypotheses about the system as well as evaluating the impact and effectiveness of an intervention. But because it is such a subjective process, reading feedback is not easy. The caseworker's skill, personal characteristics, and experience all exert an impact on how feedback is read. However, the process of reading feedback is enhanced when (1) the caseworker is better joined to the various levels and these relationships are more collaborative, (2) the caseworker receives good supervision, and (3) the caseworker has a good understanding of what constrains his or her providing service.

PREPARING AGENCIES

There are numerous areas to attend to simultaneously in the process of preparing an agency for family preservation or family reunification programs besides the issue of presenting training and consultation in an acceptable and competent fashion. These areas include the points of entry into the agency, the agenda of stakeholders for the work, and the staff's openness and capacity to accept the training and consultation.

I have faced several challenges when offering my services to an agency, but the hardest of them was trying to positively impact practice or to get caseworkers and supervisors to change the way they perform their duties. I believe that in-service training alone is not sufficient to accomplish this goal. Even the best trainer cannot insure what is being transferred into the field. In my experience, training alone helps those participants who most agree with the content. Those who disagree or do not quite understand simply return to their usual way of operating. Therefore, I think it is best if in-service training is coupled with consultation, and it is better still if the training and consultation can be offered at both caseworker and supervisory levels.

I prefer to keep these levels separated during most training events, however, so as to facilitate free group discussion among caseworkers without fear of retribution from their supervisor or to keep the supervisor from appearing uninformed to his or her staff. By combining training and consultation there is greater quality control over how concepts are being understood and how practice is being impacted. Working on both the supervisory and caseworker levels facilitates the integral establishment of the concepts into everyday practice.

The long-range effectiveness of any in-service training program rests in the understanding and support of the supervisors. Supervisors by and large set the expectations for the caseworkers. If the supervisor asks about constraints and whether the family and extended family have been seen together, then the caseworker is more likely to carry out these tasks. If the supervisor does not meet with staff or only monitors paperwork, the likelihood of unfortunate clinical mistakes may increase.

Points of Entry

The first step toward impacting practice is being hired by the agency. Usually the consultant is brought into the agency through one of three points of entry: the administration level, the management level, or the staff level. Each of these levels offers differing opportunities to the consultant as well as differing challenges. Since the administrative level is most concerned with the overall mission of the agency and smooth operation of its programs, the consultant entering through this level might be faced with the challenge of identifying how the training content promotes the agency's philosophy. On the other hand, when administration hires you and sanctions your efforts, your feedback about all aspects of the agency is likely to be valued.

For example, I was asked by a high-level administrator to provide training and consultation to the child welfare division staff. During the initial conversations with the administrator and division head, it was clear that the training was to mark a significant change in clinical orientation for staff and might encourage poor staff to leave. Once the training began, I noticed that the staff was receptive to the training concepts, but some of the supervisors were reluctant. Additional training efforts were then targeted to the supervisors. Within the context of the numerous changes in the division, of which this training was a part, a number of supervisors left the agency. This was framed as an opportunity to bring in new supervisors who would be supportive of a multisystems perspective. A year later the administrator expressed pleasure with the opportunities afforded by the training and indicated that the programs are operating more efficiently.

Managers and supervisors want the program's day-to-day operation to be efficient, productive, and effective. The consultant will be challenged to demonstrate how the proposed training and consultation will improve staff performance and meeting program goals. When I have been asked in by members of the management level, it is usually because staff are perceived to be ineffective or inefficient.

In an instance when I was brought in by a program supervisor to provide case consultation to the family preservation program in a private agency, there were few problems encountered. The supervisor enjoyed a good relationship with the agency's director, who was her immediate supervisor, and she was also liked by her staff. Consequently, her recommendation for my consultation was eagerly accepted, and the consultation occurred in accepting environment.

At the staff level, the overall emphasis is on doing a good job. The staff usually wants to be able to function autonomously and with confidence that they are doing what is correct and that they are doing it well. The challenge here will be to demonstrate how using the training concepts like the multisystems model makes their job easier. This can be particularly difficult as the multisystems model looks as if it may take more work. It is through case consultation that staff members come to appreciate how this approach can save them work.

In one instance, a staff member was behind our being hired by a community mental health center to conduct a series of workshops on the multisystems approach. This young woman had done such a splendid job of selling us to the agency that her supervisor had little need to approve the project short of arranging schedules. The staff politely received the training series, though its actual impact on practice is unknown.

Assessing the Context

At whatever point the consultant enters the agency, it is important to consider the context within which the consultation is to occur. The consultant should assess the goals for which he or she has been hired: Is it to fortify or strengthen caseworkers already considered competent, rehabilitate or improve weak or poorly trained caseworkers, or weed out and identify bad caseworkers? Is the consultation part of a new initiative or an existing program, and how do others in the agency regard it? Who is behind hiring the consultant, and what is his or her position in the agency and stake in the program?

Understanding the context includes understanding the history of previous training and recent administrative changes or upheavals. It includes understanding something of the agency's identity and its strengths and weaknesses. Last, it includes understanding the agency's place in the larger scheme of service providers or family preservation and reunification services.

In one instance, I was asked by DCFS to consult in downstate Illinois to the DCFS office and a private agency family preservation program that had gotten in trouble with the local judge over the quality of casework it performed. As I assessed the situation, DCFS and the private agency were in agreement that the program should not be terminated, as the judge wished, but should be repaired. The judge, on the other hand, was adamant that the program be closed.

It would be necessary to obtain the judge's approval of my efforts if there was any hope that my suggestions would be accepted and the agency given a chance to correct matters. It was decided that a meeting should be convened of all the parties concerned to hear specifically, and in front of everyone, what the complaints were, to ascertain if the judge would sanction my efforts and accept our recommendations for correcting the problem, and to send the judge a message that I considered his approval and sanctions vital to the success of the project. Once it was clear that the judge would tacitly accept the effort, I began the investigative process of the consultation. As part of the process, high-level DCFS administrators were advised to periodically report to the judge in order to keep the lines of communication open and to nurture his cooperation with the consultation. At the completion of my multisystems assessment, a lengthy document was written, identifying the various problems at all levels that faced the family preservation program and included specific action plans.

The agency's program was allowed to continue providing family preservation services, though the private agency administrators decided to replace the site administrator. One year later, however, the program lost its funding from DCFS and closed. Another family preservation program was funded in its place.

Reaction to the Training Program

When a consultant is newly brought into an agency, there may be reaction or resistance from any of a number of people or from different sectors of the agency. The staff may regard the consultant as helpful or as a spy for the administration. Some staff members may react negatively to the underlying philosophy of the training content. It has been my experience that, when the training program is brought in by the administration, the degree of manager and staff reactance against training is directly proportional to the disengagement between administrator and staff. On those occasions when administrator and line staff are a well organized team, the learning occurs in an exciting context. Training content is eagerly met and the training enterprise is enjoyable for all. On other occasions, though, when the administrator and staff are in conflict, there may be open reluctance to learn the material, or staff may see the task as too overwhelming.

It is important to minimize negative reaction, and a few preventive measures at the beginning can be helpful later. It is important that those individuals hiring the consultant be aware of his or her underlying practice philosophy. Without substantive agreement on the philosophical approach to child welfare and families, there is increased likelihood of negative reaction. As a consequence, the practice implications of the model should be explained to administrators and managers before beginning the consultation.

In one situation, I was asked by an agency contact to provide training on family therapy to the staff. This struck me as curious, because the agency did not provide therapy for its clients. I asked the agency contact if she wanted the staff members to become therapists and was told "no."

I then explained that family therapy training might result in staff dissatis-faction and even turnover, and instead offered to customize a training pro-gram that began with the mission of the agency and was meant to enhance staff job performance. A training and consultation program was prepared that relied upon the multisystems approach for its basic philosophy and orientation but focused the training on therapeutic casework rather than family therapy. The administrator was so pleased with the training that she instigated a 3-year training program.

Another preventive measure for minimizing resistance is to validate the strengths of the staff, in part, to facilitate joining and, in part, to minimize the hierarchy between the staff and the trainer. Caseworkers are more competent than they are often given credit for, and treating them respectfully and eliciting their ideas goes a long way toward diffusing resistance to the training. Obviously, it is also a good way to avoid con-flict between staff and trainer.

On many occasions, I have found that caseworkers are almost sur-prised when I tell them I value their ideas and then back that up with respectful behavior, questioning what they would do in a clinical situa-tion, and asking for their feedback on the training content. Most of the time the quite reserved atmosphere that I encounter at the beginning of training or consultation gives way to forthright expression, sharing, and taking risks by the caseworkers.

Dealing with Conflict

The consultant occasionally encounters personality conflicts in the process of delivering consultation. Usually it concerns some underlying conflict between persons in the agency that surfaces in front of the consultant. The consultant is advised to face the conflict directly but cautiously. For it to be of concern to the consultant, the nature of the conflict should have a directly negative impact on the training or consultation goals. Other-wise, it is really none of our business. When it is our business, then the personality conflict should be considered, and the consultant must decide if directly confronting the conflicted parties is preferable to planning around the conflict so as to minimize its influence. Sometimes the consultant may need to seek direction from the person who hired him or her and offer to engage in a problem-solving consultative role. When I have had reason to go to authorities in the agency, confidentiality of the individuals in-volved is maintained; I prefer instead to identify how the conflict is hav-ing a negative impact.

For example, one agency had a personality clash between the direc-tors of two units. One unit conducted investigations of child abuse and neglect the other provided follow-up casework services. Clearly, these two units needed each other to perform their functions within the agency, and thus the presence of the personality conflict was having severe effects on the continuity of care. I reported to the agency administrator the existence of a breakdown between the two units without identifying the personal nature of the conflict. The administrator then publicly clarified the reporting and collaboration roles between the two units and assured the unit directors that their job performance ratings would partly depend on their department's ability to operate cooperatively. In this instance each unit director was told, in essence, that the job was no place for a personal conflict with the other.

Changing Attitudes

The most basic task facing the consultant is the issue of changing attitudes. The attitude of some workers to multisystems training content is that it is too hard, too time consuming, or unnecessary. This immediate reluctance to try anything new may be explained, in part, by the fact that the public image of child welfare professionals is quite negative, so they may hear suggestions on improving clinical practice as yet more criticism of their work.

This reaction is especially likely if their strengths are not validated at the outset. Through the presentation style, the consultant should help motivate participants and build an atmosphere that stresses success and competence. A colleague I was presenting with once took a group of reluctant DCFS caseworkers and transformed them into an eager group of learners by first identifying how they loved their jobs. He had them agree to be punctual and bring food for the group if they were late to any part of the training. By that afternoon, participants were laughing and enjoying the fruit that was brought back by one late participant. Tardiness never became a problem.

Though it is a well-worn phrase, "beginning where the client is" holds true for changing caseworker attitudes as well. In order to convince caseworkers that adopting the multisystems approach would actually help them in their job, I asked a group of DCFS workers to identify who could be involved on any one case, while I noted the parties on a transparency. By the time they were finished identifying the various parties, there was no place left to write on the page. From there it was easy to describe the multisystems approach as helping them manage a large number of people, and they were more attuned to the message.

A variety of creative ways to impart content, such as role plays, discussion, and the use of video or audio presentations should be employed to encourage active participation in the learning process and to maximize the learning potential. Caseworkers should be encouraged to share their own thoughts about cases. It not only helps validate the worker as competent, but it also provides a baseline of the worker's current conceptual level. Only by knowing what a caseworker is thinking is there any opportunity to impact that thinking. Moreover, it is consistent with the multisystems approach that the ideas of a variety of participants helps the accuracy of the thinking about a case.

Beyond that, opportunities for caseworkers to explore their own values about families, family preservation and reunification, and how they see their own jobs should be built into training and consultation. Unfortunately, all too often stereotypes and prejudices, lack of self-confidence and countertransference, limited clinical or interpersonal skills, and a limited knowledge base about human development prevent caseworkers from meeting their goal of being helpful. Helping them clarify and explore values may help caseworkers overcome some of these limitations.

On the other hand, I am not suggesting that consultants support low levels of competence or skill in caseworkers. While the consultant may be the first to notice a problem worker, it is the supervisor who will ultimately have to deal with an incompetent caseworker. This highlights, again, the importance of the supervisor to the training process. Without the active support and promotion of the training content by the supervisor, all the interesting videotapes, slides, and motivational speeches will be of no avail.

CONCLUSION

When it comes to protecting our children from abuse and neglect, we have a formidable challenge. The problems of drug addiction and the presence of families with multigenerational dysfunction have made the problem of preserving families more and more difficult. And to further complicate matters, we are trying to solve the problem of children at risk in Illinois and elsewhere with an understaffed, overburdened, undertrained, and needlessly political, competitive, argumentative, and combative system—DCFS, private agencies, lawyers, and judges alike.

What is meant, then, by the notion that child welfare professionals should attempt reasonable efforts to maintain the child in the home? Those reasonable efforts should include an accurate and timely assessment of the risk of harm to the child; an accurate, in-depth, and timely assessment of the family (including the individual psychological makeup of the adult caretakers); identifying with the family and extended family the goals and objectives necessary to rehabilitate the family, if possible; and sharing information and collaborating between the professionals working with the family. A formidable challenge, indeed, but one that has no hope of being met without the use of conceptual frameworks, like the multisystems approach, that allow caseworkers to see the situation broadly and in context while also empowering them to intervene effectively and build real competencies in families in the process.

EPILOGUE

Since writing this chapter I have become a member of a small cadre of six clinicians as clinical services consultants to DCFS. We are on-site in certain DCFS offices, interacting directly with supervisors and caseworkers for the expressed purpose of supporting the supervisor's role and for offering our clinical perspective on an as-needed basis. I am the only consultant on-site in one outpost office that can best be described as a large open space cluttered with too many desks. I am contracted to spend up to 20 hours a week there and have been at it 5 months. Unfortunately, because of the demands of doctoral studies and the vagaries of life, I have rarely been able to be there 20 hours per week to this point, though that will change soon.

I regard this opportunity as a rare privilege and I am learning much. I help caseworkers interpret psychological test reports and identify the testing question when they refer clients for psychological examinations. I provide an empathic ear to a couple of "veteran" supervisors who are burned-out and too cynical after 20 years of service, because my support may have a generative effect on their functioning. A few caseworkers have asked me to share clinical impressions about their cases and I have conducted interviews of clients with some of them. I am involved in developing additional private agency resources for the out-post by facilitating collaboration between DCFS and private agency staff. I have, upon request, even furnished referrals for therapy to a few staff members. I have overheard caseworkers' anger when an adult fails to comply with a service plan and I have observed their sadness when a child is harmed. I have been touched to see caseworkers from all over the office shower attention on a young client brought to the office by one of their colleagues.

At the same time, I have witnessed some of the contraints caseworkers confront in performing their duties. Low morale is rampant. Caseworkers routinely and uniformly discuss the bad feelings they have toward administration. It appears to them that the administration believes they are incompetent by talking disparagingly about them in public and to the media.

I also hear chilling reports of judges and lawyers humiliating caseworkers in court. This happens so often, in fact, that many caseworkers are reluctant to offer their assessment on a case in court, preferring instead to rely on psychological test results or testimony from "experts," in order to avoid being criticized. In one instance, a supervisor from the outpost was called into court without warning to receive the judge's order to obtain a third psychological examination on a client in order to determine which of two conflicting psychological reports should be followed. When I asked him if he spoke up about the impropriety of such a request, I was told that this particular judge does not accept being challenged by caseworkers; to do so risks spending time in prison for contempt.

As an example of yet another constraint, I observed a caseworker leaving the outpost office to gather the belongings of a child that had been placed in the shelter from a group home the previous evening. In itself, not an unusual use of a DCFS caseworker's time. But because the private agency group home staff refused to make other arrangements to get the child his clothes, this caseworker was forced to drive over 200 miles round trip to the group home, to the shelter, and back to the office. Apparently, the caseworker's other responsibilities were regarded as unimportant by the private agency.

It is clear to me how these conditions undercut the caseworker's confidence and sabotage family preservation and reunification efforts. It is also clear that intervention into the supervisor and caseworker level alone will not be enought to remedy the situation. Here too, a multileveled approach should be undertaken that positively impacts the manner in which the DCFS administration interacts with its staff, the way judges and lawyers treat caseworkers, and whether or not private agency staff cooperate with DCFS caseworkers.

ACKNOWLEDGMENT

I wish to acknowledge the work of Lee Combrinck-Graham in developing an interview format that will empower families in the fashion described herein.

REFERENCES

Aponte, H., & Van Deusen, J. (1981). Structural family therapy. In A. S. Gurman & D. P. Kniskern (Eds.), *Handbook of family therapy* (pp. 310–360). New York: Brunner/Mazel.

Barth, R., & Berry, M. (1987). Outcomes of child welfare services under permanency planning. *Social Service Review, 61*(1), 71–87.

Bateson, G. (1972). *Steps to an ecology of mind.* New York: Ballantine Books.

Berry, M. (1992). An evaluation of family preservation services: Fitting agency services to family needs. *Social Work, 37*(4), 314–321.

Boyd-Franklin, N. (1989). *Black families in therapy: A multisystems approach.* New York: Guilford Press.

Breunlin, D. C., & Schwartz, R. C. (1986). Sequences: Toward a common denominator of family therapy. *Family Process, 25,* 67–87.

Breunlin, D. C., Schwartz, R. C., & MacKune-Karrer, B. (1992). *Metaframeworks.* San Francisco: Jossey Bass.

Bribitzer, M., & Verdieck, M. J. (1988). Home based, family centered intervention: Evaluation of a foster care program. *Child Welfare, 67*(3), 255–265.

Cimmarusti, R. A. (1989). *A multi-systems approach to family preservation: A curriculum guide.* Springfield, IL: Child Welfare Training Institute, Department of Children and Family Services.

Cimmarusti, R. A. (1990). *A curriculum for a multi-systems approach to family reunification work.* Springfield, IL: Child Welfare Training Institute, Department of Children and Family Services.

Cimmarusti, R. A. (1992). Family preservation practice based upon a multisystems approach. *Child Welfare, 71*(3), 241–256.

De Hoyos, G., & Jensen, C. (1985). The systems approach in American social work. *Social Casework, 66*(8), 490–497.

Emlen, A. C. (1981). Development of the concept of permanency planning. In S. W. Downs, L. Bayless, L. Dreyer, A. C. Emlen, M. Hardin, L. Heim, J. Lahti, K. Liedtke, K. Schimke, & M. Troychak (Eds.), *Foster care reform in the 70's: Final report of the permanency planning dissemination proiect* (pp. 1.1–1.18). Portland, OR: Regional Research Institute for Human Services, Portland State University.

Frankel, H. (1988). Family-centered, home-based service in child protection: A review of the research. *Social Service Review, 62*(1), 137–157.

Germain, C. B., & Gitterman, A. (1987). Ecological perspective. In A. Minahan (Ed.), *Encyclopedia of Social Work* (Vol. 18, pp. 488–496). Silver Spring, MD: National Association of Social Workers.

Gleeson, J. P., Smith, J. H., & Dubois, A. C. (1993). Preparing child welfare practitioners: Avoiding the single solution seduction. *Administration in Social Work, 17*(3), 21–37.

Hartman, A., & Laird, J. (1983). *Family-centered social work practice.* New York: MacMillan.

Imber-Black, E. (1988). *Families and larger systems: A family therapist's guide through the labyrinth.* New York: Guilford Press.

Ingrassia, M., & McCormick, J. (1994, April 25). Why leave children with bad parents? *Newsweek, 123*(17), 52–58.

Keeney, B. P. (1983). *Aesthetics of change.* New York: Guilford Press.

Maluccio, A., Fein, E., & Olmstead, K. (1986). *Permanency planning for children: Concepts and methods.* New York: Tavistock Publishers.

McGowan, B. G. (1983). Historical evolution of child welfare services: An examination of the sources of current problems and dilemmas. In B. McGowan & W. Meezan (Eds.), *Child welfare: Current dilemmas—future directions* (pp. 47–90). Itasca, IL: Peacock.

Miller, J., & Dore, M. M. (1991). Innovations in child protective services in service training: Commitment to excellence. *Child Welfare, 70*(4), 437–449.

Minuchin, S. (1974). *Families and family therapy.* Cambridge, MA: Harvard University Press.

Minuchin, S., & Fishman, H. C. (1981). *Family therapy techniques.* Cambridge, MA: Harvard University Press.

Norman, A. (1985). *Keeping families together: The case for family preservation,* New York: Edna McConnell Clark Foundation.

Pine, B. (1986). Child welfare reform and the political process. *Social Service Review, 60,* 339–359.

Samantrai, K. (1992). To prevent unnecessary separation of children and families: Public Law 96-272-policy and practice. *Social Work, 37*(4), 295–302.

Schuerman, J. P., & Rzepnicki, T. L. (1991). *Evaluation of the Illinois family first placement prevention programs.* Chicago: The University of Chicago, Chapin Hall Center for Children.

Seaberg, J. R. (1986). "Reasonable efforts": Toward implementation in permanency planning. *Child Welfare, 6*(5), 469–479.

Stein, T. J., & Gambrill, E. D. (1985). Permanency planning for children: The past and present. *Children and youth services review, 7,* 83–94.

Walsh, F. (Ed.). (1982). *Normal family processes.* New York: Guilford Press.

VI

CONNECTING PROGRAMS

The "connecting programs" presented in this last part are extraordinary programs in common settings. There are mothers in prison all over the country, but very few programs that strive to involve their children with them. There are mandated school counseling programs all over the country, but the one described herein is one of the few that specifically keeps the family at the center of the counseling efforts.

In searching for programs that keep families connected with incarcerated individuals I came across a group called the Family Corrections Network. This group focused almost entirely on adult family members, such as spouses and parents. It was through a more subterranean networking process that I learned about Sister Judith Falk's work. I was fascinated by Falk's observation about the importance of the transporters to the children, and I happened to mention this to a friend who lives in the area who told me that, Oh, yes, she (my friend) had been a transporter for some years. This gave some perspective to this program's presence in the community. Falk's work also demonstrates what Feinberg's program does, that many mothers are impelled to straighten out their lives by their desire to care for their children.

I met Barbara King at a conference where I had described this book. She, in turn, briefly described her program, and a chapter had to be included. Just as foster parents may side with children against their biological parents, so school personal may side with children against their parents, in situations where the children appear to be struggling and unhappy. Systems-oriented analysis of these situations would predict that the situation will become worse when these kinds of unholy alliances occur. One scenario in the school situation is that excluded parents may take out their embarassment and frustration on their child, making the situation worse. King and associates describe how a family-based school counseling system was carefully conceived and developed.

16

Project Exodus: The Corrections Connection

Judith A. Falk

PROJECT EXODUS: THE AGENCY

Introduction

Project Exodus is one of many programs of the Interreligious Council of Central New York. The Council is an incorporated, not-for-profit agency dedicated to creating and improving interreligious and interracial relations, and providing service to people in need. The mission of Project Exodus is to facilitate the transition of female ex-offenders into normal society after a period of incarceration. Most women have children, and Project Exodus works to preserve and enhance family relationships. Advocacy in the community is a necessary part of attaining these goals. Thus, there are three major components of Project Exodus: namely, case management, the Mothers' and Children's Visiting Program, and advocacy.

History and Development

The history of Project Exodus begins in 1983. The agency grew out of involvement of local clergy with prisoners at local correctional facilities. Seeing the difficult challenges that were faced by men and women being released from prison and returning to society, they realized that individuals who truly wanted to change their lives had to deal with a frightening and sometimes insurmountable array of legal, social, and practical needs, obstacles, and obligations. Exodus was to address those needs.

In the beginning, Project Exodus was a completely voluntary effort, involving the chaplains, correctional facility personnel, concerned community members, prisoners themselves, their families, and the Pastoral Care Director of the Interreligious Council of Central New York. A great deal of networking was done with other service agencies in the community and with government agencies as well.

The first funded effort was a VISTA grant in 1985. At first there was one volunteer, then two. In 1987, some funding was received from Onondaga County Department of Social Services. Later the funding stream was moved to the Department of Probation, and then to the Department of Corrections of Onondaga County. In the meantime, the Interreligious Council, the sponsoring organization, was cultivating social and financial support in the private sector, in the religious community, and with the local United Way. Linkage was formed also with the New York State Department of Social Services.

The staff of Project Exodus grew to four full-time paid members, and a part-time administrator. The staff included the director, who also did men's case management; a men's case manager; a job developer; and a women's case manager. However, the poor financial climate of the 1990s took its toll on Project Exodus, as it did on so many human service agencies. Midway through 1992, one staff member was laid off and, by the end of 1992, two other staff people were laid off. This left only the women's case manager, whose position, because of a different funding source, was secured for another year.

Philosophy: Exodus in the Bible

Project Exodus is named for the second book of the Old Testament. Our clients' situations are reminiscent of the Hebrews' release from captivity in Egypt, their journey through the wilderness, and God's covenant with them on Mount Sinai. A person leaving the captivity of incarceration does face a wilderness of starting over. In the absence of supportive friends or family, he or she has no income, housing, food, clothing or support system. A person in this position stands a good chance of breaking the law again, simply in an effort to survive. Project Exodus offers support for people in that position, helping them to create better lives for themselves.

Ms. X (names are changed throughout) was released into just such a situation. She had a friend to stay with, and that was about all. She had several medical problems that would eventually qualify her for Social

Security Disability. She also had physical mobility problems. The Exodus case manager spent a great deal of time with her, keeping parole appointments, applying for public assistance, which was needed while waiting for Social Security Income; joining pantries to supplement food in the household where she was staying; getting personal identification documented, and getting much-needed medicines when her Medicaid was not in place. This went on for weeks. At one point, Ms. X said that if it were not for Project Exodus, she would be back in prison by now. It was so difficult that she would have broken the law to get survival money. She remarked during a particularly low moment that prison looked good at that point, because at least she would have three meals and a bed. Ms. X has not returned to prison in the subsequent 3 years.

Theoretical Framework: Project Exodus

Both studies and experience show that the first days, weeks, and months after release are the most crucial in the life of the ex-offender. The first 30 days are seen as the time that, without intervention of some kind, a person is most vulnerable to rearrest and reincarceration. Other milestones are 60 days and 90 days after release. As seen on a continuum, the first day after release is the most difficult and discouraging. Each day after that gets better. It is difficult for a client in that position to see that it gets better. Exodus' mission is to intervene at the point of release and provide the extra help that is needed to get through those first difficult days.

Joy, another Exodus client, was incarcerated at Onondaga County Correctional Facility at Jamesville, New York, for 16 months on charges related to drugs. She was involved with an abusive partner who was also a drug user. Drugs were found in her apartment. Her children saw her arrested and their apartment searched and torn apart. Joy lost her apartment, her belongings, and her children, who were placed in foster care.

When Joy left Onondaga County Correctional Facility she had no income, no place to live, and little family to help her. Her sister was already caring for the four children she had lost because of the drug charges. The children's father was also in prison. Joy had left him, because of the abuse. Furthermore, her release date was Christmas Eve, and she had no gifts to give her children when they had their Christmas visit.

Joy stayed with friends for a couple of days, until the Exodus worker could set up living arrangements through the Department of Social Services. An Exodus volunteer shopped for Christmas gifts. Exodus helped with pantry food, emergency food vouchers, and emergency clothing. The Exodus case manager provided transport to medical appointments for an injured knee. Because of this knee injury, and because of the winter weather, almost total transportation was needed for apartment and furniture hunting, and for many other needs.

Exodus acted as a liaison and support for foster care issues, encouraged counseling for Joy's history of having been battered, and generally was there for support and encouragement when needed. Joy had several times when she felt that selling some drugs would be an easy way to support herself financially while waiting the several weeks it took to get a check for public assistance. She could not seek work during this time because of the knee injury.

Joy has since become involved with another abusive partner and left him. He is currently in prison. She now lives with a man who is not abusive. They love each other very much and are making a better life together. Joy has not been back to prison in the 4 years since her release. Her five children are teenagers now, and they speak with Joy about returning home. Steps are being taken in court to effect this goal. Joy hopes that the process will allow the return of one child at a time. She currently celebrates Christmas, Easter, and Thanksgiving with them, providing a festive meal and a family day at her house.

Joy has said many times that if it were not for Project Exodus, she would probably be back in prison.

Description of the Model: Project Exodus

The three parts of Project Exodus are case management, advocacy, and the mother's and children's visiting program. Case Management is at the heart of the success of Project Exodus. Participation is voluntary on the part of the client. Typically, women leaving prison have no family and friends to offer support and help. Most often they are not in stable relationships with the men in their lives. What social contacts they have may be with persons who know them only as drug users or drug sellers.

> The situation described above happened to Linda. When she was released, her biggest need was to be placed in drug treatment. She fell back into using several times. She truly knew her own weakness, but had to wait a few weeks to be evaluated and placed in treatment. She recounted how she could not even leave her apartment without someone asking her if she was "smoking today." Before her admission to a detoxification unit, the case manager was literally calling her on the telephone every hour to encourage her that she could avoid a relapse for one more hour.

Each person is different, with different needs and circumstances, unique personal limitations and problems. Each person is interviewed while still incarcerated to determine what is needed and what the person's problems and concerns are. Some groundwork can be done by the case manager before the person is released to pave the way for a more smooth transition.

Services offered to our clients have included job search and counseling, expediting public assistance applications, emergency services, temporary and long-term housing, emergency food and medical services, contact with agencies for personal and addiction counseling, help in dealing with family issues, abuse, AIDS, legal issues, and parole and probation issues. In all of this, there is the crucial element of personal support. A very significant part of what a woman in this situation needs is to know that someone is out there who cares that she improves the quality of her life.

> Jennifer had gone through a process similar to the others described. She had lost contact with us for over a year. One day, she showed up in the office asking to see me because she was pregnant and had used drugs during the early part of the pregnancy. She was worried about the baby and was asking for help with furnishings and clothing for the child. As it turned out, she kept all of her appointments for pre-natal care, and found other ways (legal ones) to provide for the physical needs of the child. The child seemed to show no ill effects from her earlier drug use. She had no supportive family, and the men in her life have been abusive. My sense was that what she needed most was someone to turn to when she felt frightened and alone. The baby is well-cared for and receives love and attention.
>
> Jennifer recently called me again because she was in an accident and broke her pelvis. She had trouble caring for herself and the baby in that condition. Exodus was able to make some contacts and facilitate some aspects of care, but Jennifer was doing most of it herself. Again, her need appeared to be mostly to know someone was there for her.

The Place of the Women's and Children's Program in the Agency

Currently, the women's case manager is the only one working in Project Exodus because of the budget cuts mentioned earlier. Men's services had to be discontinued. The total effort of the women's case manager is called the Women's and Children's Program. It consists of case management, the Mothers' and Children's Visiting Program, and advocacy. The efforts of the women's case manager have recently been more focused and limited to women who have current issues with their children. Unfortunately, the population of women in the county facility has more than doubled in 3 years' time. This means, of course, that caseloads have doubled as well, and are very large. If more personnel were available, some services could be provided that now have to be refused, and services that are now provided could be delivered in a more effective and thorough manner.

WOMEN'S AND CHILDREN'S PROGRAM

History and Development

In 1989, the Interreligious Council applied for a demonstration grant from the New York State Department of Social Services. The object of the grant was to provide services to incarcerated women and their children. It provided for a *therapist* to lead a women's support group at the prison. It also proposed and funded the convening of a *task force* to improve and coordinate community efforts on behalf of incarcerated women. Also to be hired were a *case manager* and a *children's therapist.* In a partnership agreement with the Interreligious Council, the two therapists were to be hired by Onondaga Pastoral Counseling Center.

The *therapist* was to lead a weekly support group for women at the prison, this group was not limited to women with children. This group eventually became the total responsibility of Onondaga Pastoral Counseling Center, and is no longer part of the Exodus grant.

Advocacy took the form of a task force convened by the Interreligious Council Director of Pastoral Care. It was composed of people from a broad range of positions in the community and included people from both private and government agencies, as well as private individuals. The most notable achievement of this group was the Conference on Women in the Criminal Justice System that was held in November 1991. It was very well attended, pointing up the Syracuse community's interest in the issues of women in the criminal justice system and their children.

A very effective segment of this conference was a panel consisting of an Exodus client, an incarcerated woman, and a third woman who had been incarcerated. Feedback from attendees indicated that the panel, with its personal stories and perspectives, was very enlightening. Naomi, who was introduced earlier in this chapter, was one of the panelists.

Out of this conference was formed the Women's Justice Alliance, a small group of conference attendees who chose to continue to meet to try to take some realistic action on behalf of women in the criminal justice system. The two strongest objectives that emerged from this group were the improvement and coordination of services for women in the criminal justice system and the formation of a halfway house. This halfway house would serve both as an alternative to incarceration that would allow women to keep their children while serving time, and as an intermediate step for women being released from prison, as they try to resume normal living. Efforts are currently being made to further this project.

The *case manager* was to interview referred clients at the prison to determine their goals and needs. Upon their release, she was to help them to supply their basic needs and services. She was to provide support and encouragement during the difficult time immediately following release. In addition, she was to initiate the Mothers' and Children's Visiting Program, which will be described later as it currently exists.

The *children's therapist* became part of the Mothers' and Children's Visiting Program held at Onondaga County Correctional Facility at Jamesville, New York. In the original design, the case manager was to arrange volunteer transport for the children to the prison. They were to have private visiting time with their mothers, who were incarcerated, and then take part in a children's therapy group run by the children's therapist. In addition to these duties, the case manager soon began to run a mothers support group that ran concurrently with the children's group. This continues to the present.

The program has been very popular and has been in great demand. Over time, a waiting list has developed, underscoring the need for the resources to serve more people. An assistant to the therapist has been added, so that more children could be included. The case manager has continued to build a base of volunteer transporters.

The staff also transported children to the facility. A second assistant was added in 1992, bringing the total number of staff to four.

This enables about seven women and ten children to be served in the program at any one time. The ratio of staff to children needs to be kept small if our purpose of dealing with children's feelings is to be achieved. A significant amount of individual attention is necessary to zero in on a child's feelings and problems. Also, children who are suffering often exhibit some difficult behaviors, such as that of the child who yelled out the car window as though someone were beating him, the child who spat at a staff person, and the child who hid under a table and would not come out. There are also children who are docile and delightful, who deal with or hide their feelings very well. There are children who literally have to be pulled away from Mom when it is time to leave, and who demand some personal comfort and attention. There are tears and tantrums. There are little people who feel very big responsibilities. Much, though not all of this upset is caused by the fact that the most important person in their lives has been taken away from them.

Philosophy and Theoretical Framework: Separation Is Damaging to Children

It is an observable fact that families break up when a mother goes to prison. Children go into foster care or go to new homes with relatives or friends of their mothers. Children in the same family go to separate homes in some cases. The family apartment is given up. In many cases, furniture and belongings are stolen or put out to the curb to prepare for new tenants.

This is traumatic for all involved, including extended family members, who now have extra responsibility for the children. It is difficult for the children to adjust to a new home and to lose the old one. It is also difficult to adjust to a new school. Perhaps less obviously, it is scary and unsettling for the children to be powerless as they watch their mothers, the primary caretakers, being taken away. And finally, the mother–child attachments that do exist are often simply put aside for the length of the sentence.

People who care for children in a mother's absences are generally well meaning and good-hearted. Relatives usually have a commitment to the well-being of the children. Grandparents, in particular, seem to most often take care of grandchildren in this situation. The desire seems to be to avoid giving up the children to foster care at any price. Foster care to many people means that the children will be placed into the care of strangers. It also means, at least in their perception, a long, hard effort to return the children to their families.

There are also people who agree to care for children and then use the children's public assistance money for their own purposes, leaving the children with minimal food, clothing, and necessities. There are caretakers who leave children unsupervised, even over night. There are also caretakers who mean well, but who find the extra burden just too much to bear.

Though I have met some dedicated and loving fathers who, in the mother's absence, assume the responsibility for the children, they are few and far between among the Exodus clientele.

> Joshua was one such man. He and my client, Milicent, have two young teenage children. Their daughter is mentally retarded. Their son has been accustomed to assuming a parent role with his mother and with his sister.
>
> Joshua gets up very early to care for the children and get them off to school. He then works a full day himself at a local hospital. He cooks and cleans and takes on both parental roles during Milicent's frequent trips to prison. When visiting the home, one always finds it clean and in order. The children are clean, well nourished, and cared for.
>
> Milicent is a long-time drug abuser whose prognosis is poor despite numerous resolutions and attempts at rehabilitation. Her family continues to be as supportive as possible.

Children go through the feelings associated with grief and loss, which include anger, denial, and depression. This is manifested in their moods, attitudes and behaviors. A child in this situation may become very quiet and withdrawn. He or she may act out in school or experience a drop in grades. The child may become aggressive or assaultive. Friends, relatives, and acquaintances may wonder what is happening. But what they are seeing is probably due to unresolved anger and grief because of the mother's incarceration.

The incarcerated mother goes through a similar trauma, with the constraints of prison making it impossible for her to do anything about the situation. In general, when there is a crisis, adults are so preoccupied with handling the crisis itself that the feelings of the children are largely overlooked. The Women's and Children's Program, with its components of case management, structured visiting and therapy, parenting, and advocacy tries to address the plight of the child, the mother, and the rest of the family, with a view to preserving the family relationships in the style that is best for all, with particular focus on the child.

Description of the Women's and Children's Program

The Project Exodus Women's and Children's Program includes: case management, the Mothers' and Children's Visiting Program, and advocacy. Also discussed are collaborating personnel and stakeholders, or "who benefits?"

Case Management

Case management with women and children can get very complicated and involved. Usually there are foster care and custody issues. In addition, women seem to have more serious health issues than men do. Some of these result from abortions, high-risk pregnancies, physical abuse, drugs, and AIDS.

Ms. X is now in and out of hospitals battling infections, because she is HIV positive. Joy now is documented as unable to work because of having been beaten so badly, and because of emotional and intellectual inability to function. Sandra, yet another Exodus client, was to be on psychiatric drugs for the rest of her life because of brain damage from drug use. Sandra has since died, presumably from complications resulting from drug use. She was in her 30s and leaves three young children.

The relationships that develop between a client and the case manager can become very intense and absorbing. A woman who elects to reunite her family and do it with the help of Project Exodus has a long hard road to travel—and so has the case manager. Some clients have kept in contact over a period as long as 3 years. Others are able to and prefer to be on their own after a much shorter period. Of course, there are also those who set out to do the right thing and eventually relapse into old patterns and are again incarcerated.

Mothers' and Children's Visiting Program

Most women who are in this program are referred by the counselors at the prison. Most join the program during a standard Exodus interview. One counselor at the prison acts as a liaison person between the correctional facility and Project Exodus. This counselor confers with the Exodus case manager about each family situation. She does the paperwork required by the facility to insure that each mother is cleared to participate.

The Exodus case manager then interviews the prospective participant to get necessary information about the children and those who are caring for them in the absence of the parent. Names, addresses, and phone numbers are noted. Children need to be between the ages of 5 and 12 to be eligible. Activities would not be appropriate for those older or younger. This creates the unfortunate situation in which some children in the family might be included in the visits and some not. Recently, volunteers have been recruited to transport children who are too young or too old for the program to the prison for visits during regular visiting hours.

In some cases the children are in foster care or have a court status that applies to visits with parents. Some court judgments allow a woman to see her children only if supervised by approved personnel. All of this needs to be known and discussed. The Exodus case manager seeks permission from the proper County Children's Division office to allow the family to participate.

> Jasmine applied for the visiting program and was turned down, because when contact was made with children's division, it was found out that Jasmine was allowed only supervised visits set up by that office. This was because drugs had been found in the house with her children. Jasmine was unable to take part in the program. It is necessary to accept these agency-imposed limitations and continue to do our best with those who are eligible.

The next step is to visit the home where the children are staying. The Exodus case manager goes to the home to explain the program and to arrange transportation for the children. An effort is made to get to know the children and to help them to be as comfortable as possible with the idea of going to the prison to take part in this program. Many children are familiar with the prison and with visiting procedures, and know exactly why Mom is there. For others, it is a totally new experience, and a lot of support and explanation is needed. No child is forced to go, either by Exodus or by the people who care for him or her. Sammy, for example, was an 11-year-old who went to a couple of visits and then chose not to go back; it was just too difficult for him.

Next, transportation is arranged. Sometimes the family is able to transport the children. Most often, however, the children are brought to the visit by volunteer transporters or by staff persons. Efforts are made to have the transporter call and visit the family ahead of time, so the child gets to know the person who will take him or her to the visit.

One evening a week, the transporters bring the children to the correctional facility. The children must go through the usual security measures taken when outsiders enter the prison. Children must remove jewelry, empty their pockets and go through the metal detector. At first, this frightens some children. Others treat it like a game. The staff people sign in, and a guard escorts the group into the visiting room. Mothers and children meet with hugs, kisses, laughter, and sometimes with tears. Unlike the standard visits, which take place across a table, the children can be right with their mothers, or even sit on their laps.

For the first 45 minutes or so, they just visit and catch up with each other. During this visiting time, the staff people plan the evening's activities and observe the interactions that take place. Staff, moms, and children gather in a group to discuss the plans for the evening and to welcome new people to the program.

The children then gather for their therapeutic group, and the mothers for their support group. The children do activities, play games, and make things as a way of giving them an opportunity to express their feelings and concerns about their mothers being incarcerated. The mothers' group has an assigned topic each week, but there are times when the immediate concerns of the women are so pressing that the planned topic is not discussed. Planned topics include feelings, trust, communication, and being away from your children. The following case provides an example.

> One evening, Vanessa came to the group and recounted that she had attempted suicide. Normally, prison regulations would not allow her out of her room. However, we obtained special permission for her to attend because seeing her children was so beneficial for her. Mentally and emotionally, Vanessa was not very strong. Being in prison was more than she could handle. It depressed and discouraged her beyond what she could bear. That evening in the group she received a great deal of support from the other women and from the leader. The other women had witnessed or heard about her suicied atempt, so they also needed to talk about it. Needless to say, we skipped the planned topic that night. For Vanessa, seeing her children and the rest of the group and staff seemed to lift her spirits, at least temporarily. She did not attempt to harm herself again.

At the conclusion of the mothers' group, the mothers join the children to engage with them in their activities and to discuss what they have done and learned. Separate groups help to deal with the parent's feelings on an adult level and the child's feelings on a child's level. Separate groups help to make the individuals stronger so that the relationship between them can be stronger.

The session concludes with good-byes, some very tearful. The women return to their rooms, and the transporters arrive to return the children to their homes.

It is important to note that the transporters are all volunteers, and as a measure of their dedication, we note that since there is no place for them to wait at the facility, they must make two trips each Friday evening. In addition, some transporters have done other things for the children, such as take them to the circus. One child had no winter coat, so the transporter bought one for her.

Additionally, we did not even foresee the relationships that would develop between the children and the transporters. When it is necessary for a different person to transport a child, the child sometimes reacts to it as another loss. Consistency seems important, even in this matter. It is difficult to find people with the ability and dedication to show up on one evening a week consistently to do this. We are very blessed with the volunteers we have.

> Tommy, a 12-year-old boy who had a history of antisocial behavior, is an example of a special relationship that developed between child and transporter. He had taken a knife and carved up the bathroom at his foster home; he had started several fires. And the list goes on. We all had reservations about having him participate in the program. But after two or three trips to see his mother, he said to the transporter, "I think I'm beginning to like you." This came from a child whose behavior made him seem incapable of liking anyone.

When a mother is released and the family leaves the program, there are more good-byes and, in a sense, more loss and change. Currently there are hopes and plans to form a companion program that families can join after the mother is released.

Advocacy

Since this is a small agency, staff people must wear many hats. It is necessary for all staff to join administration in public speaking and other forms of advocacy. We speak by invitation to various church groups and to other social groups in the community. We attend meetings that are geared toward uniting community service providers and coordinating their efforts.

The program specifically called for the formation of a task force to study the needs and issues of women in the criminal justice system. Named the Task Force on Women and Incarceration, it was convened by an associate Director of the Interreligious Council. It included a wide spectrum of individuals who represented political, social service, government, and educational agencies. It also included ex-offenders and other interested private citizens. This group worked on raising consciousness about the issues and problems, on trying to coordinate existing services and create new ones geared to women who are involved in the criminal justice system, and on gaining support for a halfway house for women in the community. This house would serve both as an alternative to incarceration for nonviolent offenders and as an intermediate step back into the community after release from prison.

Currently, an effort is underway to collaborate with a very successful halfway house for treatment of addictions in the Albany area. The founder and inspiration, Rev. Peter Young, will be working with us to continue our efforts to establish a halfway house for women and children in the Syracuse area.

Collaborating Personnel

Interreligious Council Staff. Staff The Interreligious Council staff is minimally involved in hands-on program activities, but they have been supportive of the efforts. The associate director in charge of Exodus has written the grants and created the basic design of the program. Fundraising and public relations efforts of this sponsoring group benefit Project Exodus as well.

Exodus Staff. Currently, the Exodus case manager is the only full-time staff person working in the program. Three other staff people are present for the 2-hour Mothers' and Children's Visiting Program. The children's therapist began with the program as a volunteer assistant. When the previous therapist could no longer continue in the program, she recommended the current therapist as a suitable replacement. The children's assistant also started with the program as a volunteer, and as the numbers of clients grew, it became evident that more staff was needed. This volunteer was asked to join as a [paid] staff person. The latest addition to our staff was hired as an assistant but, because of her background in running parenting classes and other groups, was asked to lead the mothers' support group.

There is good cohesion among the four people who work together in the visiting program. They are firmly committed to our purpose, and all have at heart the welfare of the children. Each person does extra little things, often without being asked. This shows a personal investment in the good of the clients. Good judgment and careful selection of staff is essential to a good program, particularly one like this, that has never been done before, which often needs improvisation, and which has needed to prove itself at every turn.

Stakeholders: Who Benefits?

Foster Care System. A meeting was held with administrative personnel from both Exodus and foster care. The proposed visiting program was explained to the foster care personnel. It was agreed that in families where foster care was involved, permission for the incarcerated mother to visit in the context of our visiting program would be sought. This is necessary because there are cases in which the mother has been charged with abuse or neglect and is not allowed to see the children without direct foster care supervision. Many times the charges stem from having or using drugs in the presence of the children.

Our program provided an advantage to the foster care workers because, with their heavy caseloads, they were glad to have some visits provided by us.

Prison Personnel. Correctional facilities are, of necessity, run very strictly. Security is very tight, and adherence to rules is essential. The security personnel at the prison undoubtedly provided the greatest challenge. The Mothers' and Children's' Visiting Program was held in the visiting room. Normally, during regular visiting times, inmates sit on one side of the table and visitors on the other. Noise is at a minimum, and two guards are present at all times. One guard is male, the other female. Each inmate is allowed two visitors. Children may visit only if accompanied by an adult. Infants and toddlers must be held on someone's lap and are not allowed to leave the chair or lap at any time.

Compare this with our visiting program, which also takes place in the visiting room, under the surveillance of security personnel, with children visiting mothers and staff people facilitating. No tables separate the mothers and children. Hugs and kisses abound. Laughter and noise is very evident. The energy level is very high. Mothers may read stories or help children draw pictures. They catch up on news from home and school.

Then the mothers and children separate into their groups. In one room, the mothers talk and express feelings, sometimes loudly and vehemently, sometimes joyfully, gently, and tearfully. In the large visiting room, the children sit on mats on the floor, talk, laugh, and sometimes argue. They play thoughtful card and board games. They play active games, like Follow the Leader. These activities lead into discussions of feelings and into other more quiet activities. Many of these children have been disturbed and made insecure. They do not always appear as model children.

In the beginning, security personnel understandably had difficulty adjusting to this—understandably, because if anything did get out of hand, the security personnel would be responsible.

Gradually, however, the officers became more used to us. Week after week, they saw that we could handle what was happening. Week after week, they saw our willingness to cooperate with them as far as possible. Things improved to the point where one guard agreed to wear the paper hat that one boy made just for him. Another officer no longer calls the children "rug rats" because he knows we do not approve. Now he only does it to get a rise out of us.

This program also helps to maintain discipline in the prison because the visiting program is a privilege of which an inmate can be deprived. Many women tell about times when they would have argued or caused trouble but refrained because they did not want to lose this privilege.

Volunteers. Presently, we have several volunteers who serve in various capacities. Our volunteers who transport children to visits were recruited from churches and by word of mouth. There have been several newspaper articles and a TV feature about our program. This also brought us several volunteers. Besides doing transport, volunteers work in the office, speak to groups, provide donations of clothing, housewares, and furniture, and organize these donations. We have to do very little to convince these people that what we do is worthwhile. They are already very caring people, and know the value of helping others.

One woman says, "I just can't say no to you." I tell her that this is because she isn't saying no to me, but to someone who really needs her help.

Funding Sources. The main source of funding of our program is the New York State Department of Social Services (DSS) . We have a demonstration grant from this department. Our sponsoring organization, the Interreligious Council, also secures donations from the United Way, and from churches, groups, and individuals.

We are often invited to speak to various groups, and to be interviewed for media features. This serves to get the word out, and to gain community support for what we are all about.

Clients. Participation in Exodus and in the visiting program is voluntary on the part of the client. The mother–child attachment is probably the strongest motivation anyone can have for doing anything. I believe that this relationship is a very strong reason for the success of and demand for this program.

Caretakers. Family or foster parents are contacted when a child is to participate in the visiting program. Often there are several children in these households, in addition to the person's own children. These people have numerous demands placed upon them. Some of them may know the mother who is incarcerated and disapprove of her life style. Then we must convince them that it is still a good thing for the children to have some contact with their mother. Often, these families do not have the time or the means of transportation to take children to visit at the prison. Our program fills that need.

Children. Most children want to participate in the visiting program. Some have never visited a prison before. It is a new and scary experience for some of them. Some feel duty-bound to visit, while really hating to go to the prison. Some are so used to visiting prison that it is pretty routine. It is sad to think that some children are socialized to see prison as just another part of life.

A few children have said that they wanted to stay at the prison with their mothers. Then we needed to show them that it is not really a good place to be and that what they see is only part of it.

CASE EXAMPLE: EXODUS CASE MANAGEMENT

Ruth's case provides an extended example of Exodus case management. At the recommendation of her counselor at Jamesville, Ruth applied for Project Exodus. She was interviewed by the case manager and was found to have many needs. The most immediate and pressing of these concerned her 18-month-old daughter, who had a heart defect and needed surgery. Ruth was released from prison early with probation so she could be present at the hospital during the procedure.

When Ruth was incarcerated, the child was placed in the custody of the father temporarily. He and his family looked after the child. Since the father and Ruth were now estranged, this added stress to an already tense situation. Again, it was the grandmother who provided most of the care for the child.

In going to prison, Ruth had lost everything. She left prison with the clothes on her back and little else. She had some friends who lived about 15 miles outside the city. There was no public transportation. Ruth had only one family member to help her, and he lived in another city. She had no income, food, clothing, and no support system to speak of. This is the woman who now had to, and wanted to, be a good mother to her daughter during her surgery.

She depended upon the case manager and the people she lived with for transportation to and from the hospital. She would stay at the hospital for 2 or 3 days at a time, go home briefly, and then go back. She would sleep in the pediatric waiting room when she could not be with her child.

The baby came through the surgery very well, and leads a nearly normal life with the aid of a pacemaker that may be removed in time.

Even with the best of friends, staying in someone else's house when one cannot contribute gets very stressful when it continues for any length of time. During and after the surgery, Ruth had no time or interest to look for her own apartment or to create an income for herself. It was only after the baby was through the surgery that she could put her mind to these other pressing needs.

The case manager made the 30-mile round trip with her to the hospital very often. She was there for support and encouragement as well. She connected Ruth with a pantry for emergency food. She took her to the Exodus clothing room to find clothes. She made an appointment for her to apply for public assistance. Ruth was on probation, so she also needed to go to see her probation officer once a week. Every 15-mile trip for Ruth was 30 for the case manager, who had to travel the distance to meet Ruth. Ruth also had to deal with the custody of the child being decided in court. Ruth was also in need of addiction counseling. That was completely tabled during this high-stress period.

Through all of this the relationship with the friends with whom she was staying became increasingly strained. Finally, she decided to leave that house and get the money for a motel from her uncle. This was a very short-term solution, and now housing was added to the list of needs. She could not be convinced to go to an emergency shelter. Needless to say, during this period, each day was an adventure.

She came to the Exodus office to go through the newspaper for rentals and use the phone to call about them. Then trips to see apartments began. It is very difficult to find a decent apartment on a public assistance budget, so this process was long and tedious. There was also the fact that even when an apartment was secured, there was no furniture. In looking at furnished apartments, one of our leads was successful. Ruth soon moved into a furnished apartment that seemed to be just what she needed. Then there were problems with the landlady, and Ruth was again looking for a place. She finally found one, unfurnished, and now the search began for furniture. We went to a church thrift shop and found a good deal of what she needed. The managers were very kind and, since there was an affiliation with Exodus, gave the furniture for free. They also arranged to have it delivered.

Ruth continues to deal with court, probation, and getting help for her addiction. She is also looking for work to supplement, and eventually replace, her income from public assistance.

Ruth finally lost custody of her daughter when the case was settled in family court. The father's family was seen as a more stable, established household, and a better primary environment for the child.

Though Ruth continues to assert that she does not use alcohol, it may or may not be the case. She continues to make poor judgments about the use of money and to depend heavily on other people for her basic needs. She is allowed to see her daughter, but the length of the trip to where she lives is prohibitive.

She did go back to jail to finish the short part of her term she had left and to eliminate the need to be on probation. I have not heard from her for several months; her last call was a request for money and furniture, which, at that point, I felt it best to deny.

I believe Ruth does love her child. Perhaps one day Ruth will make enough progress to gain custody. We can only hope for the best, whatever that is.

SUMMARY

Project Exodus facilitates the ongoing relationships of incarcerated mothers and their children in many ways because of the primary belief that these relationships are of central importance to both. Many times we have demonstrated that both children and their mothers can and will make significant changes in their behavior and life styles in order to be together. Our staff and the involved volunteers have found that it is well worth the considerable effort required to assist them in reaching and maintaining these goals.

17

Working with Families in the Schools

Barbara King
Lora Randolph
William A. McKay
Markus Bartell

When children enter formal schooling, they enter a world of peers and adults in which their families are often not included. While this is a valued developmental step toward personal individuation and participation in the society-at-large, it is really no time for youngsters to disconnect from their families. The institution of counseling programs for children in schools has, on the one hand, provided immediate response to painful problems that manifest themselves in school for many children. But, on the other hand, school counseling has tended to focus on the child either as the container of his or her own pathology or as the victim of an uncaring, dysfunctional, or even exploitative family. Far from assisting children to cope more effectively with their difficulties manifested in school, this approach to counseling risks accentuating difficulties and may undermine the child's access to his or her primary resource system.

This chapter is not intended as an instructional manual on family therapy in the schools, but an attempt to describe the development of a systemic program that provides family counseling within the school. Our point of view is that of an insider rather than a consultant coming from the outside.

The title of this book, *Children in Families at Risk,* says it all. How could we begin to respond to the needs of the children we serve if we did not consider the context from which the children come? Equally important is viewing the system in which we ply our trade as part of the child's context, a part that is often overlooked. The growth and development of our systemic response to the needs of the people we work with—peers, students, and families, as well as the school district—seems natural and quite logical. It is so natural, that explaining it is difficult—rather like trying to explain evolution, or how fire was discovered; there is a certain amount of spontaneity that was involved. How did we wind up with an elementary family counseling program in Hutchinson, Kansas?

Our little stroke of lightening or useful genetic mutation occurred in the spring of 1989, when a second-grader attempted to hang himself at recess with a jump rope. The superintendent and the director of special education were called to respond because the principal, the school psychologist, and the district's school social worker were not available. In the past, cases like this were typically referred for mental health services outside of the school system, but because of increased caseloads and limited time to spend on nonbillable contacts, responses to school problems were limited and were often a poor fit. In fairness to the service providers, it should be noted that they have had very little experience in dealing with the educational system on a regular basis. On the other hand, the school system typically has maintained a cautious response to outside intervention. Consequently, the interaction between the two systems has not been very smooth. Because of that lack of smoothness and the previous director of special education's personal interest in working directly with families, the school social worker was hired under the title of "home–school specialist." The focus of that position was to attend to the needs of the family and the interaction between the family and the school. Prior to the self-destructive episode by the second-grader, the district administrators were very supportive of the school social worker's efforts to work within the framework of the home–school specialist position. At the same time, they had reservations concerning the effectiveness of the typical elementary guidance programs.

In response to the crisis, it became apparent that there was a need to have on hand in each of the elementary school buildings people who would not only respond to incidents such as this one, but also be able to respond to the needs of the family. The superintendent has a master's degree in counseling, but he felt that the typical approach of the guidance counseling model would not meet the needs of today's students and the school system. The superintendent had worked closely with the school social worker and felt that the home–school specialist approach would more effectively meet the needs of the system. The dilemma was, as in most cases, how to pay for new positions in a time when there did not seem to be enough resources for the people who were currently employed.

The superintendent and school board opted to appeal to the State Board of Tax Appeals for a variance on our tax base, a procedure that did not require a vote by the public but that allowed the district to increase the tax base by one mill. The intent was to hire people based on their focus of working with families rather than based on an elementary guidance counseling degree. This variance raised over $360,000 for staff and equipment. In the interim period, several counseling programs in surrounding communities of comparable size were observed. It was found that the traditional school guidance counseling model predominated, and it was decided that the family therapy model being used by the school social worker was the model that would be expanded to provide services for all students.

The next hurdle was finding 11 qualified professionals who wanted to work with families. It seems that the interviewing process is like a courtship, in which both sides are more concerned with the process rather than content. An early mistake made during the interviewing and hiring process was the failure to define the term "working with families." The assumption was made that the people hired wanted to learn how to do family therapy and become family therapists. The functioning of the program has been affected by individual interpretations of this term. In subsequent interviews we have been clearer that the prospective counselors have a clear definition of "working with families," and have taken the approach of asking the prospective counselor about their reasons for wanting to shift from being a guidance counselor to being a systemic family therapist. This keeps the program clearly committed to the process of developing an elementary family counseling program. Services of the school social worker/home–school specialist were secured to provide training and supervision to the counselors. The need for supervision had been discussed in the interviewing process, but we didn't know how important this was to become in addressing professional differences and as an essential to ongoing professional growth.

PROGRAM DESCRIPTION

The program has strong support from central administration. The intent is to develop a family-systems-oriented school counseling program that would enhance or improve the overall experience of the participants in USD 308 (our public elementary school in Hutchinson, Kansas). Provision of services focuses on behavior as interactional rather than cause-and-effect, on what is happening or not happening rather than who is to blame, and on outcome of the behavior rather on the behavior itself. The overall effect of this approach puts the counselor in the role of observer/participant. It changes the role to one of consultant rather than fixer.

The system, rather than the individual student, becomes our client, the consumer of our services. Naturally, this approach presents a conflict between the expectations of the consumer and the service provided by the counselor. Consumers of services understandably do not expect to be seen as interactive participants in the difficulty. Their view is closer to what Cottone (1991) describes as the "psychological world view which focuses on the individual and on traits or conditions of an individual. . . . The individual is viewed as assessable and treatable, and intervention is aimed at the client rather than at social or cultural factors that might be affecting the individual" (p. 398).

This model can best be summed up as an ecological/systemic one that places emphasis on the interaction of individuals with and within an environmental context. The focus is on the interaction of the parts of the whole rather than on the parts in isolation. We believe that the sum of the parts is greater than the whole. The task is twofold: how to educate the consumer on how the systemic approach works and how to structure requests for services so that the referral can be handled in a systemic manner. Inherent in our task is to improve the quality of the relationship between home and school, and, overall, to empower all of the participants. We all need to see ourselves as interacting rather than being acted upon.

The program's theoretical framework is based on a family systems orientation. The interventions are based primarily on a structural model. Within the past 2 years, solution-focused theoretical concepts have been incorporated. Intergenerational concepts are also used to frame the interaction in a historical sense. McGoldrick's Family Life Cycle (Carter & McGoldrick, 1988) is also used to provide additional understanding of the context of the interaction. The family is viewed as an open system that functions in relation to its broader context—extended family, neighborhood, community, school, national and international issues, and economic trends—and evolves over a life cycle that is somewhat definable.

We believe that the family and systems operate in a somewhat predictable fashion in accordance with the principles of circular causality, nonsummativity, equifinality, communication, family rules, homeostasis, and morphogenesis, among others (Walsh, 1984). We have given some examples of how these concepts have been used within this program.

Circular causality, the behavior of one individual influencing the actions within the group, and *nonsummativity,* the concept that the system is more than a simple addition of the characteristics of the individual entities, can be seen in the following case.

A fifth-grade student, Andy, was referred because he refused to attend school. He reported that he was being harassed by some of his peers. The harassment was so painful for him that he refused to come to school unless he was forced to do so by his mother. She would drag her son into the school with the child screaming and pulling back. After the mother had deposited her son in his classroom, she would meet with the principal to complain about the teacher being unable to protect her son from the classroom bullies.

After this had continued for several days, the principal was able to convince the mother to come in for family counseling. It was determined by the counselor that the boy was being harassed by his classmates, but there were other factors in his context, as well. His parents had recently been divorced, and his mother was showing signs of depression. She spent most of her time grieving the loss of her marriage. On many days the only time she would stop crying and leave her bedroom was when it was necessary to force her son to attend school. After the morning confrontation with her son and the school principal, she would usually apply herself to the daily chores.

The mother was never able to identify this sequence of events, but as she met with the counselor she was able to vent her anger, assess her strengths, and find some options for her life. When this occurred, her son seemed to become free to solve his own problems and was able to respond to the classroom harassment. When the harassment diminished, he stopped refusing to attend school.

Equifinality indicates that beginning events do not necessarily determine outcomes, nor do identical outcomes originate from identical beginnings. For example, two parents of unrelated students may be involved in the school: One is there as a volunteer library aide and the other comes because of his or her child's defiant behavior. Similarly, two students come from similar situations of lower socioeconomic conditions and single-parent families, but one graduates as a honor roll student, a positive leader, and the other is involved in drugs and violence. Both came from similar backgrounds and possessed similar abilities to achieve.

Noncommunication is seen as virtually impossible. There are two parts to each piece of communication—the message, or content, and that which defines the relationship, how the information is to be taken or acted upon. An example of this two-part interaction would be a teacher making contact with a family, and through the contact making a referral to the counselor. The teacher's concern (the content) is that the student lacks motivational skills in the classroom. The parents' reaction is to the part of the message that defined them as "one down" because there is something wrong with their child. The message they received was that not only was something wrong with their child but also there was something wrong with them.

Family rules define the organizing structure for how the family interacts with each other and other systems. When approaching a family it is important to observe the interaction of family members to gain a working knowledge of these rules. The counselor is aware of who speaks to whom, who interrupts, and who speaks first. How do the family members elicit permission to speak and what to speak about? Who gives permission to speak and about what?

Homeostasis is the process by which the family maintains a balance through either negative or positive feedback. Too much or too little of a required interaction activates the homeostatic devices that correct the deviation. The task of the counselor is to tune into the system's efforts to maintain balance. For example, a single parent with children may be functioning satisfactorily until she brings in a male friend. Then the children may begin to act out until the family can settle down into a new equilibrium.

Morphogenesis is the other side of homeostasis — the flexibility required to adapt to the demands of the environment, the family life cycle. Working with the principle of morphogenesis may involve helping a family to modify family rules to develop a new balancing pattern that accounts for developmental changes. An example would be dealing with a family in which the oldest child has left home and a young sibling attempts to fill the gap left by the absent sibling. An individual's problems can be seen as the outward sign of the system's struggle to maintain a balance between homeostasis and morphogenesis.

Counselors work from a family systems orientation, but we generally follow the structural model developed by Minuchin and his colleagues in our work with families.

A goal of the Hutchinson Elementary Family Counseling Program is to provide family-oriented counseling that centers on a systemic approach to intervention in student-centered problems. In using this model, we intend to be catalysts for change in the family, in the student, in the school, and in the community. This effort may best be described as a pebble that is thrown into a pond, causing never-ending ripples in ever widening circles.

Counselors use the family systems approach to empower families to make positive adjustments. Through a flexible time option, counselors can set appointments for day or evening depending on the work schedules of the families. The family services include providing family counseling and involvement, providing family advocacy, helping families secure and receive community services, and acting as a liaison between the family, school, and other mental health service providers.

Counselors work with instructors, administrators, and other staff members on perceived areas of need. This is accomplished by helping instructors develop educational strategies to meet the needs of individual students, developing and conducting in-service programs for staff members, and acting as a liaison between staff and families.

REFERRAL

An important aspect of this program is the referral process. We generally understand that intervention begins with the referral. The attitude with which the family initiates or responds to the referral sets the climate for the intervention. Initially, we sought to simplify the access for all involved individuals. The referral process allowed principals, teachers, parents, students, and community members to initiate a referral to the counselor, and then the counselor would make the initial contact. This, though successful in a traditional guidance counseling model, created obstacles for the school family counselor. The third party referrals, ones in which the family becomes aware of the referral when the counselor contacts them with the offer to do family counseling, were generally responded to in one of two ways—anger that someone thought the family needed counseling, or minimizing, by thinking it was for a parent–teacher conference. Both responses seemed to be of a linear nature, and the families were understandably defensive. Usually the student, or the student's behavior, rather than interactions, remained the focus of meetings. The overall message for the counselor was one of "here is the problem . . . fix it." As a result, we realized that for the counseling to be effective it would be necessary for someone in the family unit to identify the need for help and for that person to make contact with the family counselor.

Effort has been made to involve teachers and principals (referral sources) in making the first contact with families and for them to advise the families that school-based family counseling was available without charge. The referral source serves as the first contact and encourages a family member to get in touch with the family counselor and gives direction on how this can be accomplished. This provides encouragement and support to the family members without diminishing the autonomy of the family. It is our belief that by following through on referrals in this manner, the family as well as the counseling process is strengthened.

Case Example: The Referral Process

Darrel's classroom teacher approached his parents concerning 6-year-old Darrel's irrational fears. These included extreme fear of storms, fear of being kidnapped, and fear of going on field trips with his classmates. The parents agreed with the teacher that Darrel's reaction to these events was inappropriate and concurred that help was needed. The teacher suggested the parents contact the school's family counselor and discuss their concerns. Darrel's mother stopped the counselor in the hallway and requested an opportunity to visit. The mother showed apprehension and embarrassment over the contact, but stated that they had been discussing the possibility of seeking professional help; however, they were embarrassed about their need and worried about the cost. After the mother was reassured by the counselor that family counseling was offered to families of the school without charge and that many parents seek consultation and help with parenting, she was willing to set an appointment. A time was arranged that would accommodate the father's work schedule.

At the first meeting it became apparent that the mother was over-solicitous toward her 6-year-old son. When asked why they were having this meeting, Darrel responded, "because of my fears." His mother supported this, describing in detail Darrel's crying and upset stomach when clouds appeared in the sky or when there was any hint that the parents might go somewhere without him. The father was quiet but protective of the mother, patting her hand when she seemed worried. His concern seemed to center more on his wife than on the son, and he stated that he was afraid she would have "a nervous breakdown" if the stress continued. When asked why he thought this, he appeared evasive and uncomfortable, making statements such as "all of this stuff with Darrel."

In the first session we gathered information about the genogram, what the family members thought it would look like if the problems were solved. They all agreed that if Darrel's fears were absent he would be free to visit and play with other children, participate in school trips without his mother accompanying him, and continue in class activities without becoming ill and demanding that his mother be called when storms came up while he was at school. Also (no surprise), Darrel's parents would be able to have a night out without Darrel becoming distraught and ill.

The counselor asked the parents to come without Darrel to the second meeting. This required negotiations between the parents and Darrel, and they finally arrived at a compromise, that Darrel would visit an older brother. When the parents came to the second meeting it was evident that they wanted to talk about their real concern that Darrel would learn from some extended family members that he was their adopted son and the biological son of an older daughter. Their fears were that he would be hurt and angry and would reject both of them and the older daughter who Darrel identified as his sister. Through the counseling process the family was able to deal with the family secret, and Darrel's fears diminished so that he was able to participate actively in school. The positive outcome of this situation can be attributed, in part, to the referral procedure utilized by the teacher.

Elementary students are allowed to make self-referrals. The counselor may interact with a student on an individual basis to discuss the child's concerns. The family is engaged in the process when it becomes apparent that this is not a temporary problem but one that involves the system-at-large in an identifiable interactive pattern. In short, if it is something more than my dog died or someone is calling me a dirty name, the counselor will quickly engage the larger system. In one such case, some students approached the counselor with concerns regarding a friend's eating habits. They had observed that one of their peers was not eating much lunch and was vomiting what food she did eat. The counselor talked to the student and then called the parent, who was not receptive to the counselor's offer of help, but acknowledged that she recognized that there was a problem and she was working with the family physician on this issue. The counselor was able to respond to the concerns of the peer group, even without the family agreeing to be seen by the family counselor. All referrals do not necessarily result in opening a case, initially, as the following case illustrates.

> A counselor received a call from a grandparent who wanted counseling for her and her grandson, Richard, who had been suspended from school. Counseling had been recommended by the suspension hearing officer as a prerequisite for returning to school. Upon further inquiry it was learned that the home was comprised of the grandparents, their son, who was the grandson's father, and the grandson's older sister. The parents were divorced and the mother was living separately. We agreed to provide counseling but stipulated that everyone would need to come in for the first session. The grandmother raised the ante at this point by saying that if the father found out that his son (her grandson) had been suspended, which was the reason for the referral, he would send the boy to live with his mother. The counselor again suggested that the best approach would be to have everyone in to sort out how best to understand this dilemma. The grandmother upped the ante yet again by saying that a psychologist had said that if the boy was forced to live with his mother he would either run away or commit suicide. It should also be noted that the contact was made by the grandmother on the fourth day of a 5-day suspension and that the father was unaware of the suspension. The counselor was supportive, but insistent, that he needed to work with the system as a unit. The grandmother refused services. The referring administrator was contacted, and the importance of beginning work with the family as a unit was explained. The administrator was supportive of the decision to provide family counseling, but because of the school's desire to meet the needs of the student, we elected to work with the student in the context of the classroom, since we were unable to engage the family system directly.

The focus of intervention at this point will be working with the classroom teachers and administrators to develop a supportive behavioral plan. According to Senge (1990), "It is vital to hold to critical performance standards through 'thick and thin' and to do whatever it takes to meet those standards. The standards that are most important are those that matter most to the customer. They usually include product quality, delivery service, service reliability and quality, and friendliness and concern of service personnel " (p. 123). Product quality, in this case, family counseling, cannot be maintained if the deliverer of the product is not able to follow the original design or intent of the program. One other critical standard for this program is that of how referrals are handled. Initial contact has to be made by the family. The counselor does not make the first contact. The school system is not always fully supportive of these two standards, and this challenges the ability of the counselor to remain flexible and open while adhering to what appear to be vital performance standards.

Parents will frequently make contact, saying that the court or the state child welfare agency ordered counseling services to be provided for their child. A typical response would be "Yes, I will work with your child but the entire family needs to come in as well." Efforts have been made to enlist the help of the family to respond to the difficulty regardless of where the referral originated. The partnership between family and counselor is vital, and if the family is at first reluctant to involve themselves in the process, the family's autonomy is acknowledged. Frequently, at a later date, the family will take the initiative to contact the counselor.

CONTINUING EDUCATION

Ten elementary school counselors were initially hired to fill the positions in the new counseling program. Counselors were interviewed with the intent of clarifying that the position would involve working with families within the school, a concept that was interpreted on an individual basis and fit into each counselor's understanding of what working with families meant. Some counselors came from previous school guidance counseling positions that focused on fixing the child, and some came directly from teaching positions and were influenced by the parent–teacher conference approach to working with families. Counselors received intensive training prior to the start of the first year. In those first sessions it was as if the trainers were speaking a foreign language. It became clear at that point, as counselors heard about genograms, ecomaps, homeostasis, triangling, and differentiation, that "working with families" took on a whole new, somewhat frightening meaning. The experience must have been something akin to what Rip Van Winkle experienced as he arose after his 20-year sleep.

Training has continued throughout these first 6 years. In-service sessions in solution-focused therapy, working with families with an incarcerated member, and in using family functioning assessment tools such as Fundamental Interpersonal Relational Orientation (FIRO; Doherty, Colangelo, & Hovander, 1991) and the McMaster Model of Family Functioning (Walsh, 1984) have been provided by instructors from Wichita State University and Friends University.

Most counselors have taken coursework in family therapy, ethics, crisis intervention, and other related subjects. The district has been supportive of counselors attending American Association for Marriage and Family Therapy state and national conferences, presenting our program to various organizations and school counseling programs, and participating in various workshops.

PERFORMANCE EVALUATION, SUPERVISION/CONSULTATION, AND FEEDBACK

Performance Evaluation

Each counselor has both a building supervisor, the principal, and a clinical supervisor or consultant. Currently, the elementary principal is the immediate supervisor of the counselor. The counselors are directly responsible to the principal at the building to which each is assigned. The building principals are the individuals who will complete the statutory performance evaluation for the counselors as stipulated in the negotiated agreement.

The document that is used for the counselor evaluation is a slightly modified form of the performance evaluation used for teachers. A cooperative effort between the principal and the counselor is necessary to make this a useful process. In some cases the principals have included the home–school specialist/social worker in this collaborative effort. Like many evaluation processes, this is still not fully satisfactory and is continuously evolving.

Supervision/Consultation

The purposes of clinical supervision of the counselors in the elementary family counseling program are (1) to provide staff development for counselors to improve their counseling techniques and expertise, (2) to monitor the quality of services provided to students and/or families, and (3) to insure that the focus on family systems remains the program emphasis.

Some common and perhaps unique training and supervision issues are created when working with school counselors who work with families. Frequently, school counselor training is in a nonsystemic approach, and retraining in systemic thinking needs to occur. Clinical supervision is an ongoing process of counselor assistance and training in which the focus of clinical supervision is to assist supervisees in identifying techniques and strategies needed to acquire or refine effectiveness in delivering a truly systemic counseling approach. Supervision for school personnel generally connotes evaluation. Therefore, asking for regular supervision with school counselors is often taken to imply that the counselor is failing. Joining with the counselor in addressing common systemic issues is critical to provide the rapport necessary for training and supervision to occur. In addition, most counselors are not accustomed to the intensity of videotaping or live supervision. Each supervisee makes videotapes of family sessions for review and analysis by the counselor as well as review, analysis, and feedback in supervision. Supervision includes working with peers in reviewing cases as well as following up with pertinent articles and books. Supervision is usually 4 hours per week and is typically accomplished in a group setting, with individual supervision done on an as-needed basis. In supervision, the counselor presents his or her case using a format (Ault-Riché, 1982) that includes a genogram, videotape, and a description of the identified patterns of interaction. Supervision guidelines follow:

   I. Identification of the family: Have a genogram showing the names, ages, dates of birth, marriages, separations, divorces, and deaths. Include the cause of death and current physical/emotional health status. List other significant events such as important moves, separations, financial changes, illness onset, accidents, and so forth.
  II. Diagram the boundaries, coalitions, alliances, and triangles.
 III. Family assessment:
     A. How did this family come to you? Referral source? Who else is involved in the process? Who is the "customer for change?
     B. What is the presenting issue/problem as the family members state it? What does each want to accomplish through family work?
     C. What is your understanding of the issue(s) in terms of structural theory—for example, hierarchy, subsystem functioning, boundaries, context, developmental stage, resonance, or flexibility.
     D. What is your understanding of the issue(s) in terms of strategic theory; that is, what is the sequence of behaviors (the dance around) the problem? What are the solutions that the family has tried so far?
     E. What is your understanding of the issue(s) in terms of systemic theory—for example, what positive function can be hypothesized for each member's behavior? What dilemma can you pose for the family?
     F. What is your understanding of the issue(s) in terns of multigenerational theory (Bowen)?
       (i) Describe the nuclear family emotional process: Which of the four options for responding to anxiety/tension is used—

spouse dysfunction, distance, marital conflict, or child function?

(ii). Describe the multigenerational transmission process, that is, the sequence of events over time as related to the four types of responses to anxiety/tension.

IV. Counselor's behavior:

A. What have you done to date with the family? What was the impact/influence of that action? How could this impact/influence have been different?

B. What difficulties are you encountering? How are you triangled? What about the family confuses, puzzles, seduces, or hooks you? What about the family's system (dance, sequence, affect) facilitates your induction into the system?

C What patterns/sequences/dances of the family are isomorphically appearing in therapy?

D. What are you asking of your supervisor?

Supervision has evolved into a collaborative effort in which the supervision group develops strategies and interventions. In the fourth year, a choice of consultation grew out of feedback from some counselors. It was expressed by some that supervision was not meeting their needs for a variety of reasons, and they preferred a less structured approach to reviewing their work. These counselors participated at a level with which they felt more comfortable. At this level there was no formal agreement about the tasks to be accomplished. Generally, participation at the consultation level was a great deal less involved than at the supervision level. After a year of working with a dual model, it was decided to return to a single approach in which all counselors participate in supervision at the same level.

Feedback

Questionnaires (see Appendix 17.1) are sent to the referral sources as well as the clients for additional feedback. The responses have been useful in that support is provided for the program. The questionnaires also provide the opportunity for the participants to voice concerns at a low-risk level.

ADVANTAGES AND DISADVANTAGES
OF THE PROGRAM

For the counselor to be available to the family within the school is advantageous because some families would not seek help outside the school.

Problems within a family affect the child in his or her larger context. Dealing with the family and the school personnel within the same frame may often stimulate a more cooperative atmosphere. When a family seeks services outside the school, there is usually limited contact between the provider and the school personnel. The situation becomes frustrating, and the productivity of counseling drops off because of less-than-effective communication between the two systems.

Another advantage of having a family systems person in the school is that he or she at times can act as a buffer between the family and the school. This can help when the family sees the school as the enemy and, for their part, the school personnel may not grasp their parts in the uncomfortable interactions. The family counselor's proximity encourages the student and family to feel comfortable seeking out services.

A strength of this program is that it brings together the family and the school. Typically, families have had concerns about what happened to their children within the realm of the school, and teachers have had concerns about what was taking place in the homes of their students. The systemic counselor can bring these concerns together in a way that facilitates growth and improves communication. In this way the development of problematic triangles between the home and school are avoided.

> This type of intervention is demonstrated in a case where the counselor overheard a teacher describing the tales told by Judy, a student. These tales depicted some frightening events that supposedly occurred in Judy's home. The counselor had worked with the family in responding to some previously prefabricated stories told by the student. With this knowledge, the counselor was able to orchestrate a meeting of the teacher, the student, and the parents that was supportive of the child but at the same time confronted the false stories. The teacher and the parents were able to reframe the stories in such a way as to build on the student's creative skills and at the same time emphasize the importance of honesty. Judy and the teacher worked together to write, edit, and type the story, which was then given to the family as an example of her creative capabilities. In this case, the counselor was able to bring the teacher and the family together to productively respond to a concern. Both the teacher and the parents were pleased with the response of the other, and this communication helped to encourage the child.

At times facilitating change within the classroom system may be exceedingly difficult and at other times may be as easy as a single effort to reframe a troubling issue or event.

> This was the case when a teacher reported that one student was very active, failing to follow instructions, and behaving unacceptably in class.

The counselor's statement that it was fortunate that the child had found a teacher who could accept that behavior as being an expression of needing structure, limits, and understanding seemed to refocus the teacher's responses. Later, when the counselor inquired about the student, the teacher reported that she and the child were getting along well, and even though the child seemed to need a great deal of structure and attention the situation had improved. Evidently, the counselor's statement created a negative feedback loop that resulted in a changed perception by the teacher. This perception allowed the teacher to tolerate some behaviors and look for productive ways to respond.

Frequently, a family feels that the school has no business meddling in the family's affairs or is resistant to seeing a family counselor within the school. Past experiences within the school environment do affect a family's attitude toward counseling in the school.

Providing family counseling within the school eliminates the economic stress of spending money for counseling. This makes counseling available to families who would not budget or have the money to budget for counseling. On the other hand, families might not be as committed to show up for appointments or as committed to change without the monetary investment.

A school-based family therapy program has its disadvantages. One disadvantage is that the counselors can find themselves in the center of triangling efforts by various parts of the systems with which they are working. For example, the family pulls to align the counselor with them, or the school personnel pull to have the counselor side with them against the family. Remaining neutral is the desirable way to deal with competing systems as they interrelate. Supervision has proven to be helpful in maintaining neutrality or recognizing that the counselor has been pulled in by one side or the other.

A related issue is the difficulty in staying differentiated, remaining systemic in the approach to dealing with the concerns expressed. Pressure can also be exerted to have the counselor fit in by covering classrooms, going on field trips, taking lunch room and recess duty, and baking cookies rather than by providing family therapy services or being a consultant to the system. It is fairly typical for the school to want counselors to perform multiple tasks. Doing these tasks defines the counselor as a guidance counselor rather than a family systems counselor. The central issue in the definition of the counselor's role grows out of how we define the area of concern. Is the concern seen from the perspective of blaming (cause and effect) or is it seen as a systemic issue? Are the patterns of interaction looked at and are interventions designed or is blame assigned? If blame is placed, then the system becomes uncomfortable with an interactive view and moves to reaffirm the original problem-solving style. Regardless of the success level, this is not unlike a family faced with the need to change but uncomfortable with the uncertainty of change. The other part of this dilemma is the counselor's own struggles with change and learning new skills. Others may not see the counselor within the school as being a "professional" counselor. Mental health service providers outside the school may look at the school-based family counselors as embodying the typical, historic guidance counseling view and think they are stepping out of their boundaries. However, through multiple interactions with various mental health providers in the community, the program and the family counselors are being seen as a viable, realistic, and competent resource in the community.

ETHICS

Dual relationships are a concern for family counselors working within the school system. Establishing roles within the school has been one of the most difficult aspects of the new position as family counselors. This position is different from any previous roles held by the counselors, whether they were teachers or guidance counselors. Counselors found themselves alone in a new position and found there were different expectations for the job than their previous ones. How were relationships to be defined with the people who just a few short years, months, or days ago were not clients, but were peers, students, or parents. One of the first steps which had to be taken was to define the position for counselors and then for those with whom they would work. Counselors soon discovered that they were no longer a part of the faculty, as they were before. Looking at the interactions that occur from such simple things as eating lunch in the teachers' lounge or baking cookies for social events, it is clear that it is too easy to get caught in a triangling conversation with staff. A remark made during supervision about sharing only information that would be helpful to the family in the therapeutic process can be used as a filter through which to let information flow before sharing it with others involved in the system. Establishing the role and how it would fit in was mostly a process of trial and error as the counselors defined their position within the school system for the themselves and others. Another aspect of dual relationships stems from the tradition that as teachers it was customary to receive gifts from the students at Christmas or at the end of the year. How does this fit into the counseling relationship? Do we eat dinner with our clients or buy products from them? Supervision has been critical in helping us define these relationships.

Confidentiality, as mentioned earlier, is a major issue in any therapeutic counseling relationship. As a transition from school guidance counseling to family systemic counseling was made, it became necessary to put new emphasis on the importance of confidentiality. The passing of information between educational staff, teachers, principals, and other educational specialists seems to happen frequently and with ease. Information is handed from one professional to the other during building team meetings, Individual Education Plan meetings, and in the faculty lounge. This handling of information with little constraint may or may not be detrimental to the student, but does present a dilemma to a family counselor working within this system. It also, quite frankly, affects the interaction between the school and outside mental health practitioners. Teachers and school personnel may think that when the therapist has relevant information that could be used in providing an appropriate educational plan for a student that information should be shared in a collaborative manner. However, clients have a right to expect information shared with a counselor to be kept confidential and not disclosed. Working within a school setting does not release a professional from conforming to legal and ethical codes. The school family counselor must work within the system, maintaining confidentiality but also expediting problem solving within the system for the client. When the counselor learns something about the family that the teachers should know, the counselor arranges for the family to pass on this information to the teachers. And vice versa, if the counselor hears a teacher expressing great frustration, hopelessness, or anger about a child or family, mediating a parent–teacher meeting would be appropriate. This requires that the family counselor be constantly aware of professional responsibility and the impact of shared information. There is not an easy answer to this situation, but it is one that requires the counselor to maintain a differentiated sense of purpose.

CASE EXAMPLES

The following vignettes depict what would pass for a typical referral and case in the elementary family counseling program. This is a composite case, to illustrate how this program functions.

> In this instance, the mother called and stated she had some concerns and would like to come in and talk with the counselor. The referral originated with the teacher, as a result of a parent–teacher conference and, as it later turned out, the juvenile court was part of the referral, as well. In the initial contact a brief structural picture of the family was gathered and an appointment was set.

Appointments are set to accommodate the family members' work schedule, so that little time is missed from work. The initial contact yielded the following structural diagram (Figure 17.1).

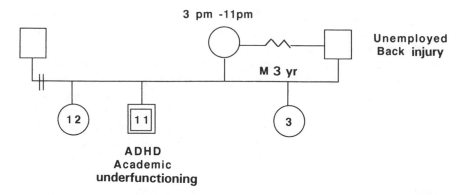

FIGURE 17.1. Depiction of initial contact.

The mother worked 3 P.M. to 11 P.M. for a janitorial service, cleaning offices. The father had been unemployed for about 1 year, due to a job-related back injury at that time. This was a blended family with two children, ages 11 and 12, from the mother's previous marriage, and one child, age 3, from the current marriage. This was the first marriage for the father. The index person was the 11-year old son, David, who was not turning in his work at school and had been diagnosed with ADHD. He had recently been arrested for shoplifting at a grocery store. The family opted to meet with the school's family counselor as a part of the juvenile court's diversion program for first-time offenders. The mother alluded to conflict with her husband over the 11-year old and asked the counselor to see the child, saying that the child would probably say more if he were seen alone. She was told that the school's approach is to meet with the entire family, to which she responded, "I will come, but I doubt that my husband will."

In these cases we offer to contact the father directly to talk about the importance of his involvement. In most cases, the mother or contact person talks with the other adult and sets up an appointment. If not, every effort is made to contact the other person and get him or her into the first session. To do otherwise has resulted in the counselor being inducted into the family on the side of the present parent against the absent parent.

In the initial contact, not only are the family members told about the school's family approach, but they are also told about the use of videotape as part of the program's approach to working with families and asked to sign the videotape consent form (Appendix 17.2) as well as the parents' rights/counselor responsibility form (Appendix 17.3).

In this session family members are asked about their understanding of the reason or reasons for having this meeting. Typically, a hierarchical order is followed in which members of the executive (parental) subsystem are asked to speak first, and since in this case the mother was spoken to first on the phone, the father was asked for his point of view first in the meeting.

> In our case, the father was also brought up to date by the counselor regarding the initial contact. The parents agreed that they were here because of the teacher's and the court's referrals but they indicated that things weren't working well at home and they had thought about coming in prior to the shoplifting incident. The father talked about the over-involvement of the mother with her son. The mother talked about the conflict between her husband and the 11-year-old. The 12-year-old shrugged and said "I don't know" about the reason for meeting. The 11-year-old complained about his father picking on him. The 3-year-old was quiet, because the family had brought toys for the child to play with. The family was asked to talk about what they would like to see changed in this family if they could have one thing changed, and they were able to establish some common general goals, such as be happier and have better communication, less fighting, more time with mom, and more time with dad. In this session more information was gathered for the genogram.

This process may vary, and this information may be gathered in the second session, after telling the family about the need to gather historical information.

> In this case, the background information showed that the ADHD diagnosis was reached shortly after the birth of the youngest sibling and that the academic problems began shortly after the father's injury. Shoplifting became the most recent concern after the parent–teacher conference.
> The structural diagram now appeared as in Figure 17.2.
> The family was asked, "How would things look if you were happier, communicated better, had less fighting, and so forth?" The family could not answer this question at the time, but as a homework assignment they were asked to go home and observe when they felt they were closest to stated goals and report back to the next session on their findings.

In supervision, connections were made between the family's transition points and the critical events in this family's life. The strengths in this family were noted to be their commitment to being a family, acceptance of each other, ability to organize around the youngest child, and ability to present some desired outcomes. The task at hand seemed to be to focus on strengthening the marital/parental subsystem, to affirm the naturalness of progression of the family life and change, and to heighten the family's awareness of the impact of the transitions that had occurred.

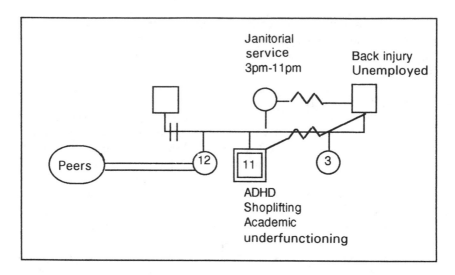

FIGURE 17.2. Structural diagram of a case family.

The initial hypothesis was that if the executive subsystem was strengthened, the other issues, such as shoplifting, ADHD, and academic nonproductivity could be resolved or worked with in an effective manner.

Subsequent sessions were spent strengthening the executive subsystem through directives in homework assignments. Particularly useful in this case was the gathering of historical data. Through those efforts, the parents were able to recapture some of the spontaneity of their early relationship and direct their energy in a cooperative way toward the family's struggles with change. Through enactments in the session, the parents were able negotiate the more sensitive issues, such as including Dad in the parenting subsystem. This left open the opportunity to present homework assignments such as family time, parental time with children, and dates for the parents.

Work with the classroom centered around notes home that focused on the positives of the 11-year-old's functioning in school. Conferences were held with the teacher after receiving permission from the family to talk about how their system functioned. As the teacher was able to focus on the positives, the mother was able to see her as an ally, a move that paralleled the move in therapy to strengthen the executive subsystem. The parents and the family counselor worked out beforehand what would be shared with the classroom teacher, so in this manner the parents felt empowered and were active participants. The teacher also felt supported and empowered, and this enabled her to remain unhooked by the 11-year-old's underproductivity and to see the function of the child's behavior in terms of the larger system. The family was also able to respond to the needs of the 11-year-old in his move into adolescence.

FUTURE CONCERNS

The goal of the program continues to be to improve the student situation through empowering the family to make useful changes. We see this goal continuing to evolve through identification of and responding to issues of professional differentiation and school system structure.

Family counselors in the schools face a number of issues that relate primarily to the area of differentiation. How will the family counselor fit into the educational system as a provider of mental health services? This relates directly to the reasons for becoming a school counselor and to professional identity as a mental health service provider. The challenge of the task is for counselors to learn to operate as consultants to other school personnel and alter the school paradigm to include a systemic approach.

Schools have their own systemic issues that will dramatically influence the counselors' ability to function as family therapists. These include control/hierarchy issues and boundary issues. The hierarchical issues relate to who defines the tasks for the counselor. Significant boundary issues for school counselors working with families have to do with who is included in counseling, where the counseling takes place, and when the sessions occur. These issues, as well as paying close attention to the hiring of systematically oriented counselors, will continue to be a priority.

ACKNOWLEDGMENTS

This program owes a great deal to Dr. William Hawver, Superintendent of Hutchinson Public Schools, without whose support and direction the program would not be a reality. A special note of thanks goes to the past and present Directors of Special Education, Dr. Robert Ash, Doug Campbell, and Dr. Ron Sarnacki, for their ongoing support and willingness to creatively use resources to provide services that transcend the usual Special Education/Regular Education boundaries. Finally, to the person who has kept this all together for these past 5 years, Dr. Shirlie Hutcherson, Assistant Superintendent, whose wisdom, humor, and administrative support has been invaluable.

REFERENCES

Ault-Riché, M. (1982). *Supervision guidelines—Marriage and family therapy training programs* [Handout]. Topeka, KS: The Menninger Clinic.

Carter, B., & McGoldrick, M. (Eds.). (1988). *The changing family life cycle: A framework for family therapy* (2nd ed.). New York: Gardner Press.

Cottone, R. (1991). Counselor roles according to two counseling world views. *Journal of Counseling and Development, 69,* 398–401.

Doherty, W. J., Colangelo, N., & Hovander, D. (1991). Priority setting in family change and clinical practice: The family FIRO model. *Family Process, 30,* 227–240.

Senge, P. M. (1990). *The fifth discipline.* New York: Doubleday/Currency.

Walsh, F. (Ed.). (1982). *Normal family processes.* New York: Guilford Press.

APPENDIX 17.1. HUTCHINSON PUBLIC SCHOOLS, ELEMENTARY FAMILY COUNSELING PROGRAM PARENT QUESTIONNAIRE

Please complete this questionnaire and return in the prepaid envelope enclosed as soon as possible.

1. How satisfied were you with the way you and your counselor got along?

   1 ——— 2 ——— 3 ——— 4 ——— 5
   Not   OK   Very
   Satisfied   Satisfied

   If you weren't satisfied, what was the primary reason?

   _____

   _____

   _____

   _____

2. How well did your counselor understand what you were feeling?

   ____ Not at all
   ____ Sometimes
   ____ Most of the time
   ____ Almost all of the time

3. How is your family now compared to how it was before you came for counseling?

   1 ——— 2 ——— 3 ——— 4 ——— 5
   Much   Unchanged   Much
   Better   Worse

4. Since coming to counseling, is your child's school work . . .

   1 ——— 2 ——— 3 ——— 4 ——— 5
   Much   Same   Much
   Better   Worse

5. Since you came to counseling, is your child's attitude about school . . .

   1 ——— 2 ——— 3 ——— 4 ——— 5
   Much   Same   Much
   Better   Worse

6. If your child had more difficulties at school, would you go to the school counselor for help?

   1 ——— 2 ——— 3 ——— 4 ——— 5
   Definitely   Unsure   Definitely
   Yes   No

7. Would you recommend that other parents go to the school counselor for help?

   1 ——— 2 ——— 3 ——— 4 ——— 5

8. How helpful was the school counselor compared to the other counselors?

   1 ——— 2 ——— 3 ——— 4 ——— 5
   Much   Same   Much
   Better   Worse

9. The reasons we came to the school counselor involve:

For each reason selected, please circle whether it is now MUCH BETTER, BETTER, the SAME, WORSE, or MUCH WORSE, since your work with the school counselor. Please circle an answer for every item which applies to your situation.

1. Behavior problem at home with one child	Much Better	Better	Same	Worse	Much Worse
2. Behavior problem at school with more than one child . .	Much Better	Better	Same	Worse	Much Worse
3. A child having difficulty with schoolwork	Much Better	Better	Same	Worse	Much Worse
4. A child not wanting to go to school	Much Better	Better	Same	Worse	Much Worse
5. A child not getting along with friends	Much Better	Better	Same	Worse	Much Worse
6. A child not getting along with brothers/sisters . . .	Much Better	Better	Same	Worse	Much Worse
7. Conflict in the family . . .	Much Better	Better	Same	Worse	Much Worse
8. Helping a child cope with a divorce	Much Better	Better	Same	Worse	Much Worse
9. Helping a child cope with a remarriage	Much Better	Better	Same	Worse	Much Worse
10. A child having emotional problems	Much Better	Better	Same	Worse	Much Worse
11. Other (what is it?)	Much Better	Better	Same	Worse	Much Worse

_____

_____

_____

11. Comments

_____

_____

_____

APPENDIX 17.2. VIDEO/AUDIO CONSENT FORM, HUTCHINSON PUBLIC SCHOOLS

(Names of Participants)

authorize _____ to make a _____
          (counselor, social worker)   (video and/or audio)

recording of _____in which I will be a participant.
       (interviews, group meetings, family meetings)

I understand that the permission for recording extends to all sessions with the family or individual members. I also understand that the permission for recording lasts until _____ or _____ until our work together has been completed. I authorize the use of these recordings for the following purpose that I have checked:

_____ 1. Counselor(s) and participant(s)

_____ 2. Supervision and/or consultation

_____ 3. USD 308 counselor in-service

Exceptions to this authorization, if any (specify exceptions):

Further, I understand that I may stop the recordings at any time and that the recordings will be erased after the above-stated purposes have been accomplished. It has been made clear that the recordings will not be used for purposes other than I have checked.

Signatures of Participants, Parents, or Legal Guardian (if participant is a minor):

_____ _____
                                                      (Date)

_____ _____
                                                       (Date)

_____ _____
                                                       (Date)

_____ _____
                                                       (Date)

_____ _____
                                                       (Date)

_____ _____
        (Signature of Counselor or Social Worker)   (Date)

APPENDIX 17.3. PARENTAL RIGHTS/COUNSELOR RESPONSIBILITIES FORM

Family counseling services are a recent addition at Hutchinson elementary schools. Therefore, the rights to which a client (parent or guardian) are entitled are listed below. For your information, the responsibilities of elementary family counselors are outlined in the document.

Parents and guardians have the following rights:
1. To know who may be informed about what occurs in counseling services
2. To know that counseling cases may be discussed in counselor supervision sessions
3. To give or withhold written permission for videotaping family sessions (Clients are strongly encouraged to permit videotaping because of the usefulness in supervision)
4. To be informed who will view taped sessions and why

Counselors are required to do the following:
1. Provide counseling services to students and families at no fee
2. Schedule family sessions at a time family members can attend
3. Report suspected child abuse or neglect to the proper authorities (required by law)
4. Serve as an advocate of the child
5. Focus counseling services on the family

The parental/guardian rights and counselors' responsibilities listed above were reviewed and explained.

| _____ | _____ | _____ | _____ |
| Parent/Guardian Signature | Date | Counselor signature | Date |

Index

WITHDRAWN

Please remember that this is a library book,
and that it belongs only temporarily to each
person who uses it. Be considerate. Do
not write in this, or any, library book.

362.7686 C536 1995

Children in families at
risk : maintaining the
c1995